Motherhood, Mental Illness and Recovery

Nikole Benders-Hadi • Mary E. Barber
Editors

Motherhood, Mental Illness and Recovery

Stories of Hope

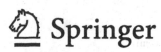
Springer

Editors
Nikole Benders-Hadi
Mary E. Barber
Rockland Psychiatric Center
Orangeburg, New York
USA

ISBN 978-3-319-01317-6   ISBN 978-3-319-01318-3 (eBook)
DOI 10.1007/978-3-319-01318-3
Springer Cham Heidelberg New York Dordrecht London

Library of Congress Control Number: 2014945647

Printed on acid-free paper

Springer is part of Springer Science+Business Media (www.springer.com)

Foreword

On May 8, 2012, at The American Psychiatric Association Annual Meeting in Philadelphia, I was honored to be invited to be the discussant for a symposium on motherhood chaired by Dr. Benders-Hadi. The research both basic and clinical by the presenters, much of which is in this book, was so well appreciated and received by attendees including myself that I strongly encouraged publication of a book to reach the world in great need of their findings and wisdom. I am pleased that this book has now come to fruition.

Dear Wise Readers: You may be mental health professionals, treatment center administrators, trainees, students in all health disciplines, educators, community leaders, including elected and appointed officials, people in care, their significant others, and their children of any age.

You are wise because the book's editors, Drs. Benders-Hadi and Barber, have identified and collected a range of scholarship and knowledge concerning mothers with mental illness and their treatment needs and issues, and you are holding this information in your hands now. You are probably holding this book because, like the authors, you realize that the needs of mothers with mental health problems must be recognized, evaluated, and appropriately treated to enable them to become the caring, competent, connected mothers to their beloved children that they want to be.

The book is divided into two parts, literally in half: Part I consists of eight chapters by leading researchers and clinicians describing their research, clinical findings, and programs to deal with issues of women psychiatric patients who become mothers by choice or violence, at all life stages from their teen years throughout senior years.

These chapters challenge some conventional assumptions. These include the assumption that women with mental health and substance problems do not have children and the assumption that they cannot be competent parents. The authors of this first half of the book provide a framework for evaluating a mother's ability to parent and for helping them to be competent as parents as they get treatment for their mental health problems. The theme of all of these chapters is the goal of recovery for the mothers, which includes functioning as successful parents.

Part II "Voices of Mothers" is divided into five sections totaling 38 very brief to more detailed chapters written by mothers who are at all stages of treatment. These sections are labeled: The Journey, Getting Help, Motivation for Healing, Multigenerational Impact, and Adult Children's Perspective. Each chapter is written by women with psychiatric diagnoses who proudly and willingly agreed to include their names as chapter authors, save for a few who chose not to.

The most important idea readers will remember after reading this section is "THERE IS HOPE" for these women. These authors/mothers display levels of insight and courage that are truly inspiring, extraordinary, and necessary for all readers to experience.

For any who might believe that mental health treatment is not helpful, or is too expensive or takes too much time, these stories show how valuable treatment can be. As story after story demonstrates, lives are saved as these women recover and can themselves contribute not only to their children's lives in all ways, but contribute to society in general. Many of the women describe becoming peer counselors as part of their recovery, so that they can help other mothers in turn.

This book should be read by everyone involved with mental health treatment. The old revolving door model where patients cycled endlessly in the mental health system represented mistreatment because of lack of knowledge. It should no longer exist, given what readers can learn from every word this precious book contains.

What is not the focus of this book, but can and should be recognized, is that men with psychiatric diagnoses are also fathers. These men can face many of the same issues described in this book and often have other gender-based sociocultural issues. Too often they are also prejudged because of gender stereotypes about their roles as fathers.

Each author's courageous sharing of seemingly unbelievable details are unforgettable and so insightful that readers will learn useful insights and techniques they can integrate into their own careers and even personal lives.

To be the best parents we must first learn about ourselves and learn to take care of ourselves. Respect for the psychiatrically compromised and/or abused victim is vital. Being a passive bystander is dangerous, whether as a victim, professional, or significant other of any degree. Be it as a friend, neighbor, teacher, or police officer, respect for the rights of those with mental health challenges should be recognized, understood, and acted upon. We can encourage others to do the same, especially as these mother-authors have demonstrated by revealing stories they may never have expected to share. We can also enable them to do so by taking the time to listen and fostering a friendly and safe environment.

As a former inner-city Brooklyn public school teacher, and psychiatrist for more than four decades, I have encountered many patients and victims of ongoing stigma which can be dangerous and deadly if it interferes with engagement or access to the correct diagnosis and treatment.

You WISE READER, must join the path to educating others about what you have learned in reading this incredible book.

Louisville, KY, USA   Leah J. Dickstein

Preface

Motherhood in the context of mental illness is a seldom discussed topic in both research and clinical circles. The assumption by the lay public and even seasoned clinicians is that women with mental illness either don't become mothers or are incapable of parenting their children. This book is intended to dispel the myth that mothers with mental illness do not exist or are not good mothers.

This book grew out of a small study we did to find out how many of the long-term hospitalized patients at the state hospital where we work are mothers. As you will read in Dr. Benders-Hadi's chapter, that number was an eye-opening 40 %. Counting the mothers we hadn't realized were right in front of us, and listening to their stories began a journey for us. The stories these women shared were compelling to us as both psychiatrists and mothers. As clinicians, we were interested in finding others who were studying mothers and how to best treat them in order to respect and maximize their capabilities. As mothers, we were inspired by the courage, strength, and willpower these women demonstrate in their everyday lives. Parenting can be a daunting task for anyone, and parenting in the midst of overcoming symptoms and challenges related to mental illness seemed to us like an awesome challenge. Yet women do it every day, as these chapters will attest.

This book is organized into two main sections. In the first section, we highlight research on mothers with mental illness and innovative programs and approaches being used to treat mothers. As readers move through these chapters, they will find useful information on topics from supporting parenting and providing adequate assessments of parenting capabilities to issues such as substance use, legal concerns for mothers, pregnancy and the perinatal period, and LGBT mothers.

The second section of this book belongs to the real experts on this topic, mothers themselves. While other books have provided personal accounts of dealing with mental illness focused on specific themes or diagnoses (Casey 2002; Taylor 2008; Van Fleteren and Van Fleteren 2008), none have focused on the successes and challenges related to motherhood. These courageous stories demonstrate that mothers with mental illness can and do become loving, amazing, caring, and wonderful parents. From the huge outpouring of interest we received when we solicited these chapters to the persistence of authors in preparing their stories for publication, we were amazed at the bravery and generosity of our mother-authors. There is clearly a great desire for mothers to have a voice so that they can convey their experiences to others. Our hope is to show the range of mothering experiences for those with mental health challenges, and within these pages you will find diverse and fascinating stories from women across the globe.

Our first goal in putting this book together was to push forward the scholarship on mothers with mental illness and programs to assist them, perhaps motivating a reader to pursue her own work or a family to advocate for better resources in their community. Our second goal was to enlighten and inspire readers with these stories of recovery. Whether you are a clinician hoping to more effectively address the needs of your patients, a mother dealing with your own struggles with mental illness, or a family member or friend who wants to know more on this subject in support of a loved one, we hope you will find something in this book that is useful to you.

We have many people to thank for helping us start and complete this book. Judith Samuels, Ph.D., at the Nathan Kline Institute in New York asked us the simple question, "How many of your patients are mothers?" that started us on this path. Jules Ranz, M.D., and the Columbia Public Psychiatry Fellowship supported us in doing the original study. Mary Jane Alexander, Ph.D., also at Nathan Kline, was our collaborator on the study and always challenged us to ask the right questions and to rethink our assumptions. Laura Miller, M.D., and Jacki McKinney, M.S.W., who were co-presenters with Dr. Benders-Hadi at the American Psychiatric Association meeting helped us to envision that this topic could become a book. Leah Dickstein, M.D., distinguished psychiatrist and all-around wonderful person, has been a terrific friend and mentor to both of us throughout this project. Finally, we want to thank our spouses and children, who provide us with daily motivation, inspiration, support, grounding, and humility that we take with us into the work we do.

Orangeburg, NY, USA   Nikole Benders-Hadi
Orangeburg, NY, USA   Mary E. Barber

References

Casey N (2002) Unholy ghost: writers on depression. HarperCollins Publishers, New York
Taylor KM (2008) Going hungry: writers on desire, self-denial, and overcoming anorexia. Random House, New York
Van Fleteren M and Van Fleteren M (2008) Different people different voices. Outsider Press, Michigan

Contents

Part I

Working With Mothers and Children

Supporting Mothers Living with Mental Illnesses in Recovery

Joanne Nicholson

Abstract

This chapter provides the rationale for a focus on mothers' recoveries, describes the family recovery model, and suggests strategies for translating family recovery principles into practice with mothers living with mental illnesses. Parenting is a significant role choice for these women. Succeeding or failing as a mother has a profound impact on a woman's mood, self-esteem, and self-efficacy; on her feelings of wellness or illness; and on her recovery. The family provides a context and motherhood provides a social role and opportunities for supporting or undermining recovery. Family recovery principles are translated into practice in key intervention concepts including: family-centered; strengths-based; family-driven and self-determined; recovery- and resilience-focused; and trauma-informed approaches, and key intervention processes including: engagement and relationship building; empowerment; availability and accessibility; and advocacy. The hope for a better quality of life for her children and family may well be at the core of a woman's recovery process.

Introduction

The goal of this chapter is to (1) provide a rationale for a focus on recovery in mothers; (2) describe the family recovery model; and (3) suggest strategies that others and we have found useful for supporting mothers in the recovery process. To our knowledge there are no supported parenting interventions developed specifically for mothers living with mental illnesses and targeting their recovery that achieve the status of evidence-based practice (i.e., that have shown positive, statistically significant impact in multiple randomized controlled trials) (David

J. Nicholson, Ph.D. (✉)
Dartmouth Psychiatric Research Center, The Geisel School of Medicine at Dartmouth,
85 Mechanic Street, Suite B4-1, Lebanon, NH 03766, USA
e-mail: Joanne.Nicholson@Dartmouth.edu

N. Benders-Hadi and M.E. Barber (eds.), *Motherhood, Mental Illness and Recovery*,
DOI 10.1007/978-3-319-01318-3_1, © Springer International Publishing Switzerland 2014

et al. 2011). However, we have had the opportunity to visit sites and study many interventions across the USA and in other countries where practitioners, parents, and family members have created innovative approaches to meet the needs of mothers and their families (Hinden et al. 2005, 2006, 2009; Nicholson et al. 2007). Efforts are underway in many sites in the USA and abroad to compile data regarding intervention participants and outcomes. This "services to science" perspective is reflected in our efforts, as we and others contribute to building the evidence base (Nicholson et al. 2009).

This chapter reflects the collaborative efforts of a large number of individuals—mothers, family members, providers, policy makers, and researchers. Our approach with mothers with mental illnesses reflects the experiences of the past two decades of conducting research and working together, and many more years of lived experience as parents, family members, providers, policy makers, and researchers. We work together to understand the experiences of mothers and families, to develop strategies and supports to meet their needs, and to create the conditions necessary for their success. Our team includes parents, individuals who live with mental illnesses, and the family members and children of parents with mental illnesses. We participate in work groups, on committees, in meetings; we plan holiday parties and school vacation activities with mothers and children; we advocate with state and federal policy makers to address the needs of our families; and we receive funding to develop and test specific interventions.

Language is powerful and important. In our work, we use the language of "parent" or "mother" because it reflects our commitment to supporting adults living with mental illnesses in the normal life roles of their choosing. Our work is geared towards meeting the needs of mothers and families in the context of their choice—whether that is in a treatment relationship with a professional provider, in a peer-to-peer support group, or as guided by a personalized action plan or power statement for achieving wellness and recovery.

Background

The majority of American women living with mental illnesses are or will be mothers and, in fact, a significant percent of mothers will experience symptoms of mental illness in their lifetimes (Nicholson et al. 2004). Motherhood may be a source of great pride to those who are successful (Benders-Hadi et al. 2013). Unfortunately, many mothers, especially those living with mental illnesses with severe daily impact and lengthy duration like schizophrenia or bipolar disorder, will be separated from their children—voluntarily or against their choosing (Nicholson et al. 2006; Park et al. 2006). These separations have profound consequences for both mothers and children. These relationships and disruptions in these relationships have numerous implications for policy and practice (Friesen et al. 2009).

Historically attention has been paid, largely through a negative lens, to the impact of maternal mental illness on children (National Research Council and

Institute of Medicine 2009). Developmental models have focused on relationships among the many risk and protective factors contributing to outcomes for children and on reducing the negative impact of parental mental illness as well as environmental characteristics and socioeconomic conditions (e.g., conflict in the family context, a limited social network, poverty) (Hosman et al. 2009). Researchers and providers have placed emphasis on intervening in the multigenerational transmission of mental illness from mother to child, with the prevention of emotional and behavioral problems in children and youth set as a priority (Beardslee et al. 2003). The notion of supporting resilience in children and youth is widely embraced (Hammen 2003). Reducing family disruption while maximizing the safety and well-being of children has long been the goal of social service and child welfare professionals (Friesen et al. 2009).

In the last 20 years or so, attention has slowly shifted to consideration of parenting as a significant and legitimate role choice and opportunity for women living with mental illnesses (Biebel et al. 2006; Nicholson and Deveney 2009; Nicholson et al. 1993; Nicholson and Henry 2003). Psychiatric rehabilitation has gained traction as a set of strategies for promoting community integration and recovery for individuals disabled by mental illnesses in one or more role domains (Salzer 2006). The consumer movement has encouraged consideration of consumer choice and voice, with individuals diagnosed with health conditions, including mental illnesses, at the heart of shared decision making and patient-centered care models (Deegan and Drake 2006). Intervention models focused on improving outcomes for individuals with mental illnesses in a variety of chosen life domains (e.g., education, employment, and housing) have been standardized, actively studied and widely disseminated (Mowbray et al. 2005; Mueser et al. 2006; Swanson and Becker 2013; Tsemberis 2010). The notion of recovery is at the center of these approaches (Deegan 1996; Onken et al. 2007). Supporting mothers in achieving their goals as parents, for themselves and their children, promotes recovery in women and undoubtedly contributes to positive outcomes for their children (Nicholson et al. 2009).

Recovery Is a Family Process for Mothers with Mental Illnesses

The course of mental illness—the emergence of symptoms, diagnosis, treatment, and recovery—is rarely linear, and prognosis and outcomes may vary depending on a variety of factors, such as gender, race, and ethnicity (U.S.D.H.H.S. 1999). Our contention is that, in addition to the most commonly studied factors (e.g., symptoms, illness severity, treatment), parenting status and success or failure in this role contribute significantly to the course of mental illness and recovery. Our experience in talking with many hundreds of mothers with mental illnesses over the years is that, regardless of their current child care giving, custody, or visitation status, mothers with mental illnesses define themselves as parents first and as psychiatric patients last. Succeeding or failing as a parent has a profound impact on a woman's mood, feelings of self-esteem and self-efficacy, and, consequently, on a mother's wellness or illness and recovery.

Psychiatric Rehabilitation

Psychiatric rehabilitation provides the theoretical underpinnings in a number of interventions in which mothers living with mental illnesses are receiving services in the USA (Hinden et al. 2006). "Psychiatric rehabilitation promotes recovery, full community integration, and improved quality of life" for individuals whose mental illnesses impair their functioning, through services that are collaborative, person directed, and individualized to promote skill development and access to resources (uspra.ipower.com/Certification/USPRA_CORE_ PRINCIPLES2009.pdf). Emphasis in psychiatric rehabilitation is placed on improving functioning in the roles and domains set as priorities by individuals. Optimal functioning is achieved through a process of identifying strengths and resources, setting relevant and meaningful goals, learning and practicing new skills, receiving appropriate feedback, and refining goals as progress is made (Salzer 2006). Practitioners, family members, or friends may facilitate a mother's access to formal and informal environmental resources and supports. A woman who is functioning optimally in a role she prioritizes is likely to feel better, and feeling better is likely to contribute to improved functioning.

Recovery

Recovery has been defined in a variety of ways by numerous authors and is considered to mean more than simply the alleviation of symptoms (Shanks et al. 2013; Whitley and Drake 2010). Superordinate dimensions of recovery proposed by authors—clinical, existential, functional, physical, and social—provide a broad framework for considering more focused components of recovery (Whitley and Drake 2010). An ecological model of recovery emphasizes the context of one's life, and in this case a focus on the family is particularly relevant to mothers. From this perspective, a woman is understood in the context of her choosing—the family. Recovery is seen as an evolving process, and participation in meaningful life roles (e.g., motherhood), community inclusion, and social integration are emphasized as desired outcomes (Onken et al. 2007).

The Value of an Ecological Model

Clearly, women who are mothers are not living in a vacuum. The context of their lives is often defined by family parameters. Families are commonly understood as systems in which members are engaged in reciprocal relationships (i.e., family members affect each other) and events are multiply determined by forces operating within and external to the family. For mothers living with mental illnesses, recovery is a dynamic process that contributes to and is influenced by family life, family experiences, and the well-being and functioning of other family members. What and how well mothers do influence other family members and vice versa; many mothers will acknowledge they are only doing as well as their children are doing at any point in time. They are encouraged when things go well with their children and may be demoralized when things go poorly.

The Family Recovery Model

The potential for understanding and supporting mothers is optimized when seen through the family lens. An ecological model of family recovery, therefore, lays out the relationships between parent and child characteristics, the family and the environment, and the interactions and transactions among them to suggest targets and pathways for recovery (Nicholson and Henry 2003). Outcomes are optimized when mothers and children are functioning as well as possible, their interactions are as positive as possible, and they have access to and benefit from resources and supports available outside the home (i.e., formal treatment and rehabilitation, relevant benefits and entitlements, informal resources like friends and family). Intervention targets suggested in the family recovery model include the mother's current functioning, her child's current functioning, their interactions, and their environmental resources and supports (Fig. 1.1).

The family provides a context and motherhood provides the opportunities for supporting or undermining recovery. Examples from conversations with mothers are readily tied to key elements of recovery (Onken et al. 2007):

- Hope and the expectation of better things in the future: *"They [her children] gave me the best. They give me love. I want to be ok for me and for them...they affected me positively."*
- A sense of agency or competence: *"having children...I've learned a lot. I have a lot of confidence in my abilities."*
- Self-determination, and the opportunity to set goals and make choices: *"I've learned my limits, I can establish boundaries. I can forgive myself for being human and for having the illness, and try to teach them [her children], educate them on mental illness, in those teachable moments."* Or *"My favorite thing in taking care of myself is to look at a day and have no plans, and just walk through it, you know. If I want to go somewhere, I go somewhere. If I want to stay in my pajamas, I stay in my pajamas."*
- Meaning and purpose: *"Before I had a child I was a binge drinker, a drug taker, and a risk taker...in abusive relationships. When I became pregnant, everything I did stopped. She [her daughter] pretty much saved my life. Because I'd be in a gutter somewhere...if I hadn't had my child."*
- Awareness and potentiality, and the belief that change is possible: *"I also try to learn from the traumatic and violent things that have happened in my life so that they don't repeat in their [her children's] lives. I'm constantly making sure that*

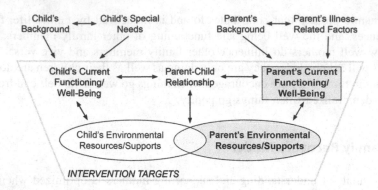

Fig. 1.1 An ecological model of family recovery

they're safe, they're ok, they think for themselves and think the correct way on a situation [rather] than just going with the crowd."

The goals of intervening with—or supporting and partnering with—mothers with mental illnesses are to acknowledge the strengths and resources women bring to the challenges of mothering, build on these to achieve their goals, facilitate access to essential environmental resources and supports, and enhance positive elements of recovery in the context of family life.

Translating Family Recovery Principles into Practice with Mothers

Psychiatric rehabilitation provides a conceptual framework for thinking about recovery. Additional theories provide suggestions for specific ways of working within this larger frame. These include: (a) attachment theory (Bowlby 2005) → the notion that relationships matter; (b) social cognitive theory (Bandura 1986) → the fact that thoughts, beliefs, and attitudes are related to behavior and can be modified; and (c) motivation/behavior change theory (Miller and Rollnick 2002) → an understanding that motivation makes a difference and is a personal thing. In addition, we embrace a number of key concepts and processes in our approach to mothers with mental illnesses and their families. These include the concepts of: (a) family-centered, (b) strengths-based, (c) family-driven and self-determined, (d) recovery- and resilience-focused, and (e) trauma-informed. Key processes include: (f) engagement and relationship building, (g) empowerment, (h) availability and accessibility, and (i) advocacy.

Key Intervention Concepts

While some agencies offer special programs for mothers living with mental illnesses, these are, in fact, rare. Individual providers or mothers themselves may piece together services and resources to support their parenting efforts and achieve parenting goals. Key intervention concepts can be incorporated into a formal intervention specifically targeted to mothers or may simply become part of the way in which an individual provider works on a daily basis with clients who are parents. We acknowledge the limitations conveyed by limited organizational resources and fiscal constraints, so encourage providers to address the needs of mothers to the extent they are able in their particular practice environment. We draw examples from the Family Options intervention, in which Family Coaches provide flexible, psychiatric rehabilitation services specifically targeted to parents living with serious mental illnesses (Nicholson et al. 2009).

Family-Centered

A family-centered approach assumes that family roles and parenting are as important to mothers living with mental illnesses, as they are to those who are well. In day-to-day practice, this suggests that women should be asked about their children (e.g., age, gender, where they are living, who is providing care for them, if they visit—when and how often), encouraged to talk about family life, and supported in setting goals in the parenting domain if that is their priority. As one mother in the Family Options intervention simply described, *"We do family activities."* If they are not yet parents, women should be asked about their reproductive goals and hopes and desires for family life.

Other family members can be involved in the recovery conversation to the extent desired by mothers; children may be included to the extent they are developmentally ready, willing, and able. Mothers may benefit from support in communicating with partners and family members as well as with children, in age- and stage-appropriate ways, about their illnesses, and recovery goals and strategies. Family members may benefit from family psycho-education about mental illnesses, treatment, and recovery.

Strengths Based

A strengths-based approach may run counter to traditional clinical training and practice that typically focus on a woman's problems or deficits. It is generally easier to engage with mothers and is typically more productive when mothers are encouraged to talk about what they do well, in addition to their areas of concern. Mothers may require coaching to identify strengths or positive attributes, particularly if they are depressed or view themselves as having failed in some way (e.g., have a history of homelessness or domestic violence or have lost custody of or contact with a child). One mother described herself as *"very down in the dumps, depressed. . .my medicine hasn't been working right. . .with the mental illness I just don't feel like I have the life I want to. . ."* It can be difficult for a mother who is profoundly depressed to see anything good at all. In fact, in this condition, they may even blame their problems on their children. For example, *"I think some days that if I didn't have kids, I also wouldn't be in the state that I'm in, like depressed, having anxiety. . ."*.

Mothers like this woman living with depression may benefit from coaching to identify strengths in their children as well as in themselves. For example, *"[The Family Coach] said he [her son] was absolutely excellent, he was helping the younger kids. They were like, 'your children are really good with other kids' so it worked out really nice."* Another mother was encouraged to talk about positive things she does with her children. *"A lot of times the kids and I will do stuff together like play board games, do karaoke together. We usually interact with the [pets] together; they're part of the family."* Mothers need to identify strengths for themselves and their children, which may help them feel more positive in these relationships.

The strengths a mother that brings to the table may include personal characteristics and resources, like good cognitive functioning or adequate symptom management, as well as external supports, such as positive relationships with partners and extended family members or a connection with a spiritual community. As one mother described her strengths, *"I do everything to encourage them [her children], nurture them. And I think that I'm a better person because I was very career minded and thought that was everything to me, and then the kids came along. My idea of what was better has changed and the kids were, like, the best thing."* Mothers must be encouraged to celebrate their own strengths and successes as well as the positive characteristics and achievements of their children to have hope for the future, which is essential to recovery.

Family-Driven and Self-Determined

Mothers set goals for family life and parenting that are family-driven and self-determined (i.e., driven by family needs and determined by mothers themselves). *"Somebody who's...saying 'What are your priorities? What is it you're trying to do? What is it you want to do that is different?'...it's very helpful."* Change is driven by what mothers identify as important to themselves and their families. As one mother suggested, *"Don't offer me a 50-min hour of psychotherapy when what I really need is a mattress for my child's bed."* Mothers often prioritize what they perceive their children to need and may not be able to focus on their own needs and recovery until at least some of their goals for their children are met.

When a mother is psychiatrically hospitalized, either voluntarily or not, she may be unable to attend to her acute treatment needs until she knows her children are safe without her and well cared for. While one mother's goal might be to care for her children 24/7, another mother may set routine, positive visits with children as a goal while they are living with another family member or in foster care. As one mother explained, who was reunited with her children after working towards this goal for a year, *"[I'm] falling in love with my kids again, once they were all back here again. And every single skill I have learned from my own life in the last year...to be able to have them here again and know they're safe has been amazing. To see them progress...I'm so thrilled to have them back with me where I can guide them..."* Understanding what motivates mothers and identifying the goals they hope to achieve will allow women to take effective steps towards recovery.

Recovery- and Resilience-Focused

A focus on recovery and resilience supports personal growth and optimal functioning. Hope fuels the belief that change is possible and allows mothers to overcome the shame, defensiveness, fear, or isolation that may hold them back from achieving their goals and enhancing their functioning. Family life and parenting may provide the context for hope and the motivation for recovery. As one mother indicated, *"They're [her children] the reason I get up out of bed every day. It's because of them."* According to another mother, *"I know I have to do the right thing because I have kids."* A third mother shared, *"I want to be ok for me and for them. I got to be strong."* Mothers may need encouragement to embrace the belief that by taking care of themselves, perhaps through effective self-care and illness management strategies, they will actually help their children, and to make the effort to do so, because it may seem counter to the notion of being a "good mother" who prioritizes her children's needs. In one mother's insight, *"They've [her children] turned me around to care more about myself because I have to care for them."*

Resilience is the process of adapting well in the face of adversity, trauma, tragedy, threats or stress (http://www.apa.org/helpcenter/road-resilience.aspx#). An individual's traits, talents, skills or interests may protect them from life's downturns. Resilience can be developed by connecting with others, modifying thoughts or attitudes about problems that arise (e.g., particularly negative thoughts), taking steps towards achieving goals, and nurturing and taking care of oneself. One mother explained, *"It can be very challenging and very difficult not being, like not being able to be the parent that I want to be. But, hopefully, I can be [the parent I want to be] if I just work at myself, you know."* This mother is working towards developing a more positive image of herself as a parent. Her resilience is fueled by hope and the belief that she can make positive changes in her life. Resilience can be built in the course of the recovery process to support and sustain positive changes and to protect a mother during times of stress and challenge.

Trauma Informed

In a trauma-informed approach, the impact of women's previous experiences on their current well-being and functioning are recognized and respected. Experiences of violence and trauma may have lifelong effects on how women feel about themselves and in their relationships with others, including their children. Past experiences may shape a mother's expectations for current and new experiences, as well as contribute to the motivation to do things differently. As one mother described, *"I've made a real effort to break those cycles and not repeat the things that my mother went through and put us through."* Another mother reported, *"I have learned a lot about what went on in my childhood to give me, um. . .I was living emotionally and I learned how not to do that. So I've been able to catch the kids in their emotions like I was trained."* This mother gained insight into the impact of her childhood experiences of abuse on the way she dealt with her children. She was able to modify her own responses as a parent and help her children learn better ways of coping in the process.

Mothers who are trauma survivors may appear overprotective of their children. For example, they may make sure their children are safe by never allowing them to play outside in the neighborhood. Alternatively, other mothers may appear disinterested in their children, depending on the approach they adopt to keeping their children safe and the ways in which they deal with their own pain. For example, as one mother indicated, *"I just try to distance myself if she's really crying and I'm irritable"* or, as spoken by another mother, *"I'll go downstairs for some distance and take a deep breath and then go back"* so as not to repeat the hurtful things their own mothers did to them. Knowing when to attend or respond to children and when to take a "time out" to monitor one's own emotional reactions is a sophisticated parenting skill. Mothers who are trauma survivors may be helped by insight into the patterns of their lives and in relationships, and the ways in which these emerge in parenting their children.

Key Intervention Processes

Recovery is built by attending to four key intervention processes that can be translated into daily practice. These processes don't necessarily happen in any given order, nor do they happen all at once.

Engagement and Relationship Building

The process of engagement and relationship building with mothers is undoubtedly influenced by their past relationship experiences. Mothers may have been disappointed or abused in relationships, personal or professional, and be quite cautious about developing a new relationship with someone who offers help. Their psychiatric diagnoses may have been used against them by family members (e.g., *Their [her children's] father has used the mental illness against me, in court and out of court…"*) or by professionals (e.g., *"…not being believed by the system, a stigma with a mental illness."*). Providers may view mothers' reluctance or inability to attend treatment appointments, perhaps because of conflicting family responsibilities or concern for the care of children, as avoidance or manipulation.

Careful consideration should be given to women's seeming ambivalence by exploring perceived obstacles to change and reported barriers to service participation, especially as they relate to motivation, parenting status, and family goals. Empathy and a nonjudgmental approach promote effective engagement and relationship building. A mother participating in our Family Options intervention described her Family Coach, *"…he's been kind of a good sounding board and is very understanding of the things that are going on in terms of what I'm dealing with."* Providers may be able to assist mothers in developing expanded, enhanced social support networks as well as positive treatment relationships by providing consistent, dependable, non-judgmental care over time. Another mother in the Family Options intervention explained, *"What's most helpful is having somebody to talk to, knowing that if things start to go wrong, I do have some place I can turn to, somebody that I can call."* A thoughtful, caring provider may be the first dependable person a mother with mental illness has had in her life.

Empowerment

Empowerment is the process of enhancing mothers' feelings of self-efficacy—the belief that they can solve problems and meet the demands of daily life. Self-efficacy is at the heart of conceptualizations of recovery (Cattaneo and Chapman 2010). Parental self-efficacy refers to a parent's feelings of competence or effectiveness in the parenting role (Kendall and Bloomfield 2005). Sometimes mothers living with mental illnesses feel powerless or hopeless in the face of their own symptoms or life circumstances and, consequently, may feel their children's behavior is more than they can handle. One disheartened mother explained, *"When they [her children] all start acting like they're 4 [years old] it drives me crazy; that'll get me, you know, going crazy. I mean I'll start yelling and screaming just like them to tell them to be quiet."* They may fear that their illnesses will be conveyed to their children through inheritance or genetics and attribute their children's misbehavior to emerging mental illnesses rather than as something they could manage or control.

The key to empowerment is success. Mothers may define success differently than providers. While providers tend to judge treatment outcomes in terms of the reduction of symptoms, mothers may have as their goal getting through the day without yelling at their children. While "reducing symptoms" and "getting through the day without yelling" are most likely related, a mother's goal and the way she frames that goal must be respected. A provider's task may be to help a mother understand the relationship between her symptoms and behavior and to identify ways of coping that allow her to achieve her goal (i.e., "getting through the day without yelling") by taking better care of herself ("reducing her symptoms").

Successes are most readily achieved by taking small steps. That is, mothers' goals must be personally relevant, realistic, and reasonably set, with steps outlined and obstacles anticipated. The necessary resources must be put into place for taking the next steps and overcoming obstacles. Providers can provide the "right" level of support to encourage self-efficacy. One mother described, *"I schedule the appointments, whether it's a doctor's appointment, a regular appointment to follow-up, and she [Family Coach] makes sure that I get there, and she'll come in if I want or wait if I want."* This is not to suggest that all providers have the capacity to transport clients to and attend meetings with them. Rather, a provider can help a mother decide on an objective and assist the mother, to the extent necessary, in mobilizing her resources to achieve her objective. This makes success more likely. According to a mother, *"It's like once you accomplish those goals, you establish and you create more, so it's like, it doesn't ever end, but it feels good to complete something I started, you know."*

An additional aspect to powerlessness is the feeling of having no choices. Providers have the opportunity to help mothers identify and assess options and make good choices by encouraging them to think about the consequences of choosing one alternative over another. Providers also have opportunities to acknowledge mothers' successes, as reported by one mother, *"My DSS [child welfare] worker said I'm doing an excellent job..."* And from another mother, *"...I wasn't expecting that they gave us a certificate of completion...just basically saying on the certificate that, um, I'm a good role model for my daughter and, um, I am successful in completing my goals...*" Even low-key acknowledgement of what might be construed by some as minor successes contributes to feelings of empowerment.

Availability and Accessibility

Mothers living with mental illnesses are likely to benefit from a flexible array of services, supports, or providers who are characterized by their availability and accessibility. Mothers' needs may well extend beyond the routine treatment session; they may benefit from access to "warm line" telephone or web-based supports at odd hours to avert bigger crises. A mother in the Family Options intervention explained, *"When I have issues going on here with the kids, trying to deal with the stress of being a single parent, she [Family Coach] talks to me on the phone; she helps me with my depression."* Mothers may prioritize very practical resources and supports that fly in the face of typical treatment recommendations or the priorities of traditional clinical providers. Mothers in the Family Options intervention initially sought help related to home and time management, conflict resolution, transportation, recreation opportunities for their children, and advocacy (Nicholson et al. 2009). *"[The Family Coach] will help with transportation and other things, get me out of the house, and get me to the clubhouse,"* according to another mother.

Mothers may benefit from facilitated access to community-based supports available to all (e.g., a food pantry, a clothing outlet, or free activities at the local recreation center or public library). Mothers and children may benefit from assistance in identifying formal and informal resources to achieve short-term family-related goals; the achievement of these goals may then allow them to address longer-term individual goals or more chronic issues. This requires a flexible approach to what is "therapeutic" or helpful versus what is typically considered to be "treatment."

Advocacy

It is extremely likely that mothers living with mental illnesses and their families will deal with a cast of characters in the community, and will benefit from advocacy role modeling and support. Most mothers have relationships with healthcare providers (e.g., pediatricians, dentists), day care or school personnel (e.g., babysitters, teachers, the school nurse, the school psychologist), friends, neighbors, and the parents of other children on the playground. Those with several children potentially have relationships with even more people. In addition, mothers may have relationships with their own health or behavioral health care providers, a care manager, an employer, and assorted friends and family members.

Mothers may benefit from support in navigating helping relationships, coordinating services for themselves and their children, and advocating effectively for their families. Providers can help in various ways through active participation or reflective involvement. They may attend meetings, role modeling effective advocacy skills for mothers in the school system or special education context, for example. As one mother described, *"I have team meetings for one of the kids and*

I know I don't have to go alone. Sitting around the table with four or five administrators can be intimidating...he [Family Coach] helped a lot with that." A provider may provide guidance in understanding complex, oftentimes confusing systems issues and service eligibility criteria. Another mother explained, *"He [The Family Coach]...helps me read it through and make sure the IEP [special education plan] has what it needs before I sign it. So that's really helpful...he breaks it down and it's much easier to understand..."* A provider can be a good sounding board, providing opportunity for reflection and feedback in dealing with challenging situations. *"I just have problems when it comes to getting letters for my landlord and getting services, so [the Family Coach is] just a support for trying to be organized and get advocacy and prioritize things."*

Mothers may find relationships challenging because of their particular configuration of mental health issues or histories of bad experiences in previous relationships. They may benefit from help in building and maintaining relationships with extended family members and key community stakeholders. Mothers may benefit from a provider's assistance in navigating issues of disclosure of mental illness to other professionals and peers. The decision to disclose a mother's illness to a schoolteacher, for example, when a child is having behavioral difficulties in the classroom, may have positive and/or negative consequences. The teacher might be more understanding of the child's issues and go "the extra mile" to provide support; or the teacher may be blaming of the parent, contributing to negative feelings and undermining the potential for a working relationship with the parent and child. Providers may be in a position to help mothers negotiate the positive, supportive community relationships every family requires.

Summary

Mothers living with mental illnesses express powerful feelings of shame, defensiveness, fear, and isolation that work against recovery, as well as great pride in motherhood and the motivation to do well as parents (Benders-Hadi et al. 2013; Nicholson et al. 1998). At the core of the recovery process is a sense of hope—that the quality of life for their children and families can and will be better. This goal sustains and motivates mothers in recovery. Recovery begins with engagement in relationships in which mothers feel they are respected, heard, and understood. Mothers report that having a plan—realistic, achievable goals with well-specified action steps—and people they can trust to help with their plan are essential to recovery. Building on strengths to achieve parenting and family goals contributes to "baby steps" on the road to success. Recovery can be a lengthy process, with progress and setbacks as mothers learn, try new strategies and skills, grapple with obstacles, and begin to see success in their efforts. Over time, mothers report feelings of increased confidence and self-efficacy—empowerment—as the recovery process repeats and reinforces positive change.

References

Bandura A (1986) Social foundations of thought and action: a social cognitive theory. Prentice Hall, Englewood Cliffs, NJ

Beardslee WR, Gladstone TRG, Wright EJ, Cooper AB (2003) A family-based approach to the prevention of depressive symptoms in children at risk: evidence of parental and child change. Pediatrics 112:119–131. doi:10.1542/peds.112.2e119

Benders-Hadi N, Barber M, Alexander MJ (2013) Motherhood in women with serious mental illness. Psychiatr Quart 84(1):65–72. doi:10.1007/x11126-012-9227-1

Biebel K, Nicholson J, Geller JL, Fisher WH (2006) A national survey of State Mental Health Authority programs and policies for clients who are parents: a decade later. Psychiatr Quart 77: 119–128

Bowlby J (2005) A secure base: clinical applications of attachment theory. Routledge, New York, NY

Cattaneo LB, Chapman AR (2010) The process of empowerment: a model for use in research and practice. Am Psychol 65(7):646–59. doi:10.1037/a0018854

David DH, Styron T, Davidson L (2011) Supported parenting to meet the needs and concerns of mothers with severe mental illness. Am J Psychiatr Rehabil 14(2):137–153. doi:10.1080/15487768.2011.569668

Deegan PE (1996) Recovery as a journey of the heart. Psychiatr Rehabil J 19(3):91–97

Deegan PE, Drake RE (2006) Shared decision making and medication management in the recovery process. Psychiatr Services 57:1636–1639

Friesen BJ, Nicholson J, Kaplan K, Solomon P (2009) Parents with a mental illness and implementation of the Adoption and Safe Families Act. In: Golden O, Macomber J (eds) Intentions and results: a look back at the Adoption and Safe Families Act. Urban Institute, Center for the Study of Social Policy, Washington, DC, pp 102–114

Hammen C (2003) Risk and protective factors for children of depressed parents. In: Luthar SS (ed) Resilience and vulnerability: adaptation in the context of childhood adversities. Cambridge University Press, New York,NY, pp 50–75

Hinden BR, Biebel K, Nicholson J, Mehnert L (2005) The invisible children's project: key ingredients of an intervention for parents with mental illness. J Behav Health Services Res 32(4):393–408

Hinden BR, Biebel K, Nicholson J, Henry AD (2006) A survey of programs for parents with mental illness and their families: identifying common elements to build an evidence base. J Behav Health Services Res 33(1):21–38

Hinden BR, Wolf T, Biebel K, Nicholson J (2009) Supporting clubhouse members in their role as parents: necessary conditions for policy and practice initiatives. Psychiatr Rehabil J 33(2):98–105

Hosman CMH, van Doesum KTM, van Santvoort F (2009) Prevention of emotional problems and psychiatric risks in children of parents with a mental illness in the Netherlands: I. The scientific basis to a comprehensive approach. Austr J Adv Mental Health 8:1–14

Kendall S, Bloomfield L (2005) Developing and validating a tool to measure parenting self-efficacy. J Adv Nursing 51(2):174–181

Miller WR, Rollnick S (2002) Motivational interviewing: preparing people to change addictive behavior (2nd ed.). Guilford Press, New York, NY

Mowbray CT, Collins ME, Bellamy CD, Megivern DA, Bybee D, Szilvagyi S (2005) Supported education for adults with psychiatric disabilities: an innovation for social work and psychosocial rehabilitation practice. Social Work 50:7–20

Mueser KT, Meyer PS, Penn DL, Clancy R, Clancy DM, Salyers MP (2006) The illness management and recovery program: rationale, development, and preliminary findings. Schizophr Bull 32:S32–S43

National Research Council and Institute of Medicine (2009) Depression in parents, parenting, and children: opportunities to improve identification, treatment, and prevention. Committee on depression, parenting practices, and the healthy development of children, board on children, youth, and families. The National Academics Press, Washington, DC

Nicholson J, Deveney W (2009) Why not supported parenting? Psychiatr Rehabil J 33(2):79–82

Nicholson J, Henry AD (2003) Achieving the goal of evidence-based psychiatric rehabilitation practices for mothers with mental illness. Psychiatr Rehabil J 27:122–130

Nicholson J, Geller JL, Fisher WH, Dion GL (1993) State policies and programs that address the needs of mentally ill mothers in the public sector. Hosp Commun Psychiatr 44:484–489

Nicholson J, Sweeney EM, Geller JL (1998) Mothers with mental illness: I. The competing demands of parenting and living with mental illness. Psychiatr Services 49:635–642

Nicholson J, Biebel K, Williams V, Katz-Leavy J (2004) Prevalence of parenthood in adults with mental illness: implications for state and federal policy, programs, and providers. In: Manderscheid RW, Henderson MJ (eds) Mental health, United States, 2002, DHHS Pub No. (SMA) 3938 Substance Abuse and Mental Health Services Administration, Center for Mental Health Services, Rockville, MD, pp 120–137

Nicholson J, Finkelstein N, Williams V, Thom J, Noether C, DeVilbiss M (2006) A comparison of mothers with co-occurring disorders and histories of violence living with or separated from minor children. J Behav Health Services Res 33(2):225–243

Nicholson J, Hinden BR, Biebel K, Henry AD, Katz-Leavy J (2007) A qualitative study of programs for parents with serious mental illness and their children: building practice-based evidence. J Behav Health Serv Res 34(4):395–413

Nicholson J, Albert K, Gershenson B, Williams V, Biebel K (2009) Family options for parents with mental illnesses: a developmental, mixed methods pilot study. Psychiatr Rehabil J 33(2): 106–114. doi:10.2975/33.2.2009.106.114

Onken SJ, Craig CM, Ridgeway P, Ralph RO, Cook JA (2007) An analysis of the definitions and elements of recovery: a review of the literature. Psychiatr Rehabil J 31(1):9–22

Park JM, Solomon P, Mandell DS (2006) Involvement in the child welfare system among mothers with serious mental illness. Psychiatr Services 57(4):493–497

Salzer MS (2006) Psychiatric rehabilitation skills in practice: A CPRP preparation and skills workbook. United States Psychiatric Rehabilitation Association, Linthicum, MD

Shanks V, Williams J, Leamy M, Bird VJ, Le Boutillier C, Slade M (2013) Measures of personal recovery: a systematic review. Psychiatr Services 64(10):974–980. doi:10.1176/appi.ps. 005012012

Swanson SJ, Becker DR (2013) IPS supported employment: a practitioner's guide. Dartmouth Psychiatric Research Center, Lebanon, NH

Tsemberis S (2010) Housing first: The pathways model to end homelessness for people with mental illness and addiction. Hazelden, Center City, MN

U.S.D.H.H.S. (1999) Mental health: A report of the Surgeon General. Substance Abuse and Mental Health Services Administration. Center for Mental Health Services, Rockville, MD

Whitley RE, Drake RE (2010) Recovery: a dimsneional approach. Psychiatr Services 61(12): 1248–50

Modes of Experience and Understanding: Parenting Assessment for Mothers with Serious Mental Illness and Child Protective Service Involvement

Teresa Ostler

Abstract

This chapter described and illustrated four modes of experience and understanding that comprise a parenting assessment for mothers with serious mental illness and child protective service involvement. The first mode introduces assessors to the immediate problems that led the child protective service to become involved with the family. The second mode seeks to understand how mothers' past experiences, their support networks, and mental illness have influenced their parenting and their ability to form and maintain relationships with others. The third mode provides information on children's attachment and developmental needs and on their experiences in being parented by their mothers. The fourth mode provides information from others who have known or treated the mother in different capacities. The assessment process involves a dialectical interplay of all four modes, each held in generative tension, each augmenting, confirming, and negating the others. Clinical illustrations are presented addressing different experiences and understanding gained from each individual mode. To formulate understandings in a new way, assessors must let go of preconceived ideas gained from one mode alone.

Tuesdays were elevator days. I walked from one building to the next, just before 8 am, through the courtyard and the glass doorways of the building into the foyer. Even at that hour, others were arriving too at the nine-story building: clients, mental health professionals, foster parents, caseworkers, and children of varying backgrounds and ages. When the elevator arrived, I entered, pressed the number 5, and waited as the doors closed. As the elevator started, I mulled over in my mind what I had read the evening before. The intake papers told me who would be arriving, what the mother's symptoms were, and why her children were in foster care.

T. Ostler, Ph.D. (✉)
School of Social Work, University of Illinois at Urbana-Champaign, Urbana, IL, USA
e-mail: ostler@illinois.edu

N. Benders-Hadi and M.E. Barber (eds.), *Motherhood, Mental Illness and Recovery*,
DOI 10.1007/978-3-319-01318-3_2, © Springer International Publishing Switzerland 2014

I was about to enter into an intense period of time where I would work with a multidisciplinary team to assess the parenting capabilities of mothers with serious mental illness who had lost custody of their children due to founded allegations of child maltreatment or risk of harm. I was part of the team, along with a psychiatrist and social worker. This chapter is about the women, their mental illnesses, about their parenting, and about assessments. I explore the idea that a parenting assessment is constituted by the dialectical interplay of four different modes of experience and understanding. They include the reasons why mothers became involved with child protective services in the first place, information about mothers' childhoods, mental illnesses, and support networks, and information about the children and from others who know the family in different capacities.

The stakes were high. Mothers we assessed had all lost custody of their children due to allegations of risk of harm or actual maltreatment. Their children had been living in foster care, often for a prolonged period of time. A legal decision now needed be made about whether interventions could ameliorate the risks in a time frame that made sense for the children, whether mothers could be immediately reunified with their children, or whether parental rights should be terminated. Erring on one side could contribute to mother and children being separated from each other forever. Erring on the other might contribute to child neglect, abuse, or risk of harm.

A developmental-clinical psychologist by training, my expertise was in children's well-being and development, psychopathology, and in bonds of caregiving and attachment. My tasks each week included meeting each mother individually and interviewing her about her children, her parenting, her childhood experiences, and her relationships with others. I observed her individually with each of her children and together as a group. I also asked mothers to complete various parenting questionnaires, then interviewed and observed each of her children, assessed their attachment and development, called foster parents, teachers, or grandparents, read records, and met with the psychiatrist and one or two social workers who were also on the team.

The team psychiatrist had expertise in how sex and gender influence the course, expression, and treatment of different psychiatric disorders. She also had expertise in assessing and treating psychiatric symptoms linked with female reproductive cycle transitions. This psychiatrist undertook a comprehensive psychiatric evaluation to make sense of the mother's symptoms, diagnose her, and to establish whether the treatment she was receiving was adequate for her condition. As part of this assessment, she interviewed each mother, obtained and read all available mental health records, contacted mental health professionals who were working with her or had known her in the past and in team discussions formulated how the mother's diagnosis and symptoms affected her parenting.

The team social worker started and ended the assessment process. As the team coordinator, she was the contact point for child protective services. She wrote up the referral notes, gathered records, maintained contact with the family, and visited the mother in her home to observe her in a natural setting with her children.

Our methodology emphasized the importance of observing mothers as they interacted with and parented their children. The methodology was also based in a review of all relevant information, past and present, we could gather on a mother's mental illness, her relationships with others, and on various facets of her parenting. In addition, we relied on both interviews and self-report measures and interviewed others about their observations and assessments. The methodology helped us to understand the impact of a variety of contexts (e.g., family, mental illness, environment and support, children) on parenting (Ostler 2008).

In our weekly meetings, team members brought in findings reflecting their areas of expertise. We discussed what each knew about a mother's parenting capabilities, past and present, and sought to understand the contributions of a mother's specific mental illness symptoms to parenting. We considered her insight into her illness (Mullick et al. Psychiatr Serv 52:488–492, 2001) and her responsiveness to and compliance with treatment. We looked at each mother's attachment experiences in childhood, how she formed and maintained supportive relationships, at stresses she was experiencing, and how her children were faring in their development and attachment.

The team met several times to discuss, analyze, and synthesize our findings about risk and resilience and to formulate recommendations. Each team member then composed an individual report summarizing their findings. The social worker also wrote a report synthesizing the team's findings on risk and protective factors and outlining recommendations for treatment.

This chapter describes the framework we used in our parenting assessment for mothers with serious mental illness and child protective service involvement. I explore and illustrate the idea that a parenting assessment is comprised of four modes of experience and understanding. The first mode involves the initial information about why a mother came to the attention of child protective services in the first place and why an assessment was needed. The second mode involves experiences with mothers: mothers' thoughts and feelings about parenting, their symptoms and mental illness, how they form and maintain relationships, and their feelings about themselves and each of their children. The third mode involves the children's attachment to and experiences with their mothers and how they are faring in their development. The fourth mode includes information from others who know mothers in different capacities.

I argue that the structure of the assessment involves a dialectical interaction between these four modes of information. Understanding results from ongoing discussions between team members, each of whom brings a different perspective and different knowledge base to the table. Part of this process involves identifying consistencies and discrepancies and actively coming to terms with biases, fears, or intrusive influences which could distort understanding. Another part involves tolerating uncertainty in order to formulate understandings in a different way.

Theoretical Approach

Before discussing each mode, I briefly review core theoretical premises from attachment, ecological, and violence risk prediction theories that undergirded the team assessment approach.

Attachment theory provides a rich basis for understanding the centrality of parenting, the bonds of love that bind parent and child to each other, and the reasons why a mother parents her children in the particular way she does (Bowlby 1988; Lyons-Ruth et al. 2005). This theory also provides a framework for understanding a child's attachment to his or her caregivers, how these bonds influence the child's ability to explore and to form relationships with others, and the effects of separation and loss on a child's bonds and his or her well-being (Bowlby 1988).

According to attachment theory (Bowlby 1988), the task of parenting is to protect a child from harm. As a child develops, a parent must be able to provide changing levels and forms of protection depending on the unique needs of each individual child as he or she develops (Solomon and George 2011). Parenting is made easier or more difficult depending on a mother's ability to form and maintain supportive relationships with others and depending on her ability to balance competing demands, including her own need for help.

Attachment theory also emphasizes that a mother's feelings for and behavior with her children are deeply influenced by experiences she has had and may still have with her own parents or caregivers. If a mother's own attachment needs were not met in childhood or if she was traumatized, she may feel helpless in the parenting role and may doubt that others will support her. In this context, she may turn to her child for support, ignore her child's needs as her own are so great, and/or may redirect anger at a child (Bowlby 1988). Current life stresses and the attitudes of a woman's partner are other important contributors to parenting.

Ecological theory provides a framework for understanding the dynamics of parenting breakdown and for isolating factors at various levels (individual, family, cultural, and societal) that contribute to parenting risk and competency. It underscores the influences of a variety of environmental and familial contexts that interact with each other over time to influence parenting (Belsky 1993). An important facet is the consideration the theory gives to protective factors that can ameliorate risk and promote more healthy parenting pathways (Cicchetti and Toth 1995).

Violence risk prediction research provides a theoretical framework for understanding when an individual with mental illness who has been violent in the past poses a substantial risk of harming others either currently or in the future (Steadman et al. 2000). It emphasizes the importance of assessing an array of empirical and theory-based risk factors in multiple domains of functioning, including a parent's own childhood experiences, their current disposition (anger, impulsiveness), and situations that could evoke risk behaviors. This theory also emphasizes the importance of looking at how specific mental illness symptoms, such as hallucinations, delusions, or violent fantasies can lead to violence, as well as at the course and prognosis of the illness, and the individual's responsiveness to treatment. Risk is viewed not as something static, but as something that can change over time and in different contexts. A risk assessment involves an estimation of probabilities: how likely it is that harm will occur now or in the near future.

In the next sections, I describe and use clinical vignettes to illustrate the four modes and the assessment process. All case examples were modified to protect confidentiality.

The First Mode: The Referral

This mode of experience and understanding was initiated when a child protective service caseworker contacted the team social worker to refer a mother for an assessment. It included the reasons why the mother came to the attention of child protective services and a dialogue in which answerable questions were formulated that could bring the case and decision making further.

Caseworkers who referred mothers often expressed concern, doubt, anger, frustration, and apprehension during the first conversation. They were relieved that a team could assess the family, but often felt overwhelmed by the complexity of a case or wanted quick advice about how to proceed. Some viewed mental illness as something frightening or dangerous, something unpredictable that needed controlling. A few viewed mental illness as incompatible with parenting. Several could see potential for a mother to change or ways that she might be able to resume a parenting role. Others were skeptical or were uncertain about the effects a prolonged separation and stay in foster care were having on children. Some did not believe the mother had a mental illness or thought her symptoms had resulted only because of the custody loss.

The referral notes summarized information gained from the first referral call for team members. It provided critical, initial information: names of each family member, date of referral, time of the first appointment, and a formulation of the referring questions. These questions were unique for each family, but they usually involved questions about what the mother's psychiatric diagnosis was, what the optimal treatment was for her condition, how her symptoms had affected or could affect her parenting, what her children's individual needs were, what their attachment to their mother was like, and whether a mother currently could meet her children needs, or, if not, whether she could change in a time frame that made sense for her children.

This mode typically revealed mothers at a time of crisis. Mrs. O, woman with schizophrenia came to the attention of child protective services after she stopped taking her psychiatric medications. The team was called when the caseworker observed that she held her 3-month-old baby son so tightly that he would cry. Ms. W was also in crisis. Diagnosed with bipolar mood disorder, Ms. W became acutely psychotic after birth. At that time, she stated that she wanted to "kill everyone, even Jenny", her 7-day-old baby. Mrs. R had borderline personality disorder, some traits of which can be associated with trauma. Her children were removed from her care after she attempted to take her own life by overdosing on pills. Mrs. N had had recurrent bouts of major depression. The child protective service agency was called after a neighbor reported that her 2-year-old had cuts and bruises on his face and body. The caseworker contacted the team as a deadline in court was approaching regarding termination of parental rights.

Reading each referral ushered in a sense of anticipation, but the content was also painful. While initiating an assessment, each referral also had the potential to contribute to over identifying with the caseworkers' viewpoint and to an early foreclosure of thinking.

The Second Mode: Mothers

My initial meeting with mothers began in the waiting room. I called out the mother's name and then introduced myself to her, her children, and to anyone else who had come, often a partner, a sibling, or foster parents. The meeting was both formal and personal. It was formal as I had not met the mother before. It was personal as I would spend the next hours with her and her children asking questions about all aspects of her life and observing her children.

Mrs. C was at the front desk when I met her for the first time. She showed little outward emotion and hardly looked at me. Mrs. R arrived for her assessment in the middle of winter. She was thin, had a black eye, and wore a thick winter coat. She looked very nervous as she hugged her six children who were gathered in the waiting room. She then had the children form a circle with her and holding hands, they prayed to the moon that they would be together soon in a new house. Mrs. R was currently homeless.

Ms. C had a different story all together. She became pregnant and voices had told her that the father was a famous football player. So she got on a bus, moved to the city he purportedly lived in, and became even more psychotic in the postpartum period. Her daughter was removed from her care at the hospital. When I met her, Mrs. C asked me if I was doing the "nesting assessment".

Almost all mothers showed great desire to resume a parenting role (Nicholson and Henry 2003). However, a few were ambivalent about parenting their child. Ambivalence was usually not easy to discern and was first evident in behavior. Ms. C, for instance, had two children. One was conceived by rape, the other from a man she loved. While stressing that she wanted to regain custody of both children, she only spent time with the child whose father she loved and ignored the other. Only over time did she tell me that she did not feel she could parent this child.

Mothers often had had painful and frightening experiences with caregivers in childhood. Some witnessed violent fights, were abused themselves, called names, were not wanted, or were left on their own for periods of time. Others were told they would be sent away. Several experienced sexual abuse or were parentified, taking care of both their own mother and siblings. Alternate caregivers were often absent. Mrs. R, a woman diagnosed with post-traumatic stress disorder who was frequently sexually abused and experienced violence in childhood, sought comfort elsewhere. She recalled hiding in a closet and putting her head on an imaginary friend's lap when she was frightened. The friend said kind things to her and helped her fall asleep.

Some mothers had parents with serious mental illness or substance abuse problems. Some were raised by a grandparent, relative, or sibling or lived with foster parents. Some mothers described their own parents as critical, blaming, rejecting, unpredictable, or showing only intermittent care. These experiences contributed to women doubting that others would be there when they needed them, not only leading to constraints in confiding in others but also to attitudes of mistrust, anger, and to fears of separation (Bifulco and Thomas 2013).

Many mothers had come to minimize their need for support. Although they sometimes longed for support, they also insisted they were self-sufficient and could manage on their own. For some women, the support networks they had were impoverished or ephemeral. One woman noted that the bible was her only support. For some women, the main support was a grandmother who had died several years prior. Others listed individuals who had harmed them or their children as their main support.

The accounts suggested that the women's own attachment needs had been chronically or intensely activated in childhood but not assuaged (Solomon and George 2011). These adverse experiences made women more prone to be highly sensitive to stress, especially in the peripartum period, and more prone to develop unfavorable attitudes about parenting and to expect and demand care from their own children by inverting the parent–child relationship.

These women became overwhelmed when their own infants or children cried. Not being able to tolerate the cries, they left the room, hit the infant, or held their hands over their infant's mouth. The behavior of other women, however, was sensitive and responsive. One woman's daughter had been sexually abused in foster care. When her daughter became extremely distraught, the mother gently held her as she cried and was able to reassure her that she was there. Mothers who had been in therapy were learning to come to terms with traumatic experiences from childhood. They were often more able to put their children's needs first and were more able than other mothers to acknowledge their own imperfections as a parent.

Mothers' childhood experiences also influenced how they felt about and understood their own children. One woman who grew up in an orphanage relied on a rigid parenting routine that she had learned by rote in childhood. During our observation, she had her own children stand in a straight line and call out their name in turn. They then needed to march in order in a circle.

Women's parenting was also strongly influenced by their mental illness, illnesses that often had their origins in childhood or adolescence. For many women, symptoms emerged in the peripartum period, a period when women are particularly prone to either developing a mental illness or for experiencing symptom exacerbation (Miller 2002). Several women we assessed had become psychotic or depressed after giving birth to their baby, who was removed at birth.

The psychiatric evaluation helped the team psychiatrist to make sense of each mother's symptoms and to establish what disorder(s) she had. She established the mother's insight into her illness and her compliance and responsiveness to treatment, as well as whether she was receiving optimal treatment. If not, recommendations for treatment were made. In Ms. P's case, the evaluation revealed that her bipolar symptoms were linked to an underlying thyroid condition. The thyroid condition was treated and her symptoms decreased. By helping her to build her support network, Ms. P was able to resume a parenting role. Obtaining information on women's symptoms both from individuals who had treated them and from records was critical as some women denied any symptoms. The psychiatrist also looked at mother's mental illness symptoms in relation to their parenting trajectory.

A few mothers were extremely depressed or manic when they arrived for the assessment. One woman heard voices and talked with someone who was not there. All mothers had had at least one if not several recent psychiatric hospitalizations. Many women, however, had been taking psychotropic medication, and their symptoms had stabilized.

Home visits by the team social worker yielded yet a different perspective on parenting and on women's lives. It added critical contextual information that helped us to understand larger contexts that influence parenting, including the neighborhood and environment, mothers' support network, and life stresses. During one home visit, a team member came to understand why one mother had kept her toddler in a cardboard box, a claim that had contributed to the mother losing custody of her child. Not having the financial resources, the mother used the cardboard box as a substitute playpen so she could supervise her child's whereabouts as she cooked.

This mode, then, added a new layer to the assessment, providing a view into contexts that ameliorated or exacerbated parenting risk. Each team member obtained information on different contexts that could influence parenting, an understanding that was informed by each team member's expertise and training. My own training had taught me the strong influence that childhood experiences can exert on parenting, but the meetings also revealed the long-term influences that chronic, untreated mental illness and the environment can exert on parenting risk.

Anxiety experienced in this mode often came from unspeakable fears of losing custody of a child forever (Ostler 2012), an anxiety that was evident only in evasive answers, mistrust, but also in denial and minimization. This unspeakable fear was often present in women who had lost prior custody of a child. In some cases, it contributed to a denial of pregnancy (Miller 1990).

The Third Mode: The Children

Observations of and interviews with children added a different layer of depth and understanding to the assessment. Children who were assessed by our team had sometimes been separated only short periods from their mothers, but many had not lived with their mother for months or even years. Some only knew their mother through visits as they had been removed at birth. Many wished to return home, but others were detached or wished to stay with foster parents. A few wished to be called by a different first name to escape into a new identity.

Children's attachment behavior is influenced by day-to-day experiences with a parent, but it is also strongly influenced by separations, something all children had experienced. During observations, many children hardly spoke with their mothers, averted eye contact, or called their mother by her first name, something that was often acutely painful to mothers. Others clung to their mothers and were unable to explore. Some older children completely adopted their mothers' perspective, and their own experiences were minimized. Many showed highly parentified behavior. One son whose mother had recurrent major depression arrived in time to help his mother with questionnaires and provided the psychiatrist with a full list of his mother's medication which he had carefully prepared. He supervised his siblings and brought them lunch. At the time, he was 11 years old. For others, the relationship with their mothers still had characteristic hallmarks of health, including an ability to use seek her out under stress.

Many children did not understand why they had been removed from their mother's care. Many blamed themselves for child protective service involvement. One 4-year-old girl constantly pinched herself in order to remind herself that she should be good. She believed that her own bad behavior had caused her mother to abuse her.

Some older children gave detailed account of experiences with their mothers, but their accounts were devoid of any personal feeling. Some of these children were highly controlling or shut down when asked about personal memories. Others, however, experienced anxiety states bordering on panic. Yet others provided fragments of information, or were unable, unwilling, or fearful to reveal more. Yet others gave a fantasized version of an idealized world that they wished to live in. These children appeared to have warded off extreme sadness, longing, and the pain of being alive by living in a state of non-experience (Ogden 2004a).

Children often came in with developmental delays, behavior and school problems, and a variety of psychiatric symptoms. Attention problems were common, but so was aggressive, angry, and helpless behavior. Several children hoarded. One small boy drank water all the time. Another soothed himself by sucking on his cheek. Some children revealed concerns they had about their own mental health, including worries that they might develop an illness like their mother's. Others showed resilience and were faring quite well. Nonetheless, children often put their own needs on a back burner and hoped for a time when life would be more normal.

Foster parents often provided a fount of information. Some had raised a foster child since birth. Others had only had the child for days or months. Foster parents varied in what they knew about children's individual needs, in their feelings about children and the children's mothers, and in how they cared for the children. Some wished to adopt a child.

The third mode exists in dialectical tension with the other modes. It provides a key perspective on a mother's caregiving abilities as it looks at how children have fared, how they respond to her, what their attachment bonds are like, and how they are developing. This mode also provides critical information on a child's individual needs and allowed team members to assess whether a mother could meet these needs in a time frame that made sense for the child.

The Fourth Mode: Others

This mode included what we gleaned from pertinent records and what we learned from others who had known or knew the mother in different capacities over the years. Interviewing others was not always straightforward. Close relatives were often defensive or reluctant to say anything negative they had observed about parenting.

This was the case with Ms. B's sister. Ms. B had been diagnosed with schizophrenia. After the birth of her first child, her symptoms worsened when she went off of her medications. Although her sister regularly brought Ms. B food and diapers for her baby, she became concerned when Ms. B would not open the door and when she heard her 2-month-old niece crying in a weak voice. When I contacted Ms. B's sister, she was reluctant to say much, noting only that her sister loved her daughter. However, as we talked more and she came to understand the baby's needs, she was more open in sharing her concerns. The assessment ultimately helped Ms. B get into treatment. Some relatives, partners, and friends were forthcoming right away with their concerns. Some felt overwhelmed or burdened by the needs of a particular family and were frustrated by the mental illness, by a mother's lack of compliance with treatment, and/or by her struggles with parenting.

Interviews with others who knew mothers in different capacities forced us to look anew at our findings and the viability of the mothers' own accounts and at the accounts of others. In many cases, we found support for a mother's or caseworker's account, but in others the contradictions were glaring. One mother, for instance, claimed that she had gone outside for 15 min to buy food when her children were removed. Our interviews with others revealed a different story. The children, ages one and three, were left alone for over 10 h before protective services were called.

On one occasion, almost all initial evidence we heard from a caseworker was extremely positive. However, as we sifted through the evidence gained from other modes, it became clear that the caseworker had overidentified with the mother's position. The children's own reports and those who knew her well revealed substantial risks. The woman had broken off repeated contact with clinicians and acquaintances and continued to have serious mental health problems.

Records provided rich information about past observations or assessments and about functioning at over time. Some records provided detailed descriptions about parenting when it was at its best and at times when a mother was under stress. Others records were less useful. Behavior was labeled as good or bad, but no details were given about what happened or the context in which the alleged behavior occurred.

Mental health professionals brought additional perspectives to the assessment. Some had worked with mothers for years and had firsthand knowledge of her illness, her response to treatment, and how she cared for her children. Some had never seen a mother with her children or were unaware that she even had children. Some had observed a mother on only one occasion. One mental health professional noted that a woman who was acutely psychotic "should never parent," although the woman was highly responsive to medication and had good parenting skills.

The Assessment Process

The above four modes comprise the structure of a parenting assessment. The process of assessment involves looking at all four modes in their singularity and at once. It compares data from the different modes to identify both inconsistencies and patterns. It considers multiple viewpoints, suspends judgment, and is closely informed both by the expertise that each team member brings and by current research on mental illness, children, and parenting. The process involves close attention to ethical issues, transparency of practices, as well as an honest brokering of knowledge and uncertainties (Gambrill 2005).

Each mode engages a different perspective and yields different understanding, and each has its own validity and flaws. Drawing on one mode alone can lead to polarized views and will preclude a sound assessment of parenting competency and risk.

The assessment process involves a dialectical interplay of all four modes, each held in generative tension, each augmenting, confirming, and negating the experiences and understanding gained from the others. In this process, discussions move between the poles of the predictable and the unpredictable, the methodical and the intuitive, the disciplined and spontaneous (cf. Ogden 2004b, p 194). Through dialogue, this dialectical interplay between modes can then contribute to a more contextual, nuanced, and comprehensive understanding of parenting competency and risk.

The following clinical vignette illustrates the experiences and understandings gained from each individual mode and the understanding achieved by considering all four modes together. The case, described in detail in Jacobsen and Miller (1998), involved a 17-year-old mother with recurrent major depression. Ms. B came to the attention of CPS after she repeatedly hit her one-year-old daughter on the body and head over a period of several months, contributing to her daughter's death. Ms. B lost custody of a first child when she was convicted and had a second child in jail.

Reading just the intake papers could contribute to a highly negative view of Ms. B's parenting as her behavior had contributed to her child's death. However, when we interviewed Ms. B herself and learned about the circumstances surrounding the abuse, our perspective on maltreatment widened. Ms. B was a young woman caring for two children under age 5. Her daughter had feeding problems and often cried inconsolably. The beatings occurred in the context of overwhelming stress. Ms. B's partner drank and beat her regularly. Ms. B's only support was her husband, but he was only intermittently present and also hit her when he drank. Her mother, who helped with Ms. B's first child, disapproved of Ms. B's partner and had maintained only sporadic contact with her daughter. Ms. B became depressed in this context and began hitting her child when her daughter could not stop crying or when she herself was hit by her partner.

The interview revealed that Ms. B was sexually abused in childhood. Her ability to form and maintain relationships with others was also largely inverted. While caring for others, she had a difficult time asking for help for herself. At the same time, Ms. B took ownership of parenting difficulties she had had and had good insight into her childhood experiences. She readily recognized circumstances that triggered her depression and had sought out treatment for her symptoms (Mullick et al. 2001). She was generally responsive to her children's needs except when overwhelmed.

Observing Ms. B's children added more depth to our understanding. The children enjoyed their mother's presence and readily sought her out for support. They both desired to return to her care, but also had developmental delays.

In interviews with therapists who had worked with her, we learned that Ms. B was highly motivated to change and was responding well to therapy. However, these sources also revealed that Ms. B maintained contact with her partner and continued to rely on his inconsistent support.

Nonlinear and dense, the assessment process looks at experiences and understanding gained from all four modes from a viewpoint of neutrality and objectivity as findings are analyzed and synthesized. In this process, it is necessary to suspend judgment and tolerate the experience of not knowing. To formulate understandings in a new way, assessors must dare to experience the tension of letting go of preconceived ideas gained from one mode alone.

Parenting assessments do not always lead to reunification. For some mothers, change may not occur in a time frame that makes sense for a particular child. Other parents, however, are able to resume a parenting role soon after an assessment or later (Jacobsen and Miller 1998).

Our assessments included recommendations that sought to address the individual concerns and needs of each mother, partner, and child, alone or together (Nicholson and Henry 2003; Ostler 2012). An assessment, then, was just the beginning of process that was aimed at furthering change and decision making. Rates of change and levels of motivation varied across mothers. When Ms. B, the young mother with depression who had killed her child, received feedback from our assessment, she completely broke off her relationship with her partner. With help, she continued to build a solid support network with family members and neighbors. When we reassessed her 6 months later, she was continuing to make steady progress in therapy and was about to regain custody of her children.

The term "assessment" can convey the idea that, in an assessment, a mother, partner, and child(ren) are relatively passive. However, if an assessment is to yield meaningful information, it should include active input from all participants. In an assessment, mothers, partners, children, and others expose themselves to considerable psychological strain. Assessors do as well, as they immerse themselves into a person's life and history. Honoring the dignity of each person, knowing that this may not be synonymous with diminishing their pain, and striving to understand what constitutes risk and resilience in the face of complex and often disturbing emotional experiences are essential aspects of the process (Ogden 2005).

References

Belsky J (1993) Etiology of child maltreatment: a developmental-ecological analysis. Psychol Bull 114:413–434

Bifulco A, Thomas G (2013) Understanding adult attachment in family relationships: research, assessment and intervention. Routledge, London

Bowlby J (1988) A secure base: clinical applications of attachment theory. Routledge, London

Cicchetti D, Toth S (1995) A developmental psychopathology perspective on child abuse and neglect. J Am Acad Child Adolesc Psychiatry 34:541–565

Gambrill E (2005) Critical thinking in clinical practice: improving the quality of judgments and decisions, 2nd edn. Wiley, Hoboken, NJ

Jacobsen T, Miller LJ (1998) Mentally ill mothers who have killed: three cases addressing the issue of future parenting capability. Psychiatr Serv 49:650–657

Lyons-Ruth K, Yellin C, Melnick S, Atwood G (2005) Expanding the concept of unresolved mental states: hostile/helpless states of mind on the adult attachment interview are associated with atypical maternal behavior and infant disorganization. Dev Psychopathol 17:1–23

Miller LJ (1990) Psychotic denial of pregnancy: phenomenology and clinical management. Hosp Commun Psychiatry 41:1233–1237

Miller LJ (2002) Postpartum depression. JAMA 287:762–765

Mullick M, Miller LJ, Ostler T (2001) Insight into mental illness and child maltreatment risk in mothers with major psychiatric disorders. Psychiatr Serv 52:488–492

Nicholson J, Henry AD (2003) Achieving the goal of evidence-based psychiatric rehabilitation practices for mothers with mental illnesses. Psychiatr Rehabil J 27(2):122–130

Ogden TH (2004a) Misrecognitions and the fear of not knowing. In: Ogden TH (ed) The primitive edge of experience. Jason Aronson, New York, pp 195–221

Ogden TH (2004b) The initial analytic meeting. In: Ogden TH (ed) The primitive edge of experience. Jason Aronson, New York, pp 169–194

Ogden TH (2005) What i would not part with. In: Ogden TH (ed) This art of psychoanalysis: dreaming undreamt dreams and interrupted cries. Routledge, London, pp 19–26

Ostler T (2008) Assessment of parenting competency in mothers with mental illness. Paul H. Brookes Publishing, Baltimore, MD

Ostler T (2012) Why weepest thou so sore? When a mother's pathway is fragile and uncertain. Zero to Three 32(6):14–19

Solomon J, George C (2011) The disorganized attachment-caregiving system: dysregulation of adaptive processes at multiple levels. In: Solomon J, George C (eds) Disorganization of attachment and caregiving, 2nd edn. Guilford Press, New York, pp 3–24

Steadman HJ, Silver E, Monahan J, Appelbaum PS, Robbins PC, Mulvey EP, Grisso T, Roth LH, Banks S (2000) A classification tree approach to the development of actuarial violence risk assessment tools. Law Hum Behav 24(1):83–100

When Your Patient Has Children: How the Clinician Can Support Good Parenting

3

Alison Heru

Abstract

Most of our patients have children. All clinicians need to know how best to support good parenting in their patients. A parent with mental illness can benefit from understanding how to talk with their children about mental illness. This chapter describes parenting and mental illness from four perspectives: the child, the parent, the child psychiatrist, and the adult psychiatrist. Children of parents with mental illness, when asked, can clearly state what they would like from the mental health system. Parents want to avoid drawing attention to their family as they are fearful of being judged negatively. Child psychiatrists have developed family-based interventions that can prevent psychiatric symptoms and illness in children. Adult psychiatrists need to encourage and support their patients in discussing mental illness as a family, and to consider the development of care plans, should the parent become ill. All clinicians should be able to provide age-appropriate family interventions to competently involve children in the office and hospital setting.

Introduction

This chapter focuses on the family as a whole: understanding that when one person in the family has mental illness, the whole family is affected. Growing up with a parent with mental illness has been written about by adult children with that experience. These first-person descriptions are cathartic for the writer and a testimony that children can survive sometimes frightening times with a parent and even do well in adulthood. However, our goal as clinicians should be to gain the confidence of struggling families in order to guide, support, and provide tools for

A. Heru, M.D. (✉)
University of Colorado School of Medicine, Denver, CO, USA
e-mail: alison.heru@ucdenver.edu

N. Benders-Hadi and M.E. Barber (eds.), *Motherhood, Mental Illness and Recovery*,
DOI 10.1007/978-3-319-01318-3_3, © Springer International Publishing Switzerland 2014

them, with the aim of minimizing difficult episodes. We want families to thrive rather than just survive.

As a family psychiatrist, my focus is on the family as a whole system. I always ask patients to bring in their family as a part of my evaluation. I explain that mental illness affects not just the person but the whole family, that patients do much better when the family receives education and support, and that family intervention can prevent illness relapse and the onset of illness in other family members. Family is defined by the patient and can include neighbors, extended family, kinship networks, church members, and othermothers (women who provide care for children who are not biologically their own, a common practice in some African-American communities; see Burton and Hardaway 2013).

This chapter highlights the perspectives of the child, parent, child psychiatrist, and adult psychiatrist. This chapter reviews age-appropriate family interventions to allow the clinician to competently involve children in the office and hospital setting. The clinician can also help parents anticipate difficulties by using planning tools such as care plans.

The Child Perspective

7-Year-Old's Perspective of Her Mother with Mental Illness
Maggie Jarry watched her mother walk around the apartment trying to catch her eyes because she believed they had floated out of her face. Her mother often locked herself in the bathroom and talked to herself in the mirror because she believed that she had telepathic powers. "We lived like this for a year, until a babysitter and her mother figured out what was going on and got professional help" for Maggie's mother.
Jarry 2009

How many of our patients are parents? How many children are their caregivers? What do we know about child caregivers? In 2005, the first large-scale American study of children providing care was released by the National Alliance for Caregiving and United Hospital Fund (NAC 2005). Through surveys and interviews with random samples of child caregivers and their parents, researchers found that over 1.3 million children between the ages of 8 and 18 are caregivers: 72 % care of a parent or grandparent, usually mother (28 %) or grandmother (31 %), and siblings (11 %). Most care recipients are over age 40 and suffer from chronic illnesses, such as dementia, heart, lung or kidney disease, arthritis, and diabetes. About 30 % of child caregivers are aged 16–18, almost 40 % are aged 12–15, and about 30 % are aged 8–11 years old. Child caregivers were interviewed by telephone for about 12 minutes and their responses compared to a controlled sample (213 caregivers and 250 non-caregivers). More than 50 % of the child caregivers helped with basic activities of daily living such as bathing, dressing, and toileting. All children helped with instrumental ADLs such as shopping, household tasks, and meal preparation. Almost all of the children (96 %) stated that they keep the care recipient company and about 75 % stated that they have someone else helping them.

Child caregivers reported more symptoms of anxiety and depression and felt that no one loved them, compared to controls. Younger children tended to have more feelings of worthless or inferiority. Children aged from 12 to 18 years old were more likely to be antisocial at school and engage in bullying. Overall, boys were twice as likely to feel it was "no use showing their feelings." Some children reported disruption in school work or activities. However, child caregivers experienced positive effects from caregiving such as feeling appreciated and were less likely to feel people expected too much from them or to feel angry about all they have to do. Overall, child caregivers were similar to peers in their views on relationships with others, level of responsibility, and school problems. Overall, child caregivers' feelings of self-esteem, sadness, loneliness, and fun were similar to non-caregivers.

Parents and clinicians may believe that children do not perceive mental illness in their parents. However, children and teens can describe very well what happens when their parent becomes ill (Cooklin 2006). In this video "When a parent has a mental illness," Dr. Alan Cooklin, a child psychiatrist from the Royal College of Psychiatry in the UK, explains what mental illness is to a group of young children. The children express their need for support and education. Support networks are found online and there are many available books such as "I'm Not Alone: A Teen's Guide to Living with a Parent Who Has a Mental Illness" by Michelle D. Sherman. According to Article 12 of the United Nations Convention on the Rights of the Child, children have a right to be listened to and have their views taken into account on matters that affect them. Table 3.1 summarizes what children want from professionals (Bilsborough 2004).

What do children understand? The following tables outline the basic levels of understanding of children and recommended approaches in three age ranges (Tables 3.2, 3.3, and 3.4).

The Parent Perspective

Most parents who have mental illness do a great job of parenting their children, given the right support and information. However societal attitudes are stacked against mothers with mental illness. Some of the common mistaken beliefs are that mothers with mental illness are unable to care for children and that a patient's desire for children, pregnancy, and motherhood should be challenged. The following barriers for patients who are parents in accessing services are individual beliefs about help-seeking, knowledge of services, fears about losing custody, stigma of mental illness, conflicting demands on parents, the presence of other stresses and difficulties, problems with access, transport, and child care (Beresford et al. 2008). Parenting is also important to fathers who deserve appropriate support and care to enable them to carry out their role (Styron et al. 2002). In November 2008, UK

Table 3.1 What children want from professionals

1. Introduce yourself. Tell us who you are and what your job is.
2. Give us as much information as you can.
3. Tell us what is wrong with our parents.
4. Tell us what is going to happen next.
5. Talk to us and listen to us. Remember, it is not hard to speak to us; we are not aliens.
6. Ask us what we know and what we think. We live with our parents; we know how they have been behaving.
7. Tell us it is not our fault. We can feel really guilty if our mum or dad is ill. We need to know we are not to blame.
8. Please don't ignore us. Remember we are part of the family and we live there too.
9. Keep on talking to us and keep us informed. We need to know what is happening.
10. Tell us if there is anyone we can talk to. MAYBE IT COULD BE YOU.

Table 3.2 3–5 year olds

• Can repeat a memorized script, but without understanding
• Communicate mostly through play and fantasy
• It is hard to understand their behaviors and moods
• Their life is centered on home and their relationship to caregiver(s) so that separation from caregiver(s) is their greatest source of stress
• Experience emotional reactions intermittently with rapid return to normal functioning
• Can experience night terrors after caregiver(s) leaves
• Can accept competent substitute caregiver (s), if adequately prepared
• Become distressed by family members' outbursts of grief and/or emotional withdrawal
• If prolonged feelings of sadness, seek formal evaluation

Children's Minister, Beverley Hughes, announced a Think Fathers campaign to dispel the myth that fathers are the "invisible parent."

The loss of child custody is a real parental concern and sorting through all the child care issues can be complex. Questions to ask are: Who is in the family system? What is the parental unit? Are extended family members or community members involved? Laws and legal and social work practice are different in each state, so enlisting the help of local experts is important.

Suitable topics to discuss with your patients who are parents are medication and pregnancy if the patient is of childbearing age, how to get more practical and emotional support, current parenting practices, what to do if you become ill, who can you trust to care for your child, and the implications of mental illness on questions of custody. Child care plans can be helpful and are discussed later in this chapter.

Table 3.3 6–8 year olds

• Highly emotional, difficulty containing emotions, with self-blame when bad things happen, may have anticipatory anxiety
• Can be overwhelmed by parent's strong anger or sadness, can make logical errors, misunderstand cause and effect
• Fear that aggressive thoughts, words, or wishes are harmful and fear rejection by peers
• Explain what child is seeing, e.g., parent's withdrawal is caused by illness, not lack of love because once children believe their own view, it is difficult to alter
• Normalize reduced school performance when stressed
• Maintain regular activities
• Encourage interest in reading or writing about illness, give permission to ask questions and express emotions, and support interest in helping with patient's care
• Prepare children to visit parent in hospital, explain what they see, make time for clarification afterward
• Communicate with teachers and other adults with regard to parent's illness, arrange substitute caregiving with people who communicate well with child, and engage others to listen to their emotional concerns
• Child should not be left in charge of parent's care
• Remind parents that coalitions and special preferences within the family may cause distress
• Consult if severe anxiety, school phobia, excessive self-blame, persistent depression, or low self-esteem

Table 3.4 9–11 year olds

• Logical thinking: understand cause and effect
• Cannot draw inferences from insufficient information
• Able to use compartmentalization and distraction to avoid strong emotion
• Outbursts of emotion followed by embarrassment/avoidance
• Benefit from being able to help with care
• Give detailed information about parent's diagnosis and include child's observations
• Assure children the illness is not their fault
• Acknowledge stress of uncertainty for every one
• Have child visit during hospitalizations, explain parent's treatment, meet medical and nursing staff
• Help child remain involved in after-school activities, sports, ongoing contact with friends

Child Psychiatrist Perspective

Over 50 % of children who have a parent with affective illness experience psychological symptoms (Beardslee et al. 1998), with three times the rates of mood or anxiety disorders reported (Halligan et al. 2007). Beardslee (2002) published a book for families and lay caregivers about the process of dealing with depression in families. It is important to highlight family factors that protect children, such as good parenting and stable relationships (Masten et al. 1999). Family interventions focus on improving family resilience and developing protective factors in the face of parental mental illness.

Family interventions, such as these described below, can reduce the incidence of childhood illness by as much as 40 %. An analysis of 13 randomized controlled trials of family interventions with parents with mental illness ($n = 1,490$ children) found that cognitive, behavioral, or psychoeducational family interventions were effective in reducing childhood illness (Siegenthale et al. 2012). Family interventions, such as Family Talk, are targeted specifically to prevent depression Beardslee et al. (2003). "Family Talk" is a program that targets families where a parent is diagnosed with a major depressive disorder or bipolar disorder and who have children aged 8 and 15 years who have never been treated for a mood disorder. Family Talk uses a cognitive psychoeducational approach of 6–10 sessions (Beardslee et al. 2007).

A related program, called "FAMpod—Families Preventing and Overcoming Depression," has received high ratings in the National Registry of Effective Programs and has been implemented in Finland, Norway, Costa Rica, and many areas in the USA. An adapted family intervention is being successfully piloted with immigrant Latina mothers with depression and their families (Valdez et al. 2013). An adaptation being implemented with military families is called Families OverComing Under Stress (FOCUS) (Beardslee et al. 2013). The core elements of FOCUS are (1) family Psychologic Health Check-in; (2) family-specific psychoeducation; (3) family narrative timeline; and (4) family-level resilience skills (e.g., problem solving). A family program that is not specific for depression is called Family Options and employs a care-coordination model tailored for individual families where a parent has a serious mental illness (Nicholson et al. 2009).

Adult Psychiatrist Perspective

Children are "invisible" to mental health professionals who provide care to adults. Adult psychiatrists feel unsure and untrained and therefore vulnerable that they may miss problems and incompetent to intervene. Additionally, adult psychiatric clinics are usually not set up to interface with child clinics and may lack a smooth referral process. For all these reasons, the reproductive activities of adult patients with mental illness are not acknowledged by either the patient who is a parent, or the adult psychiatrist. If a patient is pregnant, she may decide to drop out of treatment, or stop her medications, rather than ask her psychiatrist about parenting and mental illness.

It is important to convene a family meeting as soon as possible after accepting a new patient. The definition of family should be broad and defined by the patient. The role of others in child-rearing must be considered, for example othermothers, and invited into the family meeting (Burton & Hardaway, 2013). Othermothers are women who co-parent children that are their romantic partner's children from previous or current relationships.

Table 3.5 Visiting a parent in the hospital: guidelines for parents

• Make sure that the amount of time spent is appropriate for the age of the child. Younger children should visit for a shorter time than older children.
• Use short, focused activities such as jigsaw puzzles or books to ensure good interaction with the parent in the hospital.
• Reinforce parental role, meaning that the hospitalized parent should be well enough to act in the parental role. If they can do this for only 10 min, then the visit should be only 10 min long.
• Another parental figure should assess the situation and be responsible for detailing the routine and time spent.
• It is important to talk to children about their parent's illness. This should be ongoing and in small increments. The level of detail will be greater with older children.
• Be open, hopeful, but give realistic information. "Your mother is in hospital to get medication for her sadness. This takes a few days to a week. When she comes home, she will be able to sleep better and will feel better but she may not feel totally better for a while."
• Discuss how to help and care for ill parent. "We can help by being quiet at home, so that she can get enough sleep and rest. We can make sure she gets her favorite things to eat."
• Children need to be reassured they are cared for and loved. "Your mother loves you very much, but she needs to take care of herself right now, so she can get well."

Include children as soon as possible, in the outpatient and inpatient setting. Table 3.5 offers guidelines for parents who want to bring their children to the inpatient psychiatric setting (see Australian Infant, Child, Adolescent & Family Mental Health Association (2004) for further discussion on how to make an inpatient unit child-friendly). When you meet with the family, reassure the patient that you would like to meet their children. Offer a simple explanation such as your children might like to ask me questions or at least meet your doctor. When the children are present, tailor your comments to the developmental age of child. Statements like "Your mother has an illness that affects her thinking and feelings" can help a young child begin to understand what is going on. It is important to let them know that "She loves you just the same." Young children worry about their own care and you can reassure them that "Your father and your aunt will take care of you until she is better." It is important to give them a time frame, "That might be in 2–3 weeks." Table 3.6 offers suggestions for the first office visit.

Baby/Child Care Plans

An excellent proactive step for inpatient and outpatient settings is to develop care plans for a child or future baby. A care plan contains information to be used in the care of a baby or child, if the patient is unable to care for him/her due to illness or hospitalization. It can contain as much information as the parent wants, but usually, at a minimum, contains the names of surrogate caregivers, medication information, vaccinations, feeding, and regular activities. It should also identify who has the plan and contain signatures of the parent (s). Figure 3.1 has a care plan adapted from the Australian website for children with parents with mental illness (http://www.copmi. net.au/images/pdf/Parents-Families/baby-care-plan.pdf).

Table 3.6 Suggestions for the first office visit

Ask:
"How is your illness affecting your family?
How do the children understand your illness?
What do you explain to them?
What do they notice?"
Listen to their concerns as parents then suggest meeting with the family.
Have a helpful attitude and provide a list of support groups.
When you meet with the family, make your office child-friendly with toys, small seats, safe objects.
Treat children with respect and acknowledge the child's role in caregiving.
Ask children what questions they have.
Focus on the child's life and ask about their routine:
"How are things at home?
Do you have chores?
How do you feel when mom is not feeling well?
Who do you go to when you have a problem?
Who helps you when your mother is sick?
Do you help to take care of mom?"

Support Groups

We can encourage parents and family members to seek support in their community. Joyce Burland formed a peer support program after seeing that "family was shut out of any kind of collaborative involvement with their desperately ill family member. I simply found it unacceptable that in the USA there was this kind of prejudice against a group of people who were stepping forward to say, Help me be helpful. We were told You are not helpful" (Cunningham 2007). Her program is available nationally/internationally through the National Alliance of the Mentally Ill (NAMI) and is example of how family members can advocate for change. Maggie Jarry formed an organization called Daughters and Sons (http://www.thecrookedhouse.org) that focuses on "Facing Challenges of Growing up with a Parent with Mental Illness." The Crooked House offers a window onto a world often invisible to others. The organization offers resources for recovery for families dealing with mental illness: "You can't change the past, but perhaps you can make the path a little wider, a little clearer for tomorrow's travelers."

Summary

Preventing mental illness means identifying families at risk and intervening to reduce risk. We know that good parenting and good supports are optimal for the care of children and crucial for parents with mental illness. We must ask our patients if they are parents or prospective parents, and help them formulate

---

Baby Care Plan.

This plan is for the care of my/our baby should I/we be temporarily unable to care for him/her.

To be completed by parent/s or guardian/s:

I / We, _____, as the legal guardian of_____. (DOB   )

would like .... to stay with one of the following adults:

Name / relation to baby / contact info:

Signature_____

Important family members:

Medical (MD, vaccinations, medications, allergies):

Childcare / babysitter:

Feeding / Sleeping Routines:

If I'm hospitalized, I would like the following to occur is possible:

☐ My baby to be brought to see me when I'm well enough

☐ Regular photos/videos of my baby to be sent to me if I'm too far away for visits

☐ To speak to my baby regularly by phone when I'm well enough

☐ My baby to be shown photos of me regularly

Fig. 3.1 Baby care plan

questions that are relevant for them. We can provide illness education, develop care plans, and provide families with community supports. We can provide a list of resources for patients and their families (see below for a list of online resources). We can advocate for systems change by promoting interagency collaboration between adult child mental health services, child protection services, and social services. We can look worldwide and incorporate best practices. Australia has created a wonderful organization for children with an active online presence

(http://www.copmi.net.au). In the Netherlands, a comprehensive national prevention program focuses on children of parents with mental illness (Hosman
et al. 2009). Lastly, we must support the training of mental health professions in
working with families, talking with children, identify where prevention can occur,
and where treatment can be effective.

Resources for Patients and Their Families
The following websites contain helpful information, including the names of
support groups for families dealing with the mental illness of a loved one.
1. The Crooked House http://thecrookedhouse.org/
2. National Association for Children of Alcoholics http://www.nacoa.org/
3. The National Family Caregivers Association http://www.thefamily
   caregiver.org
4. The American Foundation for Suicide Prevention (AFSP) http://www.
   afsp.org
5. Family Connections: Coordinated by the National Education Alliance for
   Borderline Personality Disorder http://www.borderlinepersonalitydisorder.
   com/
6. Families for Depression Awareness http://www.familyaware.org
7. Families Together http://familiestogetherinc.org
8. Depression and Bipolar Support Alliance http://ww.dbsalliance.org
9. Mental Health America http://www.mentalhealthamerica.net
10. The Children's Society's Include Project http://www.youngcarer.com
11. The National Alliance on Mental: Family to Family Education Program
    http://www.nami.org
12. Support and Education Program for Families (SAFE) http://www.ouhsc.
    edu/safeprogram/
13. Network of Care http://networkofcare.org
14. Children and Adults with Attention Deficit/Hyperactivity Disorder http://
    chadd.org/
15. Active Minds on Campus http://ww.activeminds.org
16. Military Families Page: The Substance Abuse and Mental Health
    Services Administration http://www.samhsa.gov/militaryFamilies/
17. Compeer, Inc. http://www.compeer.org
18. Consumers Helping Others In a Caring Environment (CHOICE) http://
    www.choicenr.org
19. PLAN—Planned Lifetime Assistance Network (The National PLAN
    Alliance) http://www.nationalplanalliancc.org/
20. The Family Institute for Education, Practice and Research (University of
    Rochester Medical Center) http://www.nysfamilyinstitute.org/
21. World Federation for Mental Health: Center for Family Consumer Advo-
    cacy and Support http://www.wfmh.org

(continued)

22. The National Council for Community Behavioral Healthcare http://www. thenationalcouncil.org
23. What a Difference a Friend Makes http://www.whatadifference.samhsa. gov/
24. The National Federation of Families for Children's Mental Health http:// ffcmh.org/
25. National Evaluation Interactive Collaborative Network https://www. cmhs-icn.com/
26. The Technical Assistance Partnership for Child and Family Mental Health (TA Partnership) http://www.tapartnership.org/
27. Caring for Every Child's Mental Health Campaign http://www.samhsa. gov/children
28. Al-Anon Family Groups http://www.al-anon.alateen.org
29. SAMHSA's Resource Center to Promote Acceptance, Dignity and Social Inclusion Associated with Mental Health (ADS Center) http://www. allmentalhealth.samhsa.gov
30. SMART Recovery: http://www.smartrecovery.org/resources/family.htm
31. The World Fellowship for Schizophrenia and allied disorders website (http://www.world-schizophrenia.org/resources/booklist.html) has a list of recommended books for patients and their families

References

Australian COPMI baby care plan http://www.copmi.net.au/images/pdf/Parents-Families/baby-care-plan.pdf
Australian Infant, Child, Adolescent & Family Mental Health Association (2004) Checklist: is your adult mental health inpatient service family-friendly? http://www.copmi.net.au/mhw/files/MH_facilities_tips.doc
Beardslee WR (2002) Out of the darkened room: when a parent is depressed; protecting the children and strengthening the family. Little, Brown, & Company, New York
Beardslee WR, Versage EM, Gladstone TR (1998) Children of affectively ill parents: a review of the past 10 years. J Am Acad Child Adolesc Psychiatry 37:1134–1141
Beardslee WR, Gladstone TRG, Wright EJ, Cooper AB (2003) A family-based approach to the prevention of depressive symptoms in children at risk: evidence of parental and child change. Pediatrics 112(2):e119–e131
Beardslee WR, Wright EJ, Gladstone TRG, Forbes P (2007) Long-term effects from a randomized trial of two public health preventative interventions for parental depression. J Fam Psychol 21: 703–713
Beardslee WR, Klosinski LE, Saltzman W, Mogil C, Pangelinan S, McKnight CP, Lester P (2013) Dissemination of family-centered prevention for military and veteran families: adaptations and adoption within community and military systems of care. Clin Child Fam Psychol Rev 16(4): 394–409
Beresford B, Clarke S, Gridley K, Parker G, Pitman R, Spiers G (2008) Technical report for SCIE research review on access, acceptability and outcomes of services/interventions to support

parents with mental health problems and their families. Social Policy Research Unit, University of York

Bilsborough S (2004) What we want from adult psychiatrists and their colleagues: 'Telling it like it is'. In: Webster J, Seeman MV, Göpfert M (eds) Distressed parents and their families: parental psychiatric disorder. Cambridge University Press, Cambridge

Burton LM, Hardaway CR (2013) Low-income mothers as "othermothers" to their romantic partners' children: Women's coparenting in multiple partner fertility family structures. Fam Process 51:343–359

Cooklin A (2006) Being seen and heard: the needs of children of parents with mental illness (DVD). Royal college of psychiatrists: a film and training pack designed for use by staff involved in the care of parents with mental illness and their children. http://www.rcpsych.ac.uk/healthadvice/parentsandyouthinfo/youngpeople/caringforaparent.aspx

Cunningham R (2007) NAMI 2007 convention: interview with Joyce Burland (http://www.healthcentral.com/schizophrenia/c/100/12204/nami-2007)

Halligan S, Murray L, Martins C, Cooper P (2007) Maternal depression and psychiatric outcomes in adolescent offspring: a 13-year longitudinal study. J Affect Disorders 97:145–154

Hosman CMH, van Doesum KTM, van Santvoort F (2009) Prevention of emotional problems and psychiatric risks in children of parents with a mental illness in the Netherlands: I. The scientific basis to a comprehensive approach. Austr e-J Adv Mental Health 8:3

Jarry M (2009) Personal accounts: a peer saplings story: lifting the veil on parents with mental illness and their daughters and sons. Psychiatr Serv 60(12):1587–1588

Masten AS, Hubbard JJ, Gest SD, Tellegen A, Garmezy N, Ramirez M (1999) Competence in the context of adversity: pathways to resilience and maladaptation from childhood to late adolescence. Dev Psychopathol 11(1):143–169

National Alliance for Caregiving and United Hospital Fund (2005) Young caregivers in the U.S. Retrieved September 20, 2005, from http://www.caregiving.org/data/youngcaregivers.pdf

National Alliance of Caregiving http://www.caregiving.org/pdf/research/youngcaregivers.pdf

Nicholson J, Albert K, Gershenson B, Williams V, Biebel K (2009) Family options for parents with mental illnesses: a developmental, mixed methods pilot study. Psychiatr Rehabil J 33:106–114

Siegenthale E, Munder T, Egger M (2012) Effect of preventive interventions in mentally ill parents on the mental health of the offspring: systematic review and meta-analysis. J Am Acad Child Adolesc Psychiatry 51(1):8–17

Styron TH, Pruett MK, McMahon TJ, Davidson L (2002) Fathers with serious mental illnesses: a neglected group. Psychiatr Rehabil J 25:215–222

Valdez CR, Padilla B, Moore SM, Magaña S (2013) Feasibility, acceptability, and preliminary outcomes of the Fortalezas Familiares intervention for latino families facing maternal depression. Fam Process 52(3):394–410

Mothers Are Everywhere: Finding Stories of Motherhood in a State Psychiatric Hospital

Nikole Benders-Hadi

Abstract

Research and services for mothers with mental illness remain a slowly emerging field, and expanding discussion to include mothers who are also hospitalized is rare. This chapter describes a research study on the prevalence and needs of inpatient mothers at one state psychiatric hospital in suburban New York. Information on custody status, frequency of contacts, and effect of mental illness on parenting was collected, along with mothers' ideas on how the state hospital system can better serve them as parents. The idea that parenting can be tied to wellness and lead to improved treatment outcomes was not routinely acknowledged and leaves room for further research and policy changes to address this important social role among women.

Introduction

I have long known I was interested in working in the community or for a public sector agency, and that I wanted to work with families. I did my psychiatry residency training at New York University, which includes plenty of time spent in that world-renowned public hospital, Bellevue. After residency I seemed naturally led to enter the Columbia University Public Psychiatry Fellowship, a program that prepares psychiatrists for leadership roles in public and community psychiatry (Ranz et al. 1996). Fellows choose a field placement site at one of various public settings in the New York City area and take classes at Columbia 2 days a week. Fellows must also undertake a program evaluation or research project at their site.

It was during my interview at Rockland Psychiatric Center as a potential field placement that I came upon the project that became the inspiration for this book. Rockland Psychiatric Center is a large state psychiatric hospital about 20 miles

N. Benders-Hadi, M.D. (✉)
Orangeburg Service Center, Rockland Psychiatric Center, Orangeburg, NY, USA
e-mail: nikole.bendershadi@omh.ny.gov

N. Benders-Hadi and M.E. Barber (eds.), *Motherhood, Mental Illness and Recovery*,
DOI 10.1007/978-3-319-01318-3_4, © Springer International Publishing Switzerland 2014

north of New York City—not as well known as Bellevue but another institution epitomizing public sector treatment. My potential supervisor at Rockland, Dr. Mary Barber, mentioned to me during the interview that she had been asked by a colleague about how many mothers were being treated in the hospital. She had to say that she didn't know, had been thinking about the question ever since, and asked me if I would like to determine the answer. Right there, I had my chosen field placement and project for the year!

After starting at RPC I quickly realized that although a significant amount of information is collected on inpatients on admission and thereafter, parenting status appeared not to be included. The idea of acknowledging motherhood status for patients hospitalized for mental illness was almost an oxymoron for everyone I initially approached, even in a clinical setting. This study aimed to first determine the prevalence of mothers hospitalized at Rockland Psychiatric Center and second to gather information on custody, contacts, and how mental illness has impacted these patients as mothers in order to determine how the hospital could better serve these women.

While my early research on the topic revealed some studies and programs for mothers with mental illness, they almost exclusively focused on mothers in outpatient settings (Diaz-Caneja and Johnson 2004; Nicholson et al. 1993; Oyserman et al. 1994). I could not help but think that by acknowledging parenting status for those mothers who were hospitalized, we could tie parenting to wellness, positively impact treatment, and allow mothers to be discharged more quickly. Every additional day of someone not living a productive and fulfilling life of their own choosing distorts the purpose of the mental health system. My hope to garner acceptance of motherhood as an important social role among women with mental illness, and realizing the connection that could have for recovery at our facility, is what ultimately propelled this project forward.

As a mother myself, my connection to this population deepened. I realize all too well that the challenges associated with pregnancy, childbirth, and raising children can cause anyone to struggle at one time or another, and adding symptoms of mental illness into the equation may make those challenges even more pronounced. Given my personal experience, the opportunity to study the successes and challenges of mothers with mental illness, in hopes of ultimately providing a more therapeutic inpatient treatment environment, could not be overlooked. I felt confident that more than symptoms and deficits taking center stage, it would be stories of confidence, hope, and pride in parenting roles that emerged. The positive impact of acknowledging someone as a mother can enhance self-esteem, social functioning, and overall well-being, something that undeniably would be of benefit in this population as much as in the community. This chapter describes the four phases of the study as it took shape and outlines the challenges encountered in understanding the cohort at each stage.

Prevalence

The first phase of the study sought to assess the point prevalence of inpatient mothers at Rockland Psychiatric Center. At the time, there were over 400 inpatient beds at the facility, with approximately 35 % of the census comprised of women. I considered seeking the prevalence of mothers by direct inquiry of staff and informally began questioning some of staff on the unit where I held clinical responsibilities. Remarkably, it was the inconsistency of reports I found most striking. While some staff had a pretty good idea which women had children, others had no clue. This inconsistency was also not predictable by discipline, making it even more difficult to consider using this approach to get reliable results. Instead, I turned to the electronic medical record for the information I needed. In particular, I looked at the psychosocial assessment, which at this facility is completed on admission and then updated annually. Although not asking specifically about parenting status, I found this document to be the most likely place in the record for this information to be found. So I got to work. It was easy to identify the female inpatients, and then I set to reviewing the psychosocial assessment of all of these women to determine how many among them were identified as mothers.

I had ideas about what the motherhood prevalence would be. My guess was less than 20 %, given that the cohort of women were hospitalized at a typically longer-term state psychiatric facility where the median length of stay for all female patients was approximately 20 months. Most patients also had been transferred to our facility after community hospitals were unable to stabilize their symptoms. Besides being physically separated from family, the fact that they were hospitalized additionally had implications on illness impairment and current level of functioning. In actuality, the point prevalence of inpatient mothers at Rockland Psychiatric Center as of January 1, 2011 was found to be 38.5 %. That is, 50 out of 130 female inpatients were found to be mothers.

The data became even more interesting when looking at the results more closely. Out of the 130 female inpatients at that time, 49 had mention of children or their motherhood status in the medical record, and only 25 had specific mention that they were *not* mothers. A striking 43 % of the sample, or 56 women, had no mention of their parenting status either way. I thought carefully about the reasons behind this lack of documentation. Was it an indication that clinicians were not asking or did not consider it important to ask about parenting status? Alternatively, was it related to the acuity of symptoms having rendered women incapable of fully participating in a psychosocial assessment at that time? Either way, it left a gap in the data set, a hole that needed to be more understood.

For the 56 women who had no mention of motherhood status in their medical record, I went to the patients and treatment teams directly to ascertain the most accurate information possible. While some women had been discharged and were unable to be contacted, and others declined to answer any questions about their motherhood status, in the end only one additional mother among the group was identified.

The Survey

Throughout the first phase of this study, it became clear that motherhood can be a sensitive issue for women who did not or are not raising their children. Some mothers were reluctant to talk about children they did not raise or were not in contact with. For that reason, the second phase of the project involving a survey of identified mothers was introduced in a way that kept in mind such sensitivity and also left room for discussion of children even when mothers did not have current contact with them. The purpose of the survey was not only to obtain more detailed information on exactly who these mothers were, but also to address the second major question the study aimed to address—how could the hospital better serve these mothers?

Identified mothers were approached, and I sat down with 24 mothers who were found to have capacity and consented to participate in the questionnaire. Questions included information on the number of children each mother had, contact with their children, details on who was involved in raising the children, as well as open-ended questions on how their mental illness has impacted their parenting and what ideas they had on what the hospital could improve upon to address this role.

Results of the survey showed a cohort of mothers with children aging from 6 years to 52 years old. Most mothers surveyed reported having adult children, bringing into consideration the potential for ongoing guilt and loss of maternal identity. The majority of respondents also reported they served as primary caretakers of their children and had little to no involvement of child protective services. The most interesting result of the survey was related to the report of frequency of contacts with children. The majority of mothers (45.8 %) reported they had at least weekly contact with their children, some with contact multiple times a week. These contacts ranged from phone, to email, to visits to the hospital during visiting hours. The idea that hospitalization was not a deterrent to continued contact with their children only highlighted for me the importance of the relationship for both parent and child alike.

The subjective experience of sitting down to talk with these women about their parenting experience was also eye-opening. The excitement in the eyes of some women who reported to me never having been asking these sorts of questions was palpable. Everyone was given the option of stopping the interview at any point, and one mother became tearful and chose to end our discussions altogether when one of her children, who was conceived by rape, was brought up. In the end, what was clear was that the joys and sorrows of motherhood clearly existed for these women, the same as they would for any non-ill mother.

Focus Groups

The open-ended survey questions that attempted to address the impact of mental illness on parenting and get practical suggestions for how the facility could improve services provided to mothers did not garner as much data as anticipated. For that reason, the third phase of the study was started, where focus groups were held with groups of mothers to address these questions in an open forum discussion. All mothers in the facility were invited to participate and informed consent was obtained. In the end two focus groups were held, each with 5–6 participants. Each was recorded and then transcribed. As the group facilitator, I wanted my role to be as hands off as possible, to allow the mothers themselves to direct the discussion. Focus group topics that came up included how to talk to children about mental illness and empty nest syndrome, the need for ongoing parenting support groups and skills training, as well as suggestions for hospital policy change around issues of visitation.

Below is an excerpt from the transcript of one focus group. It emphasizes the guilt that can arise from physical separation as well as the feeling that a child's illness may be the mother's "fault." Names have been changed for privacy.

Jamie: *My oldest is 15 going on 16, and he lives in Florida, and my oldest sister has custody of him. I haven't seen him in about 2 years, and I really want to take a trip to see him. He can only talk to me on the phone all the time, and it's just not enough. My other son has been adopted so I haven't bonded with him at all. And that's been hard on me. The only good thing is I know who his adoptive mother is and she's very good to him, I know his adoptive sister and his grandmother, and he's in good hands. And my other son is in good hands. Um, it concerns me because I'm not there to see my oldest son, and he's having problems right now. Last summer he developed depression. He ended up overdosing on Benadryl...and in a psychiatric hospital for children for 2 days. And now my sister says he's back to being reclusive...and I'm concerned about him. I feel like if I was there I'd be able to talk to him. One thing I don't do; he's in therapy. I don't talk to him about his therapy, that's his private business. I shouldn't deal with that. So I stick to basic questions like how are you and how you doing, how's school? I feel like if I wasn't here I may be able to help him further, but it's kind of frustrating being where I am.*

Facilitator: *How do you talk to your son about depression?*

Jamie: *Its hard. And I feel responsible because I had the same problems he does. I was 15 when I first went to a psych hospital too, and I feel that somehow he inherited it from me, and that makes me feel that I did something wrong.*

Dolores: *It's not your fault. It's not your fault that you have an illness. This is something that all of us deal with, and it's not our fault that we do have a mental illness. It's how we recover from it, or how we cope with it. And I understand that your son is depressed, but as I have done with my children, I have left the door open and I tell them you can tell me anything.*

Jamie: *That's what I say to my son. I told him you can tell me anything you want, you can talk to me...I'll always be there to listen. I'll always be there to care for you, even though I might be really far away, I'm always there, you gotta remember that. And my son and I have always had a great relationship.*

Another excerpt shows the impact of having a child removed from a mother's custody. Notably, prior to the excerpt below Natalie appeared to be actively hallucinating by talking back to voices she was hearing.

Natalie: *You know...I have another kid he's 20 years old. He wasn't brought up with me, he was brought up with my cousin...I was so happy to have a baby...because this one I'm gonna grow it up as my own...well guess what happened? They put me in a chair to feed him, and all of a sudden the nurse says, Natalie, come here, you can't keep the baby, we're gonna have him adopted... I did go for treatment and everything- I could have kept the baby. I don't know why they did it, for the money or what...*

Facilitator: *Is that something that other people have experience with as well, feeling like other people are making decisions for you? Because of your mental illness?*

Natalie: *It has happened all my life. That's why I turned to drugs. You try, you try to get your kids back but he was adopted...to me he's not my son, he's my son but he's not the baby that I wanted to grow.*

Dolores: *The law is not kind to mothers who have a mental illness. They do consider this a danger to the child. So the law is pretty much against us. But, with groups like this, I believe we can put down enough ground for the future mothers who have mental illness and help them out. How to deal with the law, so that you can actually keep your child and raise your child.*

Jamie: *I was with a man for 5 years with domestic violence, he hurt me and hurt my child. And I decided to have another child who he did not hurt, but he physically hurt my oldest child and he physically hurt me. Because of that, and because of the way I was in the hospital because he was hurting me so much, they took away my children. The hardest thing was that my youngest child was nine and a half months old, I nursed him for nine and a half months, and I was still nursing and that broke my bond. And to this day, that still hurts me.*

Dolores: *No matter what happens when we are separated from our children, that bond will always be there. You are still their mother. And nobody can take that from you.*

While initial interest in the focus groups appeared to be high, attendance at each group was minimal by comparison. This led to additional questions about the awareness of clinical staff about parenting status and facility support of this issue in general which prompted the next phase of the study.

Treatment Planning

The final phase of the study aimed to determine how much motherhood status was considered in inpatient treatment planning. This was accomplished through a chart review looking at the multidisciplinary treatment plans developed for individual patients. What I found was that for nearly 21 % of surveyed mothers, there was no mention of either children or their motherhood role in the treatment plan. However for the remaining majority of surveyed mothers, there was at least passive mention of this role as important for the team to consider. While there is a distinct difference in passively mentioning a patient is in fact a mother without any elaboration and active inclusion of that role, there was at least some acknowledgment of motherhood for most mothers surveyed. Active inclusion included references to team members being in contact with children, including children in treatment and disposition planning, and/or acknowledgment of the motherhood role as important to that patient's treatment. One such record made mention that despite one mother not having had contact with her children in over 20 years, the team continued attempts to locate the family. Surprisingly, although documentation of motherhood status found in earlier phases of the study was mediocre at best, it did appear that when a mother was identified, this information was acknowledged at least to some extent in treatment.

Conclusion

In state psychiatric hospital settings in particular, no systematic information is collected on the prevalence of mothers or their contact with children. Although individualized, recovery-oriented care has become the gold standard of treatment for psychiatric patients in the state system, the special service needs of mentally ill mothers have been only rarely addressed. What I hope the description of this study accomplishes is to give readers a sense of who this group of mothers are and how much being acknowledged as a parent can mean. Rather than assuming parenting is a stressful role that is not valued by hospitalized mothers, taking the time to ask questions and inquire about our patients as individuals can impact treatment outcomes and prevent further missed opportunities to support mothers with mental illness.

References

Diaz-Caneja A, Johnson S (2004) The views and experiences of severely mentally ill mothers- a qualitative study. Soc Psychiatry Psychiatr Epidemiol 39:472–482

Nicholson J, Geller JL, Fisher WH, Dion GL (1993) State policies and programs that address the needs of mentally ill mothers in the public sector. Hosp Commun Psychiatry 44(5):484–489

Oyserman D, Mowbray C, Zemencuk J (1994) Resources and supports for mothers with severe mental illness. Health Soc Work 19(2):132–142

Ranz J, Rosenheck S, Deakins S (1996) Columbia University's fellowship in public psychiatry. Psychiatr Serv 47:512–516

Pregnancy and the Perinatal Period

5

Laura M. Polania

Abstract

Once thought to be a time of health protection and emotional well-being, pregnancy and the perinatal period is being recognized as a time of increased risk for recurrence of affective and psychotic illness. The factors contributing to this risk are numerous, and the clinical presentation can be confusing for both patient and clinician. Mental illness in the perinatal period and its risks are identifiable and predictable. Additionally, the impact of both conventional and integrative treatments on both mother and developing fetus are becoming better understood. Professionals in the field of perinatal psychiatry aim to develop and hone effective treatments of mental illness, with a focus on minimizing maternal distress and fetal risk, and preventing major adverse outcomes. We have come to understand that, in mental illness and medication treatments in pregnancy, there is no such thing as non-exposure. Our commitment is to minimize the risks of mothers' and their offsprings' exposure to acute episodes of illness, with a balanced understanding of the risks of conventional treatments. This chapter will outline current research and clinical guidelines in the treatment of mental illness during pregnancy and the perinatal period.

Once thought to be a time of health protection and emotional well-being, pregnancy and the peurperium is being recognized as a time of increased risk for recurrence of affective and psychotic illnesses (Kendell et al. 1987). With celebrities and the media giving a face to mental illness in pregnancy, the past decade has shone a public light on perinatal mental illness and need for effective treatments (Osmond 2002; Shields 2005; Paltrow 2011). Epidemiologic studies pointing to effects of mental illness on pregnancies and children, emerging data about safety/efficacy of pharmacologic and other treatments, and the urgency to address much publicized

L.M. Polania, M.D. (✉)
Audubon Clinic, New York State Psychiatric Institute, New York, NY, USA

Columbia University College of Physicians & Surgeons, New York, NY, USA
e-mail: polania@nyspi.columbia.edu

N. Benders-Hadi and M.E. Barber (eds.), *Motherhood, Mental Illness and Recovery*,   53
DOI 10.1007/978-3-319-01318-3_5, © Springer International Publishing Switzerland 2014

tragic outcomes simultaneously motivate mental health providers to develop reliable clinical guidelines. National and international organizations have been established to promote investigation into women's mental health needs (e.g., Marcé Society, North American Society for Psychosocial Obstetrics and Gynecology, Postpartum Support International), and government and public health organizations have devoted more resources to women's perinatal mental health issues (Boyd et al. 2002). These developments provide women and their care providers a backdrop for an informed discussion about mental illness in pregnancy and the postpartum period.

This chapter will outline the current wisdom regarding the prevalence and risks of depressive and anxiety disorders, bipolar spectrum disorders and major psychotic illness, and some of the literature on widely available modes of treatment. The literature and recommendations regarding mental illness in pregnancy and the perinatal period is vast and quickly expanding. Rather than providing an exhaustive review of the literature on syndromes and their treatment, this chapter aims to introduce the reader to the major factors that contribute to mental illness in the perinatal period.

Psychiatric issues in the perinatal period have historically been stratified into three major groups, the "blues," antenatal/postpartum depression, and psychosis (O'Hara 1987). Women in their reproductive years are at greatest risk for major mood disturbances. The changes in sleep, mood, energy, and appetite that accompany normal pregnancy can be difficult to distinguish from symptom collections seen in mental illness exacerbations. Before symptoms begin to affect a woman's sense of self and/or ability to care for herself and her offspring in pregnancy and postpartum periods, it is wise to seek the guidance of a mental health provider with familiarity of how mental illness presents in the perinatal period and a balanced view of effective management strategies.

Significant maternal morbidity and mortality are associated with mood disorders linked to pregnancy. At one end of the mental illness spectrum, we see the generally self-limited, culturally accepted, picture of the overwhelmed new mom supported by a network of people through her "blues." At the other, we see mothers without treatment, overwhelmed and isolated as their symptoms worsen, and put them at risk of endangering theirs and their children's lives. A study of nearly 500,000 women showed that the "relative risk" of admission to a psychiatric hospital with a psychotic illness was extremely high in the first 30 days after childbirth (Kendell et al. 1987). A substantial rate of suicide occurs postpartum, as maternal suicide accounts for up to 20 % of postnatal deaths in depressed women (Lindahl et al. 2005). Despite such high stakes, clinicians are without clear guidelines on how to best help this vulnerable population.

Although there are no empirically based treatment guidelines for the management of major mental illness during pregnancy, substantial progress has been made with improved information on the course of illness in pregnancy, the risks of recurrence during pregnancy and in the postpartum period, and the reproductive safety and efficacy of treatments. Providing balanced and individualized information about treatment options and relative risks, including the limits of current knowledge, can contribute importantly to informed family planning by women with mental illness (Viguera 2002).

The Baby Blues

The major hormonal, interpersonal, and diurnal shifts that accompany delivery can affect a new mother's mood precipitously and manifest as "baby blues," a syndrome of affective reactivity, irritability, fatigue, and general malaise generally beginning around day three after parturition. Baby blues are generally normal reactions to the hormonal changes and stress after delivery, and generally subside without medical intervention, within 2 weeks postpartum (Yalom et al. 1968). In "baby blues," suicidal ideation is not present and sad mood, worthlessness, and hopelessness are not pronounced. Although "baby blues" was previously considered benign, increasing evidence suggests that women with these symptoms are at risk of progression to postpartum major depression (Henshaw et al. 2004). All women require the support of the family and community network with a watchful eye for worsening or lack of resolution of such symptoms.

Major Depression

Though some emotionality is a frequent and normal part of pregnancy and parturition, major mood episodes affect a significant proportion of women during pregnancy and in the postpartum period. In fact, depression is the second greatest cause of morbidity for women of childbearing years, second only to HIV-AIDS in cause of disability (Mathers et al. 2006). The prevalence of depression in women's lifetimes is approximately 10–25 %, with greatest risk of depressive disorder occurring during childbearing years (Bennett et al. 2004). Studies estimate that 18 % of pregnant women will suffer from depressive symptoms and that approximately 14 % of women will meet criteria for major depression during pregnancy (Marcus et al. 2003) and postpartum (Gavin et al. 2005).

Signs and symptoms for perinatal depression are similar to those for depression in the general population: depressed mood, loss of interest or pleasure, feelings of guilt or low self-worth, disturbed sleep or appetite, low energy, and poor concentration (Lee and Chung 2007). Clinical wisdom points to depression marked by high levels of anxiety and worry about the health of the baby and the fitness of mother/patient. Prevalence of antenatal depression appears to peak in the first trimester, while postpartum depression peaks around 12 weeks after delivery (Gavin et al. 2005) with elevated risk lasting well into the first year postpartum.

Antepartum Depression

Mood and anxiety disorders profoundly affect the somatic and emotional experience of the expectant mother during pregnancy. A prospective study of nearly 1,500 patients showed significant associations between depression and/or anxiety and increased nausea and vomiting, prolonged sick leave during pregnancy, and increased number of visits to the obstetrician, specifically, visits related to fear of childbirth and those related to contractions (Andersson et al. 2004). Psychiatric diagnoses are also associated with an increased risk of inadequate prenatal care even when studies controlled for other known risk factors (Kelly et al. 1999).

Early data did not indicate that antepartum depression (depression during pregnancy) is higher at any particular trimester during pregnancy or month in the first postpartum year (Bennett et al. 2004; Gavin et al. 2005). More recent data however, shows that 43 % of women with histories of unipolar depression will relapse without treatment in pregnancy and the postpartum period, with half of such occurring by the third trimester (Vesga-López et al. 2008; Evans et al. 2001). As the patient becomes pregnant and throughout pregnancy, the clinician must closely monitor for changes in thought, diurnal, and affective patterns that can mark an abrupt worsening of mood and need for treatment adjustments.

Women who are pregnant or recently pregnant are less likely than their non-perinatal counterparts to seek mental health services (Vesga-López et al. 2008), much less comply with pharmacologic medications (Battle et al. 2006). Upon learning of their pregnancy, a significant proportion of women discontinue their psychiatric medication for fear of prenatal exposure of offspring to these agents, thereby increasing the risk of depressive relapse during pregnancy or the puerperium (Vesga-López et al. 2008). A 2006 study estimated that women who discontinue antidepressant use have a fivefold increased rate of relapse of their depression by their third trimester compared to women who maintained treatment throughout pregnancy (Cohen et al. 2006).

Anxiety and its effects on perinatal outcomes have also received increased attention. Rate of pregnant women suffering with significant anxiety symptoms is approximated at 13 % and is generally linked to comorbid depression (Heron et al. 2004). In addition, approximately one-third of all depressed women were diagnosed with comorbid Axis I disorders, most typically an anxiety disorder (panic disorder and PTSD) or, less frequently, a substance-related disorder (Battle et al. 2006). Additionally, significant prenatal anxiety has been shown to correlate to postnatal depression even after controlling for antenatal mood episodes (Austin et al. 2007; Milgrom et al. 2008).

Postpartum Depression

It appears that the postpartum period, with its disrupted sleep wake cycle, fatigue, role changes, dynamic triggers, and hormonal shifts, puts women at more of a pronounced risk for mood episodes than at any other time in their reproductive lives. Other factors that confer heightened risk for depression during pregnancy/ postpartum include a prior history of depression (O'Hara 1995), young age (Frank et al. 1990), limited social supports (Bolton et al. 1998), ambivalence about pregnancy, marital conflicts (Kumar and Robson 1984), unmarried marital status (Witt et al. 2010), and prior history of significant premenstrual symptoms (Sylvén et al. 2013). Though many medical and psychosocial factors can increase the risk of developing perinatal depression, both clinician and patient should be aware of the elevated risk for depression if risk factors such as those described above are present.

It is the task of mental health providers to help women weigh the risks of mental illness to themselves and their offspring versus the risks of pharmacologic and other treatments in the perinatal period. A woman experiencing mild symptoms of mood or anxiety disturbance, without sleep disturbance and without prior psychiatric history, may be at less risk of a severe episode than a woman with a history of past psychiatric illness, need for pharmacologic treatment, or history of suicidality or hospitalization. The risks of treatment should be considered along side of the risks of nontreatment—resulting in differing treatment plans.

Risks of Untreated Depression

Depression has been recognized as a disease that affects obstetrical and neonatal outcomes (Chung et al. 2001). Maternal depression has been shown to correlate with premature delivery (Grigoriadis et al. 2013) and preeclampsia (Kurki et al. 2000). Other studies show that significant depressive and anxiety-related symptoms in pregnancy are associated with increased risk of preterm delivery and small-for-gestational-age births (Orr 2002; Hoffman and Hatch 2000), low birth weight, intrauterine growth retardation/SGA (Steer et al. 1992; Hauck et al. 2008), and even spontaneous abortion (Boyles et al. 2000; Michel-Wolfromm 1968). Other studies have linked antenatal depression to an increased risk of operative deliveries, use of epidural anesthesia and other invasive obstetrical manipulations, increase risk of cesarean delivery, and subjective experience of length of labor (Chung et al. 2001; Andersson et al. 2004). Studies have shown that newborns of depressed mothers show a biochemical/physiological profile that mimics the physiologic changes seen in their depressed mothers, most markedly, elevated cortisol—which is linked to adverse outcomes (Field et al. 2006). It is clear that women with depression in pregnancy are at risk for complicated births and should be considered high risk. The psychiatrist and obstetrician can work with the patient to lessen these risks through early detection and effective treatment.

Perinatal depression has furthermore been associated with significant negative effects on child development. Significant depressive symptoms in pregnancy and the postpartum period have been shown to be linked to difficult infant and child-hood temperament (Britton 2011), poor or insecure attachment styles (Forman et al. 2007), and increased risk of developmental delay and lower IQ scores (Deave et al. 2008). As compared to nondepressed women and their children, these studies demonstrate the negative effects of untreated depression on infant development. It is thought that the chronic exposure to negative affective states in the mother and their effect on the dynamics between parent and child are responsible for later disruptions in interpersonal behavior (Tronick and Reck 2009). Studies on effectively treated maternal depression show that early treatment of maternal depression is directly linked to resolution of adverse behavioral and intellectual outcomes in the child (Cicchetti et al. 2000; Bigatti et al. 2001). The identification and management of depression in the perinatal period can decrease maternal suffering and optimize the health of the offspring.

Bipolar Disorder

Though most studies do not associate an increase in antenatal manic episodes relative to nonpregnant counterparts, childbirth has long been established as the precipitant in over one out of four manic episodes (Ambelas 1987; Hunt 1995). A recent observational study showed that in women having first episodes of mania/ psychosis postdelivery, the rate of subsequent non-puerperal episodes was 69 % (Brockington et al. 1981; Blackmore et al. 2013). Such results suggest that postpartum may unmask bipolar diatheses in a large proportion of women. Clinical wisdom supports these findings, and women with postpartum psychosis must be armed with an understanding that ongoing management of bipolar illness may help mitigate future episodes.

Discontinuation of medication during pregnancy occurs often in women with bipolar disorder. Although it appears to carry a high risk for antenatal and postpartum relapse. A 2007 study demonstrated an overall risk of at least one mood episode in pregnancy as high as 71 % in women with bipolar disorder who had discontinued mood stabilizer treatment. Among women who discontinued mood stabilizer treatment, recurrence risk was twofold greater than their counterparts who remained on treatment. Further, the median time to first recurrence was more than fourfold shorter, and the proportion of weeks ill during pregnancy was five times greater than subjects who continued treatment (Viguera et al. 2007). In other words, women with bipolar disturbance who stopped treatment tended to get sicker, faster, and took longer to stabilize than women who continued with their treatment.

In women diagnosed with bipolar disorder, between 25 % and 40 % of post partum periods are affected by an episode of mania or depression with psychotic features (Jones and Craddock 2001). The risk of postpartum psychosis in the general population is 1 in 1,000. This risk rises to 1 in 7 in women diagnosed with bipolar disorder and an estimated 1 in 2 in women with bipolar disorder and a family history of postpartum psychosis (Jones and Craddock 2001). Even if asymptomatic, pregnant women with family histories of bipolar disorder or postpartum mood or psychotic disturbance should be considered at significant risk for postpartum psychosis and a prophylactic plan for immediate intervention should be explicit among the treatment team.

The most frightening outcomes associated to mental illness in pregnancy have been episodes of violence associated with postpartum psychosis including filicide.

It is estimated that approximately 5 % of women with postpartum psychosis will commit infanticide (Spinelli 2009). Another case series showed that upwards of 73 % of women with psychosis who committed filicide were found to have underlying diagnoses of bipolar disorder (Kim et al. 2008). Such occurrences are tragic and terrifying, albeit rare, and harken a call to close management of all patients presenting with psychiatric symptoms in the postpartum period.

Pregnancy Risks of Bipolar Disorder

Bipolar disorder in women during pregnancy, whether treated or not, was associated with increased risks of adverse pregnancy outcomes. Studies show that pregnant women with bipolar disorder were more likely to have low birth weight infants and preterm births than pregnant women with no history of mental illness. Women with bipolar disorder are approximately two times more likely to undergo preterm delivery, and low birth weight babies, regardless of treatment status (Lee and Lin 2010; Lundgren et al. 2012).

Postpartum Psychosis

Episodes of mental illness during pregnancy generally present as predominantly depressive/dysphoric, regardless of mood disorder type (i.e., Unipolar Major Depression, Bipolar Disorder, Anxiety Disorders). Still, in the mainstream media and in the literature, increasing attention is being paid to postpartum psychosis. Postpartum psychosis is most appropriately considered a phenomenologic descriptor of the most severe of mental health disturbances that occur in perinatal period, rather than an illness of singular etiology. The illnesses that can manifest with psychosis in the postpartum period include major depression with psychotic features, bipolar I, bipolar II, schizoaffective, unspecified functional psychosis, and brief psychotic disorder. Studies since the 1980s have linked the occurrence of postpartum psychosis to underlying bipolar disorder diagnosis in over 80 % of patients (Meltzer and Kumar 1985; Kendell et al. 1987; Brockington et al. 1981). Bipolar disorder is widely accepted as the illness underlying most cases of postpartum psychosis.

Postpartum psychosis presents most commonly in the first 2 weeks of the postpartum period, often within days of delivery. Common initial symptoms include severe anxiety, restlessness, depressive mood, sleep disturbances, behavior disturbances, catatonic excitement, delusions, and hallucinations (Rohde and Marneros 1993). An early descriptive study pointed to a picture of postpartum psychosis differing from nonaffective psychoses, namely more marked reports of "delirium like" confusion and behavioral disorganization (Brockington et al. 1981). As compared with nonpuerperal counterparts, postpartum psychotic episodes present more commonly with a waxing and waning picture of thought disorganization, pronounced hallucinations and perceptual symptoms, delusions of control or influence, lack of insight, and social withdrawal (Wisner et al. 1994; Rohde and Marneros 1993). When detected, postpartum psychosis is considered a psychiatric emergency and often requires psychiatric hospitalization (Spinelli 2009).

Schizophrenia and Pregnancy

Though a significant proportion of postpartum psychosis has been linked to underlying diagnosis of bipolar spectrum illness, women with non-affective psychotic illness (i.e. schizophrenia) represent an important proportion of women who experience an exacerbation of symptoms in the perinatal period. There is a relative paucity of literature on the course of psychosis during pregnancy and the postpartum period, possibly due to a historic resistance to seeing women with chronic psychotic illness as mothers themselves. As mental health care evolves, so does our understanding of the reproductive lives of the women we treat, their potential as parents, and their unique needs as patients.

Early studies found low fertility in women with schizophrenia, when compared with rates in the general population (Slater 1971). More recent and methodologically rigorous studies show no difference in fertility between women with schizophrenia and controls (Burr et al. 1979; Miller 1997). It is posited that an increase in fertility rates in women with chronic psychosis came with the decrease in ovulatory suppression seen with atypical antipsychotics relative to first generation neuroleptics (Howard et al. 2002). Women with psychotic illnesses tend to have fewer children than nonpsychotic counterparts, yet it is estimated that up to 60 % of women in inpatient psychiatric settings are mothers (Howard 2001).

Schizophrenia is linked to behaviors that increase pregnancy-related risks. Smoking and other substance use disorders carry a 47 % lifetime prevalence in people with schizophrenia, and a 1996 retrospective study showed that up to 78 % of women admitted to substance use during their pregnancies (Miller and Finnerty 1996). In fact, in pregnant women with schizophrenia, poor self-care, poor nutrition, prenatal care, risks of substance use, poor judgment, and fetal abuse/injury have all been linked to adverse infant outcomes (Zuckerman et al. 1989; Nilsson et al. 2002).

A 2001 study showed that children of women with schizophrenia had increased risk of postneonatal death, generally attributed to an increased risk of sudden infant death syndrome (Bennedsen et al. 2001). A large 2002 study found significantly increased risks for stillbirth, infant death, preterm delivery and low birth weight, and small-for-gestational age among the offsprings of women with schizophrenia, even when controlling for adverse health behaviors (Nilsson et al. 2002; Jablensky et al. 2005). A recent study linked schizophrenia in mothers to complicated obstetrical outcomes such as preeclampsia and Eclampsia, gestational diabetes, venous thromboembolism, operative deliveries, and postpartum medical complications (Vigod et al. 2014). Children of women with schizophrenia had a marginally statistically significant increase in the risk of congenital malformations, though no control was made for smoking or other adverse pregnancy risks

(Bennedsen et al. 2001). Such findings underscore the value and need for multifaceted and intensive supports. Intensive community and treatment team supports thoroughout the reproductive years.

Psychotic symptoms can alter women's perceptions of bodily processes, leading to late detection of pregnancy and delayed postnatal care (McNeil et al. 1984). In rare cases, a psychotic denial of pregnancy can occur, particularly in women with diagnoses of chronic schizophrenia with previous custody loss and associated anticipated separation from the baby they were carrying (Miller 1997). Miller suggests that treatment for such patients should take place in a setting that integrates comprehensive psychiatric and obstetrical care and may include pharmacotherapy, supportive psychotherapy, and evaluation of the patient's parenting skills and support network to assess and optimize continued custody (Miller 1997).

More commonly, in the postnatal period, hallucinations, paranoia, and other perceputal symptoms can interfere with the mother's ability to detect and respond to nuanced cues from the baby and require supervision or help from others (Solari et al. 2009). Likewise, the negative symptoms of chronic psychosis may interfere with a mother's ability to read her baby's nonverbal cues and may reduce capacity to communicate with and appropriately stimulate the baby (Solari et al. 2009). The disturbances in object constancy observed in children of women hospitalized early in their infancy has lead researchers to follow the social and cognitive development of children of women with schizophrenia (Gamer et al. 1976). Though it is unclear that such disturbances affect later cognitive or social functioning. Early studies link impairments in object constancy to an elevated risk of development of psychosis later in life (Gamer et al. 1976). Caretakers and kin should receive guidance to be sure that the infant's needs are being met and that appropriate bonding with mother or another caretaker is provided.

Approaches to Treatment

Despite the risks outlined above, women with mental illness most often thrive as mothers. For many women, motherhood and bonding with a new baby can bring much meaning to their lives and identities. By being sensitive to the experiences of the pregnant woman with mental illness and warning signs, families and clinicians can intervene before illness exacerbations take full hold. Understanding the environment and assessing parenting capacity can guide interventions including referrals to community resources, positioning of added supports, and the introduction of psychoeducational tools to enhance parenting capacity. Lastly, the relationships between treatment team and expectant and new mother can serve as a corrective emotional experience and template for supportive healthy relationships in growing families.

There are significant challenges to the approach of treatment of the pregnant and postpartum woman with mental illness. Much fear and stigma surrounding psychiatric diagnosis continues to exist, oftentimes leading women to delay seeking care. Social, familial, and logistical barriers to care exist and are reinforced as women shift into role of primary caretaker, including pressures in early motherhood to tend exclusively to the needs of the newborn and family. Any attempts for a woman to care for or take time for herself may be seen as "selfish" or ungrateful. This is compounded with the expectation, in both mother and family, that pregnancy and the postpartum period are periods in life to be relished and enjoyed without ambivalence. Logistics in seeking care are notoriously difficult to arrange; the fear of stigma and child protection involvement likewise inhibit women from seeking care. The barriers to care are simple, multi-tiered, blatant, and nuanced—all at once.

One onerous challenge is the lack of consensus about treatment or consolidated treatment guidelines. This is generally attributable to the fact that data evaluating the safety and efficacy of treatments in pregnant/postpartum women are notoriously difficult to generalize and apply usefully. The data that exists is generally based on results of case studies, registries, and other non-empirically gathered means. There is a lack of prospective, high quality, well-controlled trials since randomized design in studies evaluating pharmacologic treatment of depression during pregnancy is generally not considered ethical. Data continues to be largely dependent on animal studies, case studies, and retrospective reviews. Historically, research in reproductive psychiatry has been predominantly observational and retrospective with small study populations, making results vulnerable to selection and recall bias, and the effects of other clinical confounders. Though imperfect, studies can provide useful information which requires the clinician's critical evaluation of both methodology and conclusions.

In 1979, the FDA adopted the Pregnancy Category System in an attempt to provide physicians and patients with a readymade analysis of the data to serve as guidance in the planning of pregnancy, before fetal exposure had occurred. This system has proven difficult to apply clinically as it rests on the assumption that pregnant women generally do not need medication, without consideration of the risks of untreated illness, or the consideration of the reality that unintended pregnancies (and hence, exposures) do occur (Feibus 2008). Further, it does not account for changes in pharmacokinetics and metabolism during differing stages in pregnancy or a sophisticated consideration of the applicability of animal data. The category system is sometimes interpreted as a grading system where the risk increases as one progresses through grades A through X, without consideration of the potential benefits of treatment. Fortunately, the FDA is currently considering a new system of reporting pregnancy and lactation data to provide clinicians and patients with a more clinically useful classification system (Boothby and Doering 2001; Law et al. 2010). Until this time, clinicians and patients are left to interpret risk using an understanding of each patient's history, the sparse literature on risk and treatment, and the current category system to address the treatment needs of patients.

An approach to consideration of treatment of mental illness in pregnancy requires a collaborative analysis between clinician and client in weighing the risk of untreated illness with the risk of medication exposure. It is favorable for exposure be kept to a minimum and if possible, to one agent at its lowest effective dose. Selection of medications must be based on an understanding of the patient's history of success with medication treatment, prior experience of the patient with exposure and illness in previous pregnancies, and available safety information. It is advisable to maximize non-pharmacologic options to help minimize exposure when possible, with an understanding of the evolving nature of mood and psychotic illness in the pregnancy and the postpartum period. Due to the enormity and complexity of the topic, the use of specific medications during pregnancy and the perinatal period will not be broached here, and readers should utilize the resources section at the end of this chapter for further information.

In approaching the evaluation and treatment of the perinatal patient, the diagnostician's task is to collect an exhaustive history and review of systems in order to separate the normal somatic symptoms of pregnancy from a major mood episode. The Edinburgh Postnatal Depression Rating Scale (Murray and Cox 1990) and the Beck Depression Inventory (Holcomb et al. 1996) can be useful tools for clinicians as they have been validated for use in the obstetric population. Special attention should be paid to family history of mood disorders as well as previous history of harm to self or others, history of psychosis, and history of symptoms linked to prior reproductive events. Further, personal or family histories should be fully explored as they may point to bipolar spectrum illness and guide treatment choices.

When discussing possible interventions, discussions should be approached from an approximation of a risk–risk ratio, the risk of exposure of the fetus or newborn to maternal illness versus the risk of exposure to the treatment that is being proposed (Yonkers et al. 2009). Discussion of medication treatment of mental illness in pregnancy and during lactation typically includes a consideration of data on risks of exposure at distinct phases in the peripartum period: teratogenic risk, neonatal risks, neurodevelopmental risk, and effects on lactation. A presentation of known data should underscore the paucity of randomized controlled trials and limitations of the available data while acknowledging that substantial data and clinical experience support the safety and efficacy of many treatments. With that in mind, non-medication interventions have shown promise in helping improve health and mitigate symptoms and should be considered as clinically appropriate.

Psychotherapy

Psychotherapy in pregnancy and the perinatal period is critical for the mother suffering from all levels of symptomatology. It is critical that clinicians aid patients in the processing of this major life event, as psychosocial stressors can often be improved with counseling and social interventions either in tandem to other treatments or as a primary approach. Ego strengths, rallying of family, promotions of healthy life choices, and validation of evolving life roles and self-concept are just some arenas where psychotherapy can help ameliorate symptoms. For instance, mild postnatal depression may be improved increasing family supports. Cognitive behavioral counseling and interpersonal therapy have been shown to be useful in treating postnatal depression (Cox et al. 1993; O'Hara 2009). Interpersonal therapy has likewise been shown to be an effective alternate or adjunct to pharmacotherapy in depression (Spinelli 1997). Psychotherapy focusing on the child–parent dyad has also shown promise in promoting maternal confidence, bonding, and child development (Cicchetti et al. 2000). Parenting support and skills groups can be especially helpful for socially isolated mothers and those with less access to educational resources, but offer all parents a social connection, valuable validation of their experiences, and the benefits associated with both teaching and learning from their peers.

Integrative Practices

More attention is likewise being given to complementary and integrative medicine and its role in pregnancy. A 2001 study showed that up to 54 % of participants with depression reported past-year use of complementary and alternative medicine. Reasons for exploring complementary approaches include, the desire for treatments to be based on a "natural approach," feeling such treatments were congruent with their own values and beliefs, and poor prior experiences with conventional approaches (Wu et al. 2007). Likewise, many integrative approaches seek to optimize health, which should be the aim of all persons involved in the care of the pregnant woman. It is therefore important for clinicians to have knowledge of complementary and integrative treatments for symptoms of mental illness in the pregnant and postpartum patient.

Several non-pharmacologic integrative treatments have shown promise as safe, effective treatments for depression in pregnancy. A small randomly controlled trial showed promise for treatment of depression with perinatal massage (Field et al. 2004) and even decreased rates of prematurity and low birth weight (Field et al. 2009). Bright light therapy has received increasing attention after an open trial showed morning light therapy to have significant antidepressant effect during pregnancy (Oren et al. 2002). Likewise, acupuncture specific to depression has been shown to be helpful in controlling symptoms in pregnant women (Manber et al. 2010). Despite encouraging data, many clinicians in practice feel that more powered systematic studies are necessary to confirm the role of complementary and alternative medicine therapies in the treatment of perinatal depression.

Conclusions

Pregnancy and the postpartum period is a time of psychiatric vulnerability for women, and both treatment and lack of treatment of mental illness carry some risk to both mother and child. Still, mental illness during this vulnerable time is predictable, identifiable, treatable, and, therefore, preventable. For the clinician treating a patient with a history of mental illness, pregnancy and postpartum period is a unique opportunity to collaborate actively with his or her patient to enhance good outcomes and help women enjoy this major life stage.

When counseling patients with mental illness regarding treatment options, it is important to elucidate the risks and benefits of treatment options for each pregnancy phase—preconception, first trimester, second trimester, third trimester, neonatal, and later in life. The risks associated with treatment change with both phases of pregnancy and the postpartum period as well as with the needs and symptom burden of the patient. Critically important is a thorough discussion of the risks both of the treatments and of untreated depression, as it evolves in pregnancy and the postpartum period (Yonkers et al. 2009).

A careful and complete assessment of and follow-up with women suffering from mental illness in pregnancy/postpartum periods should include a thorough exploration of potential psychotic symptoms and a careful safety assessment to prevent harm to both mother and child. Inquiry into the presence of bizarre delusions of influence or passivity, tactile or olfactory hallucinations, or cognitive impairment may indicate an emerging psychosis, for which psychiatric hospitalization should be strongly considered.

Mental illness itself can put women at risk for poor pregnancy outcomes, but improved research methods can help us understand the factors contributing to increased risk. Once we identify and understand the risk factors that are modifiable in treating women with mental illness, we can begin to help address such factors, with the goal of witnessing improved outcomes for both mother and child.

The goal of the mental health practitioner and patient team is to maintain mental health in women with histories of mental illness. An understanding of high risk times in pregnancy and postpartum along with identification of signs of relapse are important first steps. Clinicians and patients should be aware of relapse triggers and early warning signs (e.g., changes in sleep, hygiene, cognitive changes, affective changes). Additionally, both the clinician and patient should understand the evolving needs of the pregnant and postpartum period and adjust treatments accordingly (including but not limited to dosing of medications, timing and frequency of visits, inter-visit communication, collaboration with family, other care providers, and outside agencies). The primary medical providers and family should be contacted for collateral information about the patient and to offer psychoeducation and guidance throughout the pregnancy and postpartum period. Engagement and rallying of loved ones and caregivers can help establish a scaffolding upon which supports of the expectant and new mother can be positioned. Most cases also merit referral to high risk obstetrics for comanagement.

Many clinicians who successfully manage mental illness in pregnancy and the postpartum period expand the frame of treatment during this time of evolving needs. The clinician has a duty to collaborate with the patient's other care providers for information exchange as well as the development of a unified plan of ongoing and contingency management. Collaboration with family and medical providers can have a significant impact in maternal and fetal outcomes (Acera Pozzi et al. 2014). Similarly the rallying of family supports in the form of collaborative sessions, psychoeducation, and contacts with family members (with patient consent) is helpful. Clinicians may also serve as sounding boards for patients to better understand the normal range of reactions to the enormous life changes they face. The clinician can help navigate information, encourage patients to seek advice and help from others, provide resources and outlets, and suggest strategies to help in the care of both mother and her growing family.

General Resources for Psychiatric Disorders in Pregnancy and the Perinatal Period

- Massachusetts General Hospital Center for Women's Mental Health Web site: http://www.womensmentalhealth.org
- MedEdPPD: http://www.mededppd.org
- Postpartum support international: http://www.postpartum.net
- REPROTOX: http://www.reprotox.org
- TERIS (Teratogen Information System)
- TOXNET (TOxicology Data Network) Http://toxnet.nlm.nih.gov
- LACTMED
- Motherrisk http://www.motherrisk.org
- OTIS Organization of Teratology Information Specialists http://www. otispregnancy.org
- American Academy of neurology practice guidelines: http://www.aan.com/go/ practice/guidelines
- American psychiatric Association practice guidelines: http://www.psych.org
- National guideline clearinghouse: http://www.guideline.gov
- US FDA of Women's Health pregnancy registry: http://www.fda.gov/womens/ registries/defailt.htm
- National pregnancy Registry for Atypical Antipsychotics: http://www. womensmentalhealth.org/pregnancyregistry/
- North American antiepileptic drug pregnancy registry: http://www. aedpregnancyregistry.org

References

Acera Pozzi R, Yee LM, Brown K, Driscoll KE, Rajan PV (2014) Pregnancy in the severely mentally ill patient as an opportunity for global coordination of care. Am J Obstet Gynecol 210 (1):32–7. doi:10.1016/j.ajog.2013.07.029

Ambelas A (1987) Life events and mania: a special relationship? Br J Psychiatry 501:235–240

Andersson L, Sundström-Poromaa I, Wulff M, Aström M, Bixo M (2004) Implications of antenatal depression and anxiety for obstetric outcome. Obstet Gynecol 104(3):467–76. doi:10.1097/01.AOG.0000135277.04565.e9

Austin M-P, Tully L, Parker G (2007) Examining the relationship between antenatal anxiety and postnatal depression. J Affect Disorders 101(1–3):169–74. doi:10.1016/j.jad.2006.11.015

Battle CL, Zlotnick C, Miller IW, Pearlstein T, Howard M (2006) Clinical characteristics of perinatal psychiatric patients: a chart review study. J Nervous Mental Dis 194(5):369–77. doi:10.1097/01.nmd.0000217833.49686.c0

Bennedsen BE, Mortensen PB, Olesen AV, Henriksen TB (2001). Congenital malformations, stillbirths, and infant deaths among children of women with schizophrenia. Arch Gen Psychiatry 58(7):674–679. Retrieved from http://www.ncbi.nlm.nih.gov/pubmed/11448375

Bennett HA, Einarson A, Taddio A, Koren G, Einarson TR (2004) Prevalence of depression during pregnancy: systematic review. Obstet Gynecol 103(4):698–709. doi:10.1097/01.AOG.0000116689.75396.5f

Bigatti SM, Cronan TA, Anaya A (2001) The effects of maternal depression on the efficacy of a literacy intervention program. Child psychiatry and human development 32(2):147–62, Retrieved from http://www.ncbi.nlm.nih.gov/pubmed/11758880

Blackmore ER., Rubinow DR, O'Connor TG, Liu X, Tang W, Craddock N, Jones I (2013) Reproductive outcomes and risk of subsequent illness in women diagnosed with postpartum psychosis. Bipolar Disorders 394–404. doi:10.1111/bdi.12071

Bolton H, Hughes PM, Turton P, Sedgwick P (1998) Incidence and demographic correlates of depressive symptoms during pregnancy in an inner London population. J Psychosom Obstet Gynaecol 19(4):202–209, Retrieved from http://informahealthcare.com/doi/abs/10.3109/01674829809025698

Boothby LA, Doering PL (2001) FDA labeling system for drugs in pregnancy. Ann Pharmacother 35(11):1485–1489. doi:10.1345/aph.1A034

Boyd RC, Pearson JL, Blehar MC (2002) Prevention and treatment of depression in pregnancy and the postpartum period: summary of a maternal depression roundtable: a U.S. perspective. Arch Women Mental Health 4:79–82

Boyles SH, Ness RB, Grisso JA, Markovic N, Bromberger J, CiFelli D (2000) Life event stress and the association with spontaneous abortion in gravid women at an urban emergency department. Health Psychol 19(6):510–4, Retrieved from http://www.ncbi.nlm.nih.gov/pubmed/11129353

Britton JR (2011) Infant temperament and maternal anxiety and depressed mood in the early postpartum period. Women Health 51(1):55–71. doi:10.1080/03630242.2011.540741

Brockington IF, Downing AR, Cernik KF, Schofield EM, Francis AF, Keelan C (1981) Puerperal psychosis phenomena and diagnosis. Arch Gen Psychiatry 38(7):829–833. doi:10.1001/archpsyc.1981.01780320109013

Burr WA, Falek A, Strauss LT, Brown SB (1979) Fertility in psychiatric outpatients. Hosp Commun Psychiatry 30(8):527–531

Chung TK, Lau TK, Yip AS, Chiu HF, Lee DT (2001) Antepartum depressive symptomatology is associated with adverse obstetric and neonatal outcomes. Psychosom Med 63(5):830–834

Cicchetti D, Rogosch FA, Toth SL (2000) The efficacy of toddler-parent psychotherapy for fostering cognitive development in offspring of depressed mothers. J Abnorm Child Psychol 28(2):135–48, Retrieved from http://www.ncbi.nlm.nih.gov/pubmed/10834766

Cohen LS, Altshuler LL, Harlow BL, Nonacs R, Newport DJ, Viguera AC, Stowe ZN (2006) Relapse of major depression during pregnancy in women who maintain or discontinue antidepressant treatment. JAMA 295(5):499–507. doi:10.1001/jama.295.5.499

Cox JL, Murray D, Chapman G (1993) A controlled study of the onset, duration and prevalence of postnatal depression. Br J Psychiatry 163(1):27–31. doi:10.1192/bjp.163.1.27

Deave T, Heron J, Evans J, Emond A (2008) The impact of maternal depression in pregnancy on early child development. BJOG 115(8):1043–51. doi:10.1111/j.1471-0528.2008.01752.x

Evans J, Heron J, Francomb H, Oke S, Golding J (2001) Cohort study of depressed mood during pregnancy and after childbirth. BMJ 323(7307):257–60, Retrieved from http://www.pubmedcentral.nih.gov/articlerender.fcgi?artid=35345&tool=pmcentrez&rendertype=abstract

Feibus KB (2008) FDA's proposed rule for pregnancy and lactation labeling: improving maternal child health through well-informed medicine use. J Med Toxicol 4(4):284–288

Field T, Diego MA, Hernandez-Reif M, Schanberg S, Kuhn C (2004) Massage therapy effects on depressed pregnant women. J Psychosom Obstet Gynaecol 25(2):115–22, Retrieved from http://www.ncbi.nlm.nih.gov/pubmed/15715034

Field T, Diego M, Hernandez-Reif M (2006) Prenatal depression effects on the fetus and newborn: a review. Infant Behav Dev 29(3):445–55. doi:10.1016/j.infbeh.2006.03.003

Field T, Diego M, Hernandez-Reif M, Deeds O, Figueiredo B (2009) Pregnancy massage reduces prematurity, low birthweight and postpartum depression. Infant Behav Dev 32(4):454–60. doi:10.1016/j.infbeh.2009.07.001

Forman DR, O'Hara MW, Stuart S, Gorman LL, Larsen KE, Coy KC (2007) Effective treatment for postpartum depression is not sufficient to improve the developing mother-child relationship. Dev Psychopathol 19(2):585–602. doi:10.1017/S0954579407070289

Frank E, Kupfer DJ, Perel JM, Cornes C, Jarrett DB, Mallinger AG, Grochocinski VJ (1990) Three-year outcomes for maintenance therapies in recurrent depression. Arch Gen Psychiatry 47:1093–1099

Gamer E, Gallant D, Grunebaum H (1976) Children of psychotic mothers: an evaluation of 1-year-olds on a test of object permanence. Arch Gen Psychiatry 33(3):311–317, Retrieved from http://dx.doi.org/10.1001/archpsyc.1976.01770030029004

Gavin NI, Gaynes BN, Lohr KN, Meltzer-Brody S, Gartlehner G, Swinson T (2005) Perinatal depression: a systematic review of prevalence and incidence. Obstet Gynecol 106(5 Pt 1):1071–83. doi:10.1097/01.AOG.0000183597.31630.db

Grigoriadis S, VonderPorten EH, Mamisashvili L, Tomlinson G, Dennis C-L, Koren G, Ross LE (2013) The impact of maternal depression during pregnancy on perinatal outcomes: a systematic review and meta-analysis. J Clin Psychiatry 74(4):e321–41. doi:10.4088/JCP.12r07968

Hauck Y, Rock D, Jackiewicz T, Jablensky A (2008) Healthy babies for mothers with serious mental illness: a case management framework for mental health clinicians. Int J Ment Health Nurs 17:383–391

Henshaw C, Foreman D, Cox J (2004) Postnatal blues: a risk factor for postnatal depression. J Psychosom Obstet Gynecol 25(3–4):267–272. doi:10.1080/01674820400024414

Heron J, O'Connor TG, Evans J, Golding J, Glover V (2004) The course of anxiety and depression through pregnancy and the postpartum in a community sample. J Affect Disorders 80(1):65–73. doi:10.1016/j.jad.2003.08.004

Hoffman S, Hatch MC (2000) Depressive symptomatology during pregnancy: evidence for an association with decreased fetal growth in pregnancies of lower social class women. Health Psychol 19(6):535–43, Retrieved from http://www.ncbi.nlm.nih.gov/pubmed/11129356

Holcomb WL, Stone LS, Lustman PJ, Gavard JA, Mostello DJ (1996) Screening for depression in pregnancy: characteristics of the Beck depression inventory. Obstet Gynecol 88:1021–1025

Howard LM (2001) Psychosocial characteristics and needs of mothers with psychotic disorders. Br J Psychiatry 178(5):427–432. doi:10.1192/bjp.178.5.427

Howard LM, Kumar C, Leese M, Thornicroft G (2002) The general fertility rate in patients with psychotic disorders. Am J Psychiatry 159:991–997

Hunt N (1995) Does puerperal illness distinguish a subgroup of bipolar patients? J Affect Disord 34(2):101–107. doi:10.1016/0165-0327(95)00006-9

Jablensky AV, Morgan V, Zubrick SR, Bower C, Yellachich LA (2005) Pregnancy, delivery and neonatal complications in a population cohort of women with schizophrenia and major affective disorders. Am J Psychiatry 169:79–91

Jones I, Craddock N (2001) Familiality of the puerperal trigger in bipolar disorder: results of a family study. Am J Psychiatry 158(6):913–7, Retrieved from http://www.ncbi.nlm.nih.gov/pubmed/11384899

Kelly RH, Danielsen BH, Golding JM, Anders TF, Gilbert WM, Zatzick DF (1999) Adequacy of prenatal care among women with psychiatric diagnoses giving birth in California in 1994 and 1995. Psychiatr Serv 50(12):1584–90, Retrieved from http://www.ncbi.nlm.nih.gov/pubmed/10577877

Kendell R, Chalmers J, Platz C (1987) Epidemiology of the peurperal psychosis. Br J Psychiatry 150:662–668

Kim J-H, Choi SS, Ha K (2008) A closer look at depression in mothers who kill their children: is it unipolar or bipolar depression? J Clin Psychiatry 69:1625–1631

Kumar R, Robson KM (1984) A prospective study of emotional disorders in childbearing women. Br J Psychiatry 144:35–47, Retrieved from http://www.ncbi.nlm.nih.gov/pubmed/6692075

Kurki T, Hiilesmaa V, Raitasalo R, Mattila H, Ylikorkala O (2000) Depression and anxiety in early pregnancy and risk for preeclampsia. Obstet Gynecol 95(4):487–90, Retrieved from http://www.ncbi.nlm.nih.gov/pubmed/10725477

Law R, Bozzo P, Koren G, Einarson A (2010) Motherisk update FDA pregnancy risk categories and the CPS do they help or are they a hindrance? Can Fam Physician 56:239–241

Lee DTS, Chung TKH (2007) Postnatal depression: an update. Best practice & research. Clin Obstet Gynaecol 21(2):183–91. doi:10.1016/j.bpobgyn.2006.10.003

Lee H-C, Lin H-C (2010) Maternal bipolar disorder increased low birthweight and preterm births: a nationwide population-based study. J Affect Disorder 121(1–2):100–5. doi:10.1016/j.jad.2009.05.019

Lindahl V, Pearson JL, Colpe L (2005) Prevalence of suicidality during pregnancy and the postpartum. Arch Women Mental Health 8(2):77–87. doi:10.1007/s00737-005-0080-1

Lundgren M, Brandt L, Reutfors J, Andersen M, Kieler H (2012) Risks of adverse pregnancy and birth outcomes in women treated or not treated with mood stabilisers for bipolar disorder: population based cohort study. Br Med J 7085(November):1–10. doi:10.1136/bmj.e7085

Manber R, Schnyer RN, Lyell D, Chambers AS, Gress JL, Huang MI, Martin-okada R (2010) Acupuncture for depression during pregnancy. Obstet Gynecol 115(3):511–520

Marcus SM, Flynn HA, Blow FC, Barry KL (2003) Depressive symptoms among pregnant women screened in obstetrics settings. J Women Health 12(4):373–80. doi:10.1089/154099903765448880

Mathers C, Lopez A, Murray C (2006) The burden of disease and mortality by condition: data, methods, and results for 2001. In global burden of disease and risk. World Bank, Washington, DC

McNeil TF, Kaij L, Malmquist-Larsson A (1984) Women with nonorganic psychosis: mental disturbance during pregnancy. Acta Psychiatr Scand 70:127–139

Meltzer ES, Kumar R (1985) Puerperal mental illness, clinical features and classification: a study of 142 mother-and-baby admissions. Br J Psychiatry 147:647–54, Retrieved from http://www.ncbi.nlm.nih.gov/pubmed/3830326

Michel-Wolfromm H (1968) The psychological factor in spontaneous abortion. J Psychosom Res 12(1):67–71, Retrieved from http://www.ncbi.nlm.nih.gov/pubmed/5663947

Milgrom J, Gemmill AW, Bilszta JL, Hayes B, Barnett B, Brooks J, Buist A (2008) Antenatal risk factors for postnatal depression: a large prospective study. J Affect Disorder 108(1–2):147–57. doi:10.1016/j.jad.2007.10.014

Miller LJ (1997) Sexuality, reproduction, and family planning in women with schizophrenia. Schizophr Bull 23(4):623–35, Retrieved from http://www.ncbi.nlm.nih.gov/pubmed/9365999

Miller LJ, Finnerty M (1996) Sexuality, pregnancy, and childrearing among women with schizophrenia-spectrum disorders. Psychiatr Serv (Washington, DC) 47(5):502–6, Retrieved from http://www.ncbi.nlm.nih.gov/pubmed/8740491

Murray D, Cox J (1990) Screening for depression during pregnancy with the Edinburgh depression scale (EPDS). J Reproduct Infant Psychol 8:99–107

Nilsson E, Lichtenstein P, Cnattingius S, Murray RM, Hultman CM (2002) Women with schizophrenia: pregnancy outcome and infant death among their offspring. Schizophr Res 58(2-3):221–9, Retrieved from http://www.ncbi.nlm.nih.gov/pubmed/12409162

O'Hara MW (1987) Post-partum "blues", depression, and psychosis: a review. J Psychosom Obstet Gynecol 7(3):205–227. doi:10.3109/01674828709040280

O'Hara MW (1995) Postpartum depression: causes and consequences. Springer, Heidelberg, pp 168–194

O'Hara MW (2009) Postpartum depression: what we know. J Clin Psychol 65(12):1258–1269. doi:10.1002/jclp

Oren DA, Wisner KL, Spinelli M, Epperson CN, Peindl KS, Terman JS, Terman M (2002) An open trial of morning light therapy for treatment of antepartum depression. Am J Psychiatry 159(4):666–9, Retrieved from http://www.ncbi.nlm.nih.gov/pubmed/11925310

Orr ST (2002) Maternal prenatal depressive symptoms and spontaneous preterm births among African-American women in Baltimore, Maryland. Am J Epidemiol 156(9):797–802. doi:10.1093/aje/kwf131

Osmond M (2002) Behind the smile. Grand Central Publishing, New York

Paltrow G (2011). I felt like a Zombie. *Good Housekeeping*

Rohde A, Marneros A (1993) Psychoses in puerperium: symptoms, course and long-term prognosis. Geburtshilfe Frauenheilkd 53(11):800–10. doi:10.1055/s-2007-1023730

Shields B (2005) Down came the rain. Hyperion, New York

Slater (1971) Marriage and fertility of psychiatric patients compared with national data. Sociol Biol s18:s60–s73

Solari H, Dickson KE, Miller L (2009) Understanding and treating women with schizophrenia during pregnancy and postpartum. Can J Clin Pharmacol 16(1):23–32

Spinelli MG (1997) Interpersonal psychotherapy for depressed antepartum women: a pilot study. Am J Psychiatry 154(7):1028–30, Retrieved from http://www.ncbi.nlm.nih.gov/pubmed/9210760

Spinelli MG (2009) Postpartum psychosis: detection of risk and management. Am J Psychiatry 166:405–408

Steer RA, Scholl TO, Hediger ML, Fischer RL (1992) Self-reported depression and negative pregnancy outcomes. J Clin Epidemiol 45(10):1093–9, Retrieved from http://www.ncbi.nlm.nih.gov/pubmed/1474405

Sylvén SM, Ekselius L, Sundström-Poromaa I, Skalkidou A (2013) Premenstrual syndrome and dysphoric disorder as risk factors for postpartum depression. Acta obstetricia et gynecologica Scandinavica 92(2):178–84. doi:10.1111/aogs.12041

Tronick E, Reck C (2009) Infants of depressed mothers. Harvard Rev Psychiatry 17(2):147–56. doi:10.1080/10673220902899714

Vesga-López O, Blanco C, Keyes K, Olfson M, Grant BF, Hasin DS (2008) Psychiatric disorders in pregnant and postpartum women in the United States. Arch Gen Psychiatry 65(7):805–15. doi:10.1001/archpsyc.65.7.805

Vigod S, Kurdyak P, Dennis C, Gruneir A, Newman A, Seeman M, Ray JG (2014) Maternal and newborn outcomes among women with schizophrenia: a retrospective population-based cohort study. Br J Obstet Gynaecol 1:1–9. doi:10.1111/1471-0528.12567

Viguera AC (2002) Reproductive decisions by women with bipolar disorder after prepregnancy psychiatric consultation. Am J Psychiatry 159(12):2102–2104. doi:10.1176/appi.ajp.159.12.2102

Viguera AC, Whitfield T, Baldessarini RJ, Newport DJ, Stowe Z, Reminick A, Cohen LS (2007) Risk of recurrence in women with bipolar disorder during pregnancy: prospective study of mood stabilizer discontinuation. Am J Psychiatry 164(12):1817–24. doi:10.1176/appi.ajp.2007.06101639, quiz 1923

Wisner KL, Peindl K, Hanusa BH (1994) Symptomatology of affective and psychotic illnesses related to childbearing. J Affect Disorder 30(2):77–87, Retrieved from http://www.ncbi.nlm.nih.gov/pubmed/8201128

Witt WP, DeLeire T, Hagen EW, Wichmann MA, Wisk LE, Spear HA, Hampton J (2010) The prevalence and determinants of antepartum mental health problems among women in the USA: a nationally representative population-based study. Arch Women Mental Health 13(5):425–37. doi:10.1007/s00737-010-0176-0

Wu P, Fuller C, Liu X, Lee H-C, Fan B, Hoven CW, Kronenberg F (2007) Use of complementary and alternative medicine among women with depression: results of a national survey. Psychiatr Serv (Washington, DC) 58(3):349–56. doi:10.1176/appi.ps.58.3.349

Yalom ID, Lunde DT, Moos RH, Hamburg DA (1968) Postpartum blues" syndrome. A description and related variables. Arch Gen Psychiatry 18(1):16–27, Retrieved from http://www.ncbi.nlm.nih.gov/pubmed/5634686

Yonkers KA, Wisner KL, Stewart DE, Oberlander TF, Dell DL, Stotland N, Lockwood C (2009) The management of depression during pregnancy: a report from the American Psychiatric Association and the American College of Obstetricians and Gynecologists. Gen Hospital Psychiatry 31(5):403–13. doi:10.1016/j.genhosppsych.2009.04.003

Zuckerman B, Amaro H, Bauchner H, Cabral H (1989) Depressive symptoms during pregnancy: relationship to poor health behaviors. Am J Obstet Gynecol 160(5 Pt 1):1107–11, Retrieved from http://www.ncbi.nlm.nih.gov/pubmed/2729387

Substance Use Disorders and Motherhood

6

Abigail J. Herron and Melodie Isgro

Abstract

Substance abuse is a growing problem among women. They have unique characteristics in terms of their patterns of drug use, risk factors, and the physiologic effects of use compared to men. Special populations within this group, especially women who are pregnant and/or parenting, have distinctive risks, barriers, and needs. Recognition of these distinct features is vital to establishing effective treatment systems and an essential feature of the recovery process. Additionally, pregnancy and motherhood can often result in decreased or altered patterns of substance use to allow for caregiver responsibilities and can be a strong motivator in seeking and completing substance abuse treatment. Tailored and comprehensive treatment programs for this unique group show improved outcomes both for the women and their children.

Several components of treatment have been shown to correlate with improved outcomes: (1) child care, (2) prenatal care, (3) women-only programs, (4) supplemental services and workshops for women, (5) mental health treatment, and (6) comprehensive programming. With appropriate interventions, mothers with substance use disorders are able to not only achieve abstinence from alcohol and drugs of abuse, but can demonstrate improved mental health, increased socioeconomic functioning, and more effective parenting. Though some programs offer comprehensive services that incorporate these areas, there is still a great need for development and empirical study in this area.

A.J. Herron, D.O. (✉) • M. Isgro, M.D.
Addiction Institute of New York at Mt. Sinai, St. Luke's and Roosevelt Hospitals,
New York, NY, USA
e-mail: aherron@chpnet.org; misgro@chpnet.org

N. Benders-Hadi and M.E. Barber (eds.), *Motherhood, Mental Illness and Recovery*, 73
DOI 10.1007/978-3-319-01318-3_6, © Springer International Publishing Switzerland 2014

Introduction

Substance abuse continues to be a growing problem among women, with estimates that up to 6.5 % of females aged 12 and older currently abuse alcohol or illicit drugs (National Survey on Drug Use and Health (NSDUH), 2011). Women have unique characteristics in terms of their patterns of drug use, risk factors, and the physiologic effects of use compared to men. This subsequently affects their screening, assessment, and treatment considerations. Special populations within this group, especially pregnant women and women with children, have distinctive risks, barriers, and needs. In this chapter, we will further explore these various issues to help best determine strategies for optimal care of this vulnerable population.

Patterns of Use and Risk Factors

Women tend to place a high value on their interpersonal relationships and may subsequently be more easily influenced by them compared to men. Often they are first introduced to substance use through a close relationship such as from a romantic partner, family member, or friend. Although initial use may be in an occasional social context, women may continue to use or even escalate their use as a way to maintain or deepen their relationships, particularly if the partner is a heavy user. Women with substance use disorders are more likely to have addicted partners than their male counterparts, and these relationships can directly influence their progression to high-risk drug use behaviors, especially their faster acceleration to IV drug use compared to men (Center for Substance Abuse Treatment (CSAT), 2009). Frequently, women will end up becoming dependent on their partners to supply their illicit drug. While marriage can sometimes be a protective factor against development of substance abuse, women who are divorced, separated, or never married tend to have higher incidences of substance use disorders.

Aside from interpersonal factors, other reasons for initiation of substance use can be varied, but some women report a desire to lose weight or have more energy as their initial goal. Because of this, women tend to abuse over-the-counter medications such as laxatives, diuretics, emetics, diet pills, and cough and cold preparations more often than men. Some women may have use precipitated by stressors or negative affect. This can result in initial overuse progressing to abuse of prescription drugs such as pain medications or anxiolytics. The younger women are when they first begin to use, the higher the risk of the development of dependency and the correlation to severity (Marcenko et al. 2000). Although women tend to begin substance abuse at an older age compared to men, they become dependent more quickly and suffer the consequence of their abuse sooner, a phenomenon known as telescoping (National Center on Addiction and Substance Abuse at Columbia University 2003).

Co-occurring mental health disorders are another significant risk factor for drug abuse, and these are more prevalent in women compared to men, with anxiety and depressive disorders experienced most commonly. These disorders may be present prior to initiation of substance abuse, develop as a consequence of use, or develop independently and concurrently. Some substance abuse development may stem from an effort by the woman to self-medicate symptoms of mental illness. Other times, inadequate dosing of prescription medications for a diagnosed mental health disorder leads to self-adjustment of medication with increasing dosages, more frequent use, or addition of illicit substances to ameliorate symptoms. Personality disorders are also commonly seen in women with substance use disorders, most notably borderline personality disorder.

Women with substance use disorders also have high rates of trauma and interpersonal violence, with some studies estimating that up to 30–75 % of women in substance abuse treatment programs having been victims of sexual abuse and rape (Marcenko et al. 2000; Finkelstein 1993). A history of trauma, especially childhood sexual abuse, has been found to correlate directly with female drug use and its severity (Marcenko et al. 2000; Kendler et al. 2000). Substance abuse may stem from an effort to self-medicate symptoms caused by the trauma. In turn, substance abuse may further increase a woman's risk of trauma by decreasing her ability to defend herself, altering her judgment, or leading her to have high-risk behaviors.

Individual personality factors may also put a woman at greater risk for substance abuse. Novelty seeking, frequently seen in youth but often extending into adulthood, has been associated with increased initiation of use. Other risk factors include a tendency toward obsessiveness, chronic low levels of anxiety, and difficulty in regulating affect (CSAT 2009). Certain risk factors such as depression, low self-esteem, and peer pressure have been shown to increase the susceptibility of younger women to substance abuse (National Center on Addiction and Substance Abuse at Columbia University 2003).

Familial influence can carry significant risk in the development and course of substance use disorders in women. A history of substance abuse in either parent increases the risk of abuse in their children whether through genetic influences, environmental influences, or both. The prevalence of alcohol dependence is 10–50 times higher in women who have a parent with a substance abuse disorder compared with the general population (CSAT 2009). Women who have to take on adult responsibilities in childhood, or were raised in chaotic, argumentative, blame-oriented, or violent households, are more likely to develop substance abuse. Various socioeconomic factors can also increase risk. Those who face employment or educational discrimination may use substances as a way of coping. Women who have less education, lower incomes, and higher rates of unemployment are more likely to have substance use disorders.

Physiologic Effects of Use

Women are more susceptible to the short- and long-term effects of drugs and alcohol, in part due to having proportionately more body fat and lower volumes of body water compared to men. This results in a more rapid progression from initial use to the development of health-related problems. Women use substances for shorter periods of time before seeking treatment, but they report a greater severity of psychiatric, medical, and employment complications (CSAT 2009). Women can become more quickly intoxicated from smaller quantities of alcohol than men. They are more susceptible to alcohol-related organ damage including damage to organs/organ systems such as the liver, heart, bone, nervous, and reproductive systems. Other drugs classes, such as opiates and stimulants, have similar increased physiological effects on women compared to men, often causing higher rates of disease regardless of degree of drug use or intensity.

Effects on Pregnancy

All substances have at least some effect on a woman's pregnancy, the fetus in utero, and the infant at birth. An extensive discussion of the perinatal effects of substance use is outside the scope of this chapter, but we will briefly discuss the consequences of some of the more frequently abused drugs during pregnancy. Tobacco, marijuana, alcohol, opiates, sedatives, and stimulants can all lead to various degrees of pregnancy complications including increased incidences of preeclampsia, abruptio placenta, spontaneous abortion, premature delivery, intrauterine death, and stillbirths. In utero complications from drug abuse can manifest themselves as birth defects, intrauterine growth retardation, brain development retardation, hypoxic encephalopathy, intracranial hemorrhage, and other physical and developmental abnormalities. At birth, many infants suffer from withdrawal symptoms secondary to extended prenatal drug abuse. Neonatal Abstinence Syndrome resulting from prenatal opiate use is a well-documented withdrawal syndrome with symptoms such as tremors, sweating, jitteriness, hypertonia, poor feeding, and watery stools. These infants typically require postnatal treatment with morphine for their symptoms resulting in extended hospital stays, and prolonged withdrawal symptoms can persist well into the neonatal period. Prenatal drug use has also been shown to have both obvious and sometimes subtle lifelong detrimental effects on an individual born to an addicted mother. One example of this is Fetal Alcohol Syndrome resulting from in utero alcohol exposure. Individuals affected by this syndrome can have lifelong complications including learning and memory deficits and social/emotional impairments, as well as a characteristic physical appearance.

Pregnant substance abusers are often aware of the potential negative consequences to their baby from continued use during their pregnancy, which can result in a decrease in use during this period. In the case of adolescent mothers, a decline in drug use and an increase in quit rates during pregnancy and just after delivery, sometimes extending into early childrearing years, have been shown (Flanagan and Kokotailo 1999). During pregnancy, young women are less likely to smoke, drink, or engage in substance abuse, mostly due to concerns about the risk to their pregnancies and unborn children (Flanagan and Kokotailo 1999). Women who continue to use drugs after becoming pregnant tend to have greater severity of their substance abuse, greater likelihood of substance use among family and friends, less prenatal care, and a higher number of pregnancies.

Effects of Motherhood on Substance Use

Approximately one-third of those with substance use disorders are women of childbearing age (WHO World Health Organization 2008). Rates of substance abuse in pregnancy and extending into early motherhood have seen gradual increases over time with 5 % of pregnant women aged 15–44 currently using illicit drugs (SAMHSA 2012). It is further estimated that 9 % of children have at least one parent who is dependent on alcohol or illicit drugs (SAMHSA 2003). Conversely, up to 80 % of substance abusing women are mothers of at least one child (Center on Addiction and Substance Abuse 1996) and 70 % of women in substance abuse treatment programs have children (US Dept. HHS 1999).

Motherhood has its own set of interconnecting risk factors for substance abuse. These include single parenthood, poverty, unstable living conditions, minimal social resources and support, ongoing and past violence and abuse, and mental health problems (Marcenko et al. 2000; Daro and McCurdy 1992). Women who are gainfully employed may have fewer economic concerns, but are not exempt from stressors such as work–family conflict. This has been shown to be a risk factor significantly related to increased cigarette use and heavy alcohol use among employed mothers (Frone et al. 1994).

Young mothers appear to be a particularly vulnerable patient population. A report from the National Survey on Drug Use and Health (2011) shows that mothers aged 15–17 have a higher likelihood of using tobacco and marijuana products than their counterparts who are not mothers. Usage rates show that among young mothers, 35 % smoked cigarettes, 30 % used alcohol, and 11.7 % used marijuana in the past month. This early use increases the risk of developing future dependence to these and other illicit drugs. Furthermore, they have not been found to "grow out" of substance use as they pass into adulthood. Early substance abuse among teen mothers has been shown to negatively impact their parenting capabilities, as well as increase the risk of drug abuse in their children.

Mothers with substance use disorders can experience low self-esteem, feel socially isolated, and have greater levels of life stress. Although they are able to recognize the negative consequences of their substance abuse on their children, they may feel powerless over their addiction. Substance abusing mothers list their children's well-being as a major area of concern and tend to have guilt about their drug abuse as it relates to possible negative outcomes for their children (Luthar and Walsh 1995). They are also more likely to temporarily alter their pattern of use to allow for caregiver responsibilities than men. Reunification with their children often proves to be a strong motivator in seeking substance abuse treatment (Marcenko and Striepe 1997).

Effects of Substance Abuse on Parenting

Studies show that substance abusing mothers tend to have more problematic interactions with their children throughout their childhood and into adolescence compared to non-substance abusing mothers (Mayes 1995). Bonding, mutual arousal/enthusiasm, and ego development in early maternal–infant interactions can be negatively affected by the substance abuse (Burns et al. 1997; Fineman et al. 1997). As children progress to school-age, addicted mothers are frequently less emotionally involved and have poorer parenting attitudes than non-addicted mothers (Ammerman et al. 1999; Kettinger et al. 2000). Their parenting practices can dramatically swing from one extreme to another, from increased failure to set limits (Bernardi et al. 1989) to punitive, threatening disciplinary measures (Bauman and Dougherty 1983; Hien and Honeyman 2000). They have an increased tendency to use an authoritarian type of discipline with greater potential for child abuse than their non-addicted cohorts (Kelley 1998; Bauman and Dougherty 1983).

Parenting capabilities of mothers with substance disorders are not significantly different than other non-using mothers with similar life circumstances such as poverty, trauma, or oppression (Bauman and Dougherty 1983). Addicted mothers often have limited parenting knowledge and misconceptions about parenting practices (Velez et al. 2004). Many mothers in substance treatment programs show concern about their parenting abilities and express a desire to increase their level of competency, confidence, and satisfaction in their parenting (Hien et al. 2009). This suggests that substance abusing mothers have the *capacity* for good parenting that the substance abuse interferes with, particularly as the addiction progresses. As the addicted mother becomes increasingly preoccupied with her drug use, her physical and emotional health deteriorate, money and resources that could support her children are re-prioritized to her drug habit, and she is less available for her children on all levels (Wasserman and Leventhal 1991). Gradually the daily activities and responsibilities of parenting fall away. Despite this, research has shown that addicted mothers highly value their parental role, continue to love their children, and seek reunification if separated. They often feel guilty that they are not meeting their children's or their own expectations of themselves as parents (Baker and Carson 1999).

Effects on Children of Addicted Mothers

Children of substance abusing mothers are at increased risk for physical, academic, and socio-emotional problems. From the time they are conceived and continuing throughout their childhood, they are exposed to an accumulation of factors all known to contribute to biological, developmental, and behavioral problems. One of the initial risk factors includes prenatal exposure to alcohol and other drugs including tobacco, which result in approximately one-quarter of these children having health problems at birth (Conners et al. 2003). After birth, further risk factors often include maternal mental illness, low maternal education, low-income status, instability in caregivers, child abuse and neglect, little paternal involvement, residential instability, and experiences in foster care (Conners et al. 2003). Each of these risk factors has been shown to independently result in negative outcomes for children, although alone are unlikely to result in a major developmental problem. However, it is the accumulation of these risks that makes the child of a substance abusing parent most vulnerable. The accrual of the environmental risk factors by themselves over time can outweigh the adverse consequences of any prenatal substance exposure (Conners et al. 2003). As these children progress through adolescence, the risk of developing a substance abuse problem of their own is also markedly increased. Substance use among youths aged 12–17 increase 93 % when the mother uses substances herself (NSDUH 2005).

Compounding the problem is that these children also have limited opportunities to develop the relationships and skills that might help buffer them from these risks. Given the instability in their lives, they may have difficulty forming stable and supportive relationships with caring adults. This further limits their ability to acquire good skills for social interaction and emotional regulation. Often they will not have sufficient access to stimulating encounters that help to bolster knowledge and a sense of achievement. Thus the cycle tends to repeat itself inter-generationally with these children having a high risk for substance abuse and following in their addicted parents' footsteps, many of whom were themselves children growing up in the same environment (Conners et al. 2003).

Substance Abuse and the Child Welfare System

Estimates suggest that up to 50–80 % of parents who are involved with the child welfare system have substance abuse problems (SAMHSA 2001; USDHHS 1999). Children living in homes with substance abuse have a higher risk of maltreatment and neglect due to parental inability to provide adequate shelter, care, and economic stability for their children (Bays 1990). Substance abusing parents often have impaired judgment and emotional dysregulation contributing to increased child abuse potential (Ammerman et al. 1999). This combination of factors results in a greater likelihood that addicted mothers involved with the child welfare system will lose their parental rights compared with their non-addicted cohorts (Marcenko et al. 2000).

Substance abusing mothers with child welfare system involvement present for treatment with a different clinical profile than other substance abusing mothers. They often present with less severity, likely because it is earlier in the course of their illness, but have a greater level of employment and economic problems and higher likelihood of referral through the criminal justice or other systems. These women also tend to be younger and have a greater number of children than other substance abusing mothers (Grella et al. 2006).

Substance Abuse and Child Placement

Many children who are placed outside of their home by the child welfare system come from biological parents who abuse drugs. Additionally, these children are disproportionately likely to stay in substitute care (Besharov 1994). Increasingly, placement with relatives, also known as relative foster care, kinship care, relative family care, or home-of-relative care, has become more commonplace. Studies show that children in kinship care typically remain longer than children placed in non-relative foster care (Berrick et al. 1994). Relative foster care families also tend to get less supportive services than non-related foster care families (Berrick et al. 1994). One study (Tyler et al. 1997) showed no differences in the quality of caregiving behaviors provided by the biological substance abusing mother in treatment compared with relative caregivers, although the quality was below optimal in both groups. This finding is concerning given that the quality of early caregiving has been linked to long-term developmental outcomes (Wachs and Gruen 1982) especially among biologically high-risk children such as those born with prenatal exposure to alcohol and illicit drugs.

Several characteristics of addicted mothers correlated with foster care placement of their children. The severity of their addiction was highly correlated with child placement (Marcenko et al. 2000). It was also found that children whose mothers had a history of sexual abuse in childhood, or ongoing abuse, were more likely to get placement, although maternal physical abuse as a child or adult without sexual abuse was not a factor (Regan et al. 1987). Women with co-occurring mental health disorders are more likely to drop out of substance abuse treatment programs, and dropout of treatment negatively correlates with reunification of the child with the parent (Rockhill et al. 2007). Those mothers who are able to have more treatment and mental health service needs met during their treatment program, and are able to stabilize their lives as defined by longer periods of abstinence, secure housing, higher income, and social support, had higher rates of reunification with their children (Grant et al. 2011).

Treatment Services

Women face unique obstacles to treatment, encountering barriers at both personal and system levels that keep them from accessing services, including fear of losing custody of their children, guilt, lack of transportation and child care, and unemployment (Bloom et al. 2003; Brady and Ashley 2005). Treatment that provides comprehensive services and support is associated with increased rates of abstinence, better overall health, and improved parenting skills whereas treatment that is limited to addressing substance use alone may contribute to a higher potential for relapse (CSAT 1994). The provision of integrated treatment to meet these needs is a key factor in engagement, retention, decreased substance use, improved functioning, and increased client satisfaction (Choi and Ryan 2007).

Table 6.1 Elements of the comprehensive treatment services model

Clinical treatment services	Clinical support services	Community support services
• Outreach and engagement	• Primary health care	• Transportation
• Screening and assessment	• Life skills	• Child care
• Crisis intervention	• Child care	• Housing
• Treatment planning	• Advocacy	• Employment
• Case management	• Community recovery supports	services
• Substance abuse counseling	• Housing	• Faith-based
• Drug monitoring	• Parenting supports	organizations
• Pharmacotherapies	• Family programs	• Mutual help
• Mental health services	• Educational support	societies
• Medical care	• Employment readiness and	• Recovery
• Trauma-informed and trauma-	vocational services	management
specific services	• Linkages with legal and child	
	welfare systems	

Gender-specific factors influencing treatment and recovery include relationships and the family, high prevalence of trauma, and co-occurring mental health disorders. CSAT's Comprehensive Treatment Model (1994, 2009) describes elements of care that are categorized as follows: (1) Clinical treatment services which are necessary to address the medical and biopsychosocial issues of addiction, (2) Clinical support services which assist clients in their recovery, and (3) Community support services which are outside of treatment but available within a community support system for clients (See Table 6.1).

While services that address the full range of needs should be provided to all women, mothers deserve increased attention to their unique roles as parents, and their children also require services and supports. Among women with substance use disorders, the most frequent source of referral to treatment was self-referral followed by the criminal justice system and other community referrals, including child protective services (Brady and Ashley 2005). Furthermore, referral or involvement with the criminal justice system or child protective services is associated with longer lengths of treatment (Brady and Ashley 2005). Children are a significant factor influencing treatment engagement, retention, and outcomes, and regaining or reestablishing the role of primary caregiver can be a major motivating force for women.

Beginning in the 1980s and 1990s, an increasing number of programs were developed to specifically provide treatment to mothers with substance use disorders, helped by SAMHSA's Pregnant and Postpartum Women and their Infants (PPWI) Grant Program, the Residential Women and Children (RWC), and the Pregnant and Postpartum Women (PPW) Demonstration Program which provided funding to many projects in the 1990s. Evaluation of these programs found that women reported decreased substance use and adverse pregnancy outcomes, reduced criminal involvement, and improved retention of custody (SAMHSA 2001).

While more programs have recognized the need for treatment that addresses women's specific substance abuse-related needs, considerable variability remains in both outpatient and residential treatment settings. No universally accepted definition for what constitutes substance abuse programming for women exists. In addition to substance abuse counseling, programs for women often incorporate one or more of the following: (1) services intended to increase access such as child care or transportation, (2) services addressing specific needs of women such as prenatal and mental health care, HIV risk reduction, and trauma services, and (3) services provided in a women-only setting (Brady and Ashley 2005).

Comprehensive treatment has been shown to be highly effective, offering advantages over traditional substance use treatment, in decreased substance use, increased program retention, decreased prenatal and birth complications, and positive psychosocial outcomes. The following components were particularly correlated with improved outcomes: (1) child care, (2) prenatal care, (3) women-only programs, (4) supplemental services and workshops for women, (5) mental health treatment, and (6) comprehensive programming (for review, see Ashley et al. 2003). Gender-specific, or women-only, treatment has been shown to be highly effective, particularly when incorporating prenatal and/or child care, with improved outcomes in substance use, mental health, employment, birth outcomes, and physical health (Ashley et al. 2003; Greenfield et al. 2007; Najavits et al. 2007). Niv and Hser (2007) found that women in gender-specific programs had a greater severity of problems, including substance abuse, medical conditions, and psychiatric illness, but were more likely to receive services with better drug and legal outcomes at follow-up compared to women in mixed programs. Additionally, women are more likely than men to use services available in comprehensive programs (Grella et al. 2000; Ashley et al. 2003; Marsh and Cao 2005) and more likely to benefit from them (Greenfield et al. 2007).

Parenting Interventions in Substance Abuse Treatment

A woman's relationship with her children and her identity as a mother play a vital role in her sense of self. Many women view parenting as the central purpose in their lives (Substance Abuse and Mental Health Services Administration 2000). Improving parenting improves outcomes for mother and child. Evidence shows that effective parenting skills may also improve the mother's self-esteem and sense of competence (Bauman and Dougherty 1983; Zweben et al. 1994). By improving parenting skills through comprehensive treatment, the risks to children of women with substance use disorders can be minimized. In a review of studies with female substance abusers who were pregnant and/or parenting and receiving parenting treatment in addition to substance use counseling, Niccols et al. (2012) found that integrated treatment programs helped women to strengthen bonds with their children, use more positive discipline techniques, and gain influences into intergenerational influences on parenting.

A number of substance abuse programs incorporate parenting interventions into treatment. The *Strengthening Families Program* (Kumpfer 1987) is a 12–14 session behavioral and cognitive skills training program originally designed to reduce vulnerability to drug abuse in 6–12 year old children of substance abusing parents, which has now been modified to include 10–14 year olds. The program consists of parent training, which focuses on limit-setting, developmental characteristics of children, conflict management and sharing expectations about using substances, children's skills training, and family skills training. It has been shown to be effective in several populations, including children of substance users, abused and neglected children, and low-income urban minority families (Kumpfer and Alvarado 1995; Kumpfer et al. 1996).

The Nurturing Program for Families in Substance Abuse Treatment and Recovery (Camp and Finkelstein 1997) is a parent training program developed for pregnant and parenting women in substance abuse treatment. In the initial part of this project, pregnant and parenting women with substance use disorders received specialized individual and group services including a structured parenting skills group based on the curriculum of The Nurturing Program for Parents of Children Birth to Five years old for two and a half hour weekly sessions over 23 weeks. Interventions focused on improving parenting skills and reducing the risk of child maltreatment (Bavelok and Bavelok 1989). Findings showed that women who completed the skills training made improvements in self-esteem and parenting skills (Camp and Finkelstein 1997). The program was later modified to become the Nurturing Program for Families in Substance Abuse Treatment and Recovery (Moore and Finkelstein 2001). The curriculum was expanded to include information about the recovery process and parenting development, as well as intergenerational patterns of substance abuse and child maltreatment, and has been implemented in multiple substance abuse treatment programs.

An additional program which incorporates parenting skills into substance abuse treatment is the Relational Psychotherapy Mother's Group (RPMG), a 24-week manualized treatment that was introduced in methadone maintenance as a supplement to treatment for heroin-addicted mothers and their children (Luthar and Suchman 2000). RPMG uses an interpersonal psychotherapy model to address deficits in parenting, focusing on specific issues such as conflict resolution, limit setting, and effective parenting style through modeling effective parenting and communication. In a randomized treatment trial the 37 heroin-addicted mothers assigned to RPMG showed greater child involvement and greater reductions in opioid use as well as more positive psychosocial adjustment than women who received methadone and drug counseling alone. This suggests that addressing the psychological and interpersonal issues of substance abusing women can have substantial beneficial influence on their substance use (Brunswick et al. 1992).

Conclusion

Women, especially those who are pregnant or parenting, have unique characteristics of substance use which demand treatment to meet their specialized needs. Recognition of these distinct features is vital to establishing effective treatment systems and an essential feature of the recovery process. Several components of treatment have been shown to correlate with improved outcomes: (1) child care, (2) prenatal care, (3) women-only programs, (4) supplemental services and workshops for women, (5) mental health treatment, and (6) comprehensive programming. With appropriate interventions, mothers with substance use disorders are able to not only achieve abstinence from alcohol and drugs of abuse, but can demonstrate improved mental health, increased socioeconomic functioning, and more effective parenting. Though some programs offer comprehensive services that incorporate these areas, there is still a great need for development and empirical study in this area.

References

Ammerman RT, Kolko DJ, Kirisci L, Blackson TC, Dawes MA (1999) Child abuse potential in parents with histories of substance abuse disorder. Child Abuse Negl 23(12):1225–1238

Ashley OS, Marsden ME, Brady TM (2003) Effectiveness of substance abuse treatment programming for women: A review. Am J Drug Alcohol Abuse 29(1):19–53

Baker PL, Carson A (1999) "I take care of my kids": Mothering practices of substance-abusing women. Gender Soc 13:347–363

Bauman P, Dougherty F (1983) Drug-addicted mothers: parenting and their children's development. Int J Addict 18:291–302

Bavelok S, Bavelok JD (1989) Nurturing program for parents and children birth to five years: activities manual. Family Development Resources, Park City, UT

Bays J (1990) Substance abuse and child abuse: Impact of addiction on the child. Pediatr Clin North Am 37:881–904

Bernardi E, Jones M, Tennant C (1989) Quality of parenting in alcoholics and narcotics addicts. Br J Psychiatry 154:677–682

Berrick JD, Barth RP, Needell B (1994) A comparison of kinship foster homes and foster family homes: Implications for kinship foster care as family preservation. Children Youth Serv Rev 16:33–63

Besharov DJ (1994) When drug addicts have children: reorienting child welfare's response. Child Welfare League of America, Inc.; American Enterprise Institute, Washington, DC

Bloom B, Owen B, Covington S (2003) Gender-responsive strategies: research, practice and guiding principles for women offenders. National Institute on Corrections, Washington, DC

Brady TM, Ashley OS (eds) (2005) Women in substance abuse treatment: results from the Alcohol and Drug Services Study (ADSS) (DHHS Publication No. SMA 04–3968, Analytic Series A-26). Rockville, MD: Substance Abuse and Mental Health Services Administration, Office of Applied Studies

Brunswick A, Messeri P, Titus SP (1992) Predictive factors in adult substance abuse: a prospective study of African-American adults. American Psychological Association, Washington, DC

Burns KA, Chethik L, Burns WJ, Clark R (1997) The early relationship of drug abusing mothers and their infants: an assessment at eight to twelve months of age. J Clin Psychol 53(3):279–287

Camp JM, Finkelstein N (1997) Parenting training for women in residential substance abuse treatment. Result of a demonstration project. J Subst Abuse Treat 14:411–422

Center for Substance Abuse Treatment (1994) Practical approaches in the treatment of women who abuse alcohol and other drugs. HHS Publication No. (SMA) 94–3006. U.S. Government Printing Office, Washington, DC

Center for Substance Abuse Treatment (2009) Substance abuse treatment: addressing the specific needs of women. Treatment improvement protocol (TIP) series 51. HHS Publication

No. (SMA) 09–4426. Substance Abuse and Mental Health Services Administration, Rockville, MD

Center on Addiction and Substance Abuse (1996) Substance abuse and the American woman. The National Center on Addiction and Substance Abuse at Columbia University, New York

Choi S, Ryan JP (2007) Co-occurring problems for substance abusing mothers in child welfare: matching services to improve family reunification. Children Youth Serv Rev 29:1395–1410

National Center on Addiction and Substance Abuse at Columbia University (2003) The formative years: pathways to substance abuse among girls and young women ages 8–22

Conners NA, Bradley RH, Mansell LW, Liu JY, Roberts TJ, Burgdorf K, Herrell JM (2003) Children of mothers with serious substance abuse problems: an accumulation of risks. Am J Drug Alcohol Abuse 29(4):743–758

Daro D, McCurdy K (1992) Current trends in child abuse reporting and fatalities: the results of the 1991 annual state survey (Working Paper No. 808). National Committee for Prevention of Child Abuse, Chicago, IL

Fineman NR, Beckwith L, Howard J, Espinosa M (1997) Maternal ego development and mother-infant interaction in drug-abusing women. J Subst Abuse Treat 14(4):307–317

Finkelstein N (1993) Treatment programming for alcohol and drug dependent pregnant women. Int J Addict 28:1275–1310

Flanagan P, Kokotailo P (1999) Adolescent pregnancy and substance use. Clin Perinatol 26(1): 185–200

Frone MR, Barnes GM, Farrell MP (1994) Relationship of work-family conflict to substance use among employed mothers: the role of negative affect. J Marriage Family 56(4):1019–1030

Grant T, Huggins J, Graham JC, Emst C, Whitney N, Wilson D (2011) Maternal substance abuse and disrupted parenting: distinguishing mothers who keep their children from those who do not. Children Youth Serv Rev 33:2176–2185

Greenfield SF, Brooks AJ, Gordon SM, Green CA, Kropp F, McHugh RK, Lincoln M, Hien D, Miele GM (2007) Substance abuse treatment entry, retention, and outcome in women: a review of the literature. Drug Alcohol Depend 86(5):1–21

Grella CE, Joshi V, Hser Y (2000) Program variation in treatment outcomes among women in residential drug treatment. Eval Rev 24(4):364–383

Grella CE, Hser YI, Huang YC (2006) Mothers in substance abuse treatment: differences in characteristics based on involvement with child welfare services. Child Abuse Negl 30:55–73

Hien D, Honeyman T (2000) A closer look at the maternal substance abuse-violence link. J Interpers Violence 15(5):503–522

Hien DA, Litt LC, Cohen LR, Miele GM, Campbell A (2009) Trauma services for women in substance abuse treatment: an integrated approach. American Psychological Association Press, New York, NY

Kelley SJ (1998) Stress and coping behaviors of substance abusing mothers. J Soc Pediatr Nurs 3:103–110

Kendler KS, Bulik CM, Silberg J, Hettema JM, Myers J, Prescott CA (2000) Childhood sexual abuse and adult psychiatric and substance use disorders in women: an epidemiological and co twin control analysis. Arch Gen Psychiatry 57(10):953–959

Kettinger LA, Nair P, Schuler ME (2000) Exposure to environmental risk factors and parenting attitudes among substance-abusing women. Am J Drug Alcohol Abuse 26(1):1–11

Kumpfer KL (1987) Special populations: etiology and prevention of vulnerability to chemical dependency in children of substance abusers. In: Brown BS, Mills AR (eds) Youth at high risk for substance abuse (DHHS Publication ADM 90–1537). National Institute on Drug Abuse, Washington, DC, pp 1–71

Kumpfer KL, Alvarado R (1995) Strengthening families to prevent drug use in multi-ethnic youth. In: Botvin G, Schinke S, Orlandi M (eds) Drug abuse prevention with multi-ethnic youth. Sage, Newbury Park, CA, pp 253–292

Kumpfer KL, Molgaard V, Spoth R (1996) The Strengthening Families Program for the prevention of delinquency and drug. In: Peters RD, McMahon RJ (eds) Preventing childhood disorders, substance abuse, and delinquency, vol 3, Banff international behavioral science series. Sage, Thousand Oaks, CA, pp 241–267

Luthar SS, Suchman N (2000) Relational psychotherapy mother's group: a developmentally informed intervention for at-risk mothers. Dev Psychopathol 12:235–253

Luthar SS, Walsh KG (1995) Treatment needs of drug-addicted mothers: Integrated parenting psychotherapy interventions. J Subst Abuse Treat 12:341–348

Marcenko MO, Striepe MI (1997) A look at family reunification through the eyes of mothers. Commun Alternat 9:33–48

Marcenko MO, Kemp SP, Larson NC (2000) Childhood experiences of abuse, later substance use, and parenting outcomes among low-income mothers. Am J Orthopsychiatry 70(3):316–326

Marsh JC, Cao D (2005) Parents in substance abuse treatment: implications for child welfare practice. Children Youth Serv Rev 27(12):1259–1278

Mayes LC (1995) Substance abuse and parenting. In: Bornstein MH (ed) Handbook of parenting, vol 4, Applied and practical parenting. Erlbaum, Mahwah, NJ, pp 101–1266

Substance Abuse and Mental Health Services Administration (2012) Results from the 2011 national survey on drug use and health: summary of national findings, NSDUH Series H-44, HHS Publication No. (SMA) 12–4713. Substance Abuse and Mental Health Services Administration, Rockville, MD

Moore J, Finkelstein N (2001) Parenting services for families affected by substance abuse. Child Welfare 80(2):221–238

Najavits LM, Rosier M, Nolan AL, Freeman MC (2007) A new gender-based model for women's recovery from substance abuse: results of a pilot outcome study. Am J Drug Alcohol Abuse 33: 5–11

National Survey on Drug Use and Health (2005) Mother's serious mental illness and substance use among youths. The NSDUH Report, May 13, 2005

National Survey on Drug Use and Health (2011) Substance use among young mothers. The NSDUH Report, March 10, 2011

Niccols A, Milligan K, Sword W, Thabane L, Henderson J, Smith A (2012) Integrated programs for mothers with substance abuse issues: a systematic review of studies reporting on parenting outcomes. Harm Reduction J 9:14

Niv N, Hser YI (2007) Women-only and mixed-gender drug abuse treatment programs: service needs, utilization and outcomes. Drug Alcohol Depend 87:94–201

Regan DO, Ehrlich SM, Finnegan LP (1987) Infants of drug addicts: at risk for child abuse, neglect, and placement in foster care. Neurotoxicol Teratol 9:315–319

Rockhill A, Green BL, Furrer C (2007) Is the adoption and safe families act influencing child welfare outcomes for families with substance abuse issues? Child Maltreat 12(1):7–19

Substance Abuse and Mental Health Services Administration (2003) Children living with substance-abusing or substance-dependent parents. National Household Survey on Drug Abuse Office of Applied Studies, Rockville, MD

Substance Abuse and Mental Health Services Administration (SAMHSA) (2000) Cooperative agreement to study children of women with alcohol, drug abuse and mental health (ADM) disorders who have histories of violence. (No. TI 00–006). US Department of Health and Human Services, Rockville, MD

Substance Abuse and Mental Health Services Administration, Office of Applied Studies (2001) Benefits of residential substance abuse treatment for pregnant and parenting women: highlights from a study of 50 demonstration programs of the center for substance abuse treatment. Substance Abuse and Mental Health Services Administration, Rockville, MD

Tyler R, Howard J, Espinosa M, Doakjzs SS (1997) Placement with substance-abusing mothers vs placement with other relatives: infant outcomes. Child Abuse Neglect 21(4):337–349

U.S. Department of Health and Human Services (1999) A report to Congress on substance abuse and child protection. United States Government Printing Office, Washington, DC

Velez ML, Jansson LM, Montoya ID, Schweitzer W, Golden A, Svikis D (2004) Parenting knowledge among substance abusing women in treatment. J Subst Abuse Treat 26:215–222

Wachs TD, Gruen GE (1982) Early experience and human development. Plenum Press, New York, NY

Wasserman DR, Leventhal JM (1991) Maltreatment of children born to cocaine dependent mothers. Am J Dis Children 145:410–411

World Health Organization (2008) Principles of drug dependence treatment. World Health Organization, Geneva, Switzerland

Zweben JE, Clark WH, Smith DE (1994) Traumatic experiences and substance abuse: mapping the territory. J Psychoactive Drugs 26(4):327–344

Legal Issues Regarding Children

7

Nancy S. Erickson

Abstract

Mothers with mental illnesses are sometimes threatened with loss of custody of their children to the father or another relative simply because of stereotypes about mental illness and incorrect assumptions that if a mother has a mental illness, she cannot be an adequate parent. Some people even assume that any parent with a mental illness will be dangerous to a child. The mental and physical health of each parent is a factor the court is always concerned about, but it is only one of many factors. Custody evaluators who are appointed to assist courts are obligated to base their recommendations not on stereotypes but on expert knowledge. The guidelines applicable to evaluators mandate that they look not simply at diagnostic labels but at actual parenting skills and the interactions between the parent and the child, which can be very positive. Scientific knowledge concerning mental illness has expanded exponentially in the past few decades. There has been significant research on the effects of mental illness on parenting, which demonstrates that diagnostic labels often lead to incorrect assumptions regarding parental abilities. The Americans with Disabilities Act of 1990 prohibits discrimination against persons with disabilities, and the ADA Amendments Act of 2008 made it clear that not only persons with physical disabilities but also persons with psychiatric or psychological disabilities are protected by the law. Additionally, some state custody statutes specifically prohibit discrimination based on parental disability.

N.S. Erickson, J.D., LL.M., M.A. (Forensic Psychology) (✉)
Law Offices of Nancy S. Erickson, Brooklyn, NY, USA
e-mail: nancyserickson@earthlink.net

N. Benders-Hadi and M.E. Barber (eds.), *Motherhood, Mental Illness and Recovery*,
DOI 10.1007/978-3-319-01318-3_7, © Springer International Publishing Switzerland 2014

Introduction

For many mothers with mental disorders, one of their biggest fears is that the legal system may separate them from their children. If the child's father is in the picture, the mother may fear that he will seek custody and then keep her from participating in the child's life by claiming that she is unfit because of her disorder. The mother may also fear that her mental disorder may cause her to do something that may come to the attention of child protective services (CPS) and might lead to CPS attempting to terminate her parental rights (Jenuwine and Cohler 2009; Busch and Redlich 2007).

All mothers may have such fears from time to time. However, it is likely that, even prior to having children, women with mental disorders have suffered discrimination based on stereotypes about mental illness. Therefore, fears about being stereotyped as bad mothers may be activated when they give birth.

Fortunately, discrimination based on disabilities—including mental disorders—appears to be waning, albeit not quickly enough. The average person seems to be more knowledgeable about mental disorders now than in the past, possibly because of increased access to information through the media, including the Internet.

Another reason for a decrease in the stigma of mental illness may be the fact that understanding of the causes and consequences of many mental illnesses has dramatically increased in the past several decades, and medications have been developed that can cure or at least control the symptoms of many mental disorders.

Additionally, to the extent that discrimination against people with disabilities (PWD) still exists, the Americans with Disabilities Act (ADA) and the ADA Amendments Act of 2008 (ADAAA) may help to protect PWD against discrimination in the courts as well as in other areas (LaFortune and DiCristina 2012; Hurder 2002).

Despite the advances of modern psychiatry and psychology and the requirements of the ADA and other anti-discrimination laws, discrimination against parents (especially mothers) with mental disorders continues. Family court judges and others often still make a knee-jerk assumption that parents with mental disorders will be incapable of properly parenting their children. It is unfair that such parents are often "presumed guilty until proven innocent," but they and their attorneys must recognize that, realistically, they do have an uphill battle and must prepare well to overcome such a reaction.

History of the Treatment of Mothers in the Legal System

Historically, women have not fared well with regard to legal issues concerning custody of their children (Mason 1994). Mothers with mental illness have fared particularly poorly. Under the common law of England, from which the United States gained its original laws, mothers who were married had no right to custody of their children. If the father wanted custody, he had the right to have custody of marital children. A mother who was not married usually did not have to worry about losing custody to the father, because most often he did not want to acknowledge the child, but she also had no right to get child support. If the father wanted custody, she sometimes was forced to give up custody so that the child could be fed and otherwise cared for.

The common law rules also viewed married women as having virtually no legal existence or legal rights apart from their husbands. The legal doctrine of "coverture" viewed the husband and wife as one person, and the one was the husband. The husband had the right and duty to control the wife, even to the point that if a husband believed his wife was mentally ill, he had the power to have her institutionalized (Chesler 2005). He also could take charge of her "treatment" outside of an institution, so that some women were confined by their husbands to their homes under conditions that were hardly better than institutionalization or even imprisonment (Gilman 1892).

In the early twentieth century, the concept that custody should be decided on the "best interests of the child" (BIC) began to take hold. Custody decisions started to improve for some mothers, but only for mothers of very young children, as the "tender years" doctrine developed as part of the BIC standard. Under that doctrine, a child of "tender years" (approximately seven or younger) was thought to be better off with his or her mother, unless the mother was "unfit" (Herman 1999; Mason 1994).

However, older children were still viewed as belonging to the father, who was supposedly better able to guide them—especially boys—into adulthood. Older children were also less of a burden. In fact, until child labor laws were in place and enforced, an older child could actually be a financial benefit to a parent. So mothers got priority when children were physical and financial burdens and fathers got priority when the children were financially valuable. During the period when the "tender years" presumption was in effect, mental illness sometimes, but not always, was equated with automatic unfitness. If the evidence presented indicated that the mother had "recovered," she still had the presumption in her favor (Annotation (2013), pp. 27–28).

By the 1970s, legislative change and court cases under the Equal Protection Clause of the Constitution made the BIC doctrine sex neutral in most states, at least on its face—fathers and mothers were supposed to be on an equal footing in terms of custody, with no presumption to one or the other regardless of the age of the child. Mothers still got custody of children in the majority of cases, however, because fathers did not contest custody and simply agreed that the mother could have custody. Child support laws encouraged such a result, because there were few guidelines for determining the correct amount of child support, orders were unrealistically low, and enforcement was extremely difficult. Consequently, fathers could avoid both the burden of physically caring for the children and most of the burden of financially supporting them by leaving them with their mothers.

If the mother suffered from a mental illness, the father could decide to contest custody or to leave the children with her (despite any disadvantages to the children that might have been caused by her mental disorder). On the other hand, if the father decided to contest custody based on her mental disorder, his likelihood of gaining custody probably was enhanced by the stigma attached to mental illness. However, if the evidence showed that medications and/or other treatment brought her condition under control, she sometimes could retain custody, especially if she had been the primary caretaker parent (Annotation (2013), pp. 34–36).

During the 1970s and early 1980s, domestic violence was not yet recognized as the scourge that we know it now to be, and the law failed to protect battered women. In fact, psychologists often assumed that if a woman was abused, she must have a preexisting mental disorder—perhaps depression, Dependent Personality Disorder, or even masochism (Brown 1992). Judges often made those same assumptions. There was a failure to recognize that if a battered woman had a mental disorder, it was possible—even likely—that the mental disorder was caused by the abuse, not a cause of the abuse.

We now know that Posttraumatic Stress Disorder (PTSD), depression, and other mental disorders are common sequelae of domestic abuse (Morrell and Rubin 2001; Seighman et al. 2011). Unfortunately, the law still has not fully caught up with the research on this issue. However, cases have recognized that mental disorders that are transient and situational—caused by the crisis in the marital relationship—should not preclude an award of custody to the individual with such a condition, and there are even cases where an abused mother who attempted suicide was granted custody upon her recovery (Annotation (2013), pp. 35–37).

Regardless of the cause of a mother's mental disorder, the court is supposed to look at the mother's relationship to the child and her parenting abilities and practices, not simply the diagnosis or diagnoses that may have been given to her. The question to be answered is whether she in fact parents the children in an acceptable manner and whether the children will be better served by being in her custody rather than in the custody of their father. She may have a diagnosis that appears very serious, but if she is still able to parent her children well, that is what should be considered, not the diagnostic label.

This chapter will take a more in-depth look at the question of determining the BIC in the context of "private" custody cases (where two private individuals are vying for custody—usually the mother and the father).

There are many other important legal issues regarding pregnant women and mothers who have mental disorders—in particular, under what circumstances Child Protective Services may remove a child from a mother who has a mental disorder or terminate her parental rights, and issues regarding mentally ill pregnant women and mothers in the criminal justice system—that this chapter will not address. Mothers (and fathers) in private custody cases may have—or may have had in the past—contact with child protective agencies or the criminal justice system, so advocates for mothers with disabilities may need to educate themselves on these issues as well.

Custody: Mothers Versus Fathers

The Meaning of "Custody"

Legal custody (sometimes just "custody" for short) is the authority to make decisions regarding the child, such as decisions concerning education, religion, medical care, etc. Legal custody may be sole (to one parent) or joint (both parents make decisions). If legal custody is joint and the parents do not agree, then one parent may have to go back to court to get a ruling on the disputed issue. Clearly joint custody is not appropriate for parents who cannot communicate civilly, and it is especially inappropriate where there has been domestic abuse.

Residential custody is physical custody, i.e., the residential custody determination governs with whom the child will live. Sometimes a court orders "sole" residential custody to one parent and "visitation" or "access" to the other. Sometimes a court order states that residential custody is "joint " or "shared," which simply means that the child spends some time living with one parent and some time with the other parent. However, in situations in which one parent has "sole" residential custody and the other has overnight visitation, it could also be said that they are "sharing" residential custody. Therefore, the term "shared" or "joint" residential custody may be really meaningless, except that the noncustodial parent may prefer the label of "shared" or "joint" custody.

Legal Standards for Determining Custody and Visitation Issues

The current standard for custody throughout the country when a court must decide between two parents is the "best interests of the child" (BIC). That is a very vague concept. A judge could interpret it in many different ways, many of which could be subjective values and biases of the judge. In order to give the court more guidance as to what BIC means, many states' custody statutes list factors for the court to consider (Elrod and Spector 2011). Factors often listed in state statutes include the following:

1. The love, affection, and other emotional ties existing between the parties involved and the child.
2. The capacity and disposition of the parties involved to give the child love, affection, and guidance and to continue the education and raising of the child in his or her religion or creed, if any.
3. The capacity and disposition of the parties involved to provide the child with food, clothing, medical care, or other remedial care recognized and permitted under the laws of this state in place of medical care and other material needs.
4. The length of time the child has lived in a stable, satisfactory environment and the desirability of maintaining continuity.
5. The permanence, as a family unit, of the existing or proposed custodial home or homes.
6. The moral fitness of the parties involved.

7. The mental and physical health of the parties involved.
8. The home, school, and community record of the child.
9. The reasonable preference of the child if the court considers the child to be of sufficient age to express preference.
10. The willingness and ability of each of the parties to facilitate and encourage a close and continuing parent/child relationship between the child and the other parent or the child and the parents.
11. Domestic violence, regardless of whether the violence was directed against or witnessed by the child.
12. Any other factor considered by the court to be relevant to a particular child custody dispute.

Factor 7—the mental and physical health of the parties involved—is a factor the court is likely to be especially concerned about when a parent has a mental illness. However, it should be stressed that this factor is only one among many and that it speaks of "health," not diagnosis.

When parental custody is being challenged by a non-parent, the BIC standard is not used in most states because the United States Supreme Court has held that parents have constitutional rights to the care and custody of their children which are superior to those of others. Even grandparents do not stand on the same footing as parents (*Troxel v. Granville*, 2000). Therefore, most states require the non-parent to prove that the parent is in some way clearly unfit or that other extraordinary circumstances exist before the BIC comes into play. A parent's mental (or physical) illness does not automatically equal unfitness.

Custody Evaluations

It is the job of the judge to determine the BIC. However, most states allow judges to appoint individuals—usually mental health professionals but sometimes attorneys or others—to conduct custody evaluations to assist the courts to make their determinations. It is important to remember that the evaluator is not permitted to make the BIC determination. The evaluator may only provide data—and sometimes, but not always, recommendations—that may assist the court in making that determination.

In most states, the evaluator must be an "expert," which generally means that the evaluator must have relevant knowledge that is beyond what is known by the average person (the judge is viewed as an average person). Sometimes state statutes, court rules, or case law specify which professionals may be used as custody evaluators and what training they must have (e.g., California Court Rules).

When mental health professionals were first used in custody cases, each parent would hire her or his own "expert," and a "battle of the experts" would ensue. Currently, most courts prefer to appoint a so-called "neutral" evaluator to report to the court, but some also allow each parent to hire her or his own (although that evaluator might or might not be given access to interview all members of the family).

Each state differs (and often each judge differs) in how custody evaluators are expected to approach custody evaluations. For example, the Office of the Professions of the New York State Education Department has promulgated "Guidelines for Child Custody Evaluations," but the guidelines are not detailed, leaving much room for divergent practices (NYSED 2009). Organizations of mental health professionals, such as the American Psychological Association, have also promulgated guidelines, but they are "aspirational," not legally binding.

With regard to assessment of mental health of the parents, both the 1994 and the 2009 American Psychological Association (APA) guidelines concerning custody evaluations for the courts stress that it is not a mental health diagnosis that matters but the functional abilities of the parent to perform the duties of a parent in an acceptable manner.

The 1994 APA guidelines state (APA 1994, 526):

> The focus of the evaluation is on parenting capacity, the psychological and developmental needs of the child, and the resulting fit. In considering psychological factors affecting the best interests of the child, the psychologist focuses on the parenting capacity of the prospective custodians in conjunction with the psychological and developmental needs of each involved child. This involves (a) an assessment of the adult's capacities for parenting ...; (b) an assessment of the psychological functioning and developmental needs of each child and of the wishes of each child where appropriate; and (c) an assessment of the functional ability of each parent to meet these needs, including an evaluation of the interaction between each adult and child,..., Psychopathology may be relevant to such an assessment, insofar as it has impact on the child or the ability to parent, but it is not the primary focus (emphasis added).

The 2009 APA guidelines, published in 2010, state (APA 2010, 864):

> The evaluation focuses upon parenting attributes, the child's psychological needs, and the resulting fit.... From the court's perspective, the most valuable contributions of psychologists are those that reflect a clinically astute and scientifically sound approach to legally relevant issues.... The most useful and influential evaluations focus on skills, deficits, values and tendencies relevant to parental attributes and a child's psychological needs. Comparatively little weight is afforded to evaluations that offer a personality assessment without attempting to place it in the appropriate context. Useful contextual considerations may include the availability and use of effective treatment, the augmentation of parenting attributes through the efforts of supplemental caregivers, and other factors that affect the potential impact of a clinical condition upon parenting (emphasis added).

Clearly from 1994 to 2010 the emphasis has shifted even farther away from mere diagnoses to functional abilities, including abilities enhanced by effective treatment and other assistance to a parent (see also National Council on Disability 2012).

In line with the APA guidelines, the "Practice Parameters" of the American Academy of Child and Adolescent Psychiatry state (AACAP 1997):

> The evaluator should note each parent's health status, including any physical ailments or unhealthy habits.... The evaluator should assess whether either parent abuses drugs or alcohol.... Another common issue arises when one parent has (or is alleged to have) a psychiatric illness. Herman (1999) emphasizes that the issue is not a diagnosis per se but, instead, is the effect of psychiatric impairment on the parent-child relationship....

It is not necessary to render a *DSM-IV* diagnosis in a custody dispute. The process is an evaluation of parenting, not a psychiatric evaluation. However, some clinicians give diagnoses, if appropriate, after obtaining a complete psychiatric history and recording results of a mental status examination....

If parties are given diagnoses, the clinician should explain the ramifications (if any) of the diagnosis for custody. Otherwise, providing a diagnosis confuses the court and provides fodder for attorneys (emphasis added).

Similarly, the APA Specialty Guidelines for Forensic Psychology, like the APA and AACAP guidelines quoted above, also caution against using clinical diagnoses, stating: "Forensic practitioners are encouraged to consider the problems that may arise by using a clinical diagnosis in some forensic contexts, and consider and qualify their opinions and testimony appropriately" (APA Committee on Ethical Guidelines for Forensic Psychology 2013).

Additionally, advocates for mothers with mental disabilities should consult the APA "Guidelines for Assessment and Intervention with Persons with Disabilities," which stresses the need to look for strengths as well as weaknesses when working with persons with disabilities (APA 2012; see also National Council on Disability 2012).

Thus, the significant relevant guidelines in the fields of psychiatry and psychology all emphasize that attention should be directed to parenting ability, not the label of any disorder(s). Researchers have come to the same conclusion:

Ultimately, the literature suggests that the determination of the effect of a mental illness is based, not on a particular parental condition or diagnosis, but on how that condition affects the daily personal and parental functioning of the parent affected and on the effects of that functioning on the child (Raub et al. 2013).

Most researchers agree that forensic evaluators should be cautioned against "the predisposing bias that [psychiatrically diagnosed] individuals are incapable of adequate parenting, are not amenable to parenting interventions, and will remain "unfit" even if their diagnostic status changes" and recommend the evaluation of functional parenting competency (Benjet et al. 2003, pp. 246).

Functional parenting is always the appropriate focus, but because bias against people with mental disorders still exists, that fact may have to be repeated throughout the custody case to make sure the evaluator and the judge do not lose sight of it.

Custody evaluators are usually mental health professionals—psychiatrists, social workers, and psychologists—and their training is in diagnosing and treating disorders. The role of a custody evaluator, on the other hand, is a forensic role, not a treatment role. The forensic role is to assist the court in arriving at a legal conclusion. Sometimes a custody evaluator finds it difficult to maintain the more unfamiliar forensic stance and falls back into the more familiar treatment role. The custody evaluator may need to be reminded of the important role distinction (Greenberg and Shuman 1997).

Typically an evaluation consists of interviews with each parent (and the child, if old enough), contacts with "collaterals," such as teachers, employers, doctors, and other witnesses to the relationships between the parents and the children, and consideration of relevant documents, such as court documents, medical records, school and employment records, etc.

If the evaluator is a psychologist, the evaluator may also wish to conduct some psychological "tests." The MMPI-2 and the Rorschach (ink blot) test are the most commonly used "tests" (Bow et al. 2005). Use of tests in a situation involving a parent who is mentally ill is especially likely to lead to biased recommendations (National Council on Disability 2012). A judge or custody evaluator is supposed to look for the relative strengths and weaknesses of the competing parents. Tests look for mental weaknesses but not strengths. Tests are likely to find mental weaknesses, even in parents who are excellent parents. Tests will therefore usually tip the scales against the parent who has a mental illness, even though that parent could have strengths that allow her to be an excellent parent. Tests can also come up with inaccurate results. A good example of that is the tendency of psychological tests to inaccurately assess battered mothers (Erickson 2005; Rosewater 1988).

Judges are very heavily influenced by custody evaluations, which leads to the concern that custody cases are being decided by the mental health professionals rather than the judges. Evaluations are also being increasingly criticized as unscientific and often unnecessary (Kelly and Ramsey 2009; Krause and Sales 2000; Melton et al. 2007; O'Connell 2009; Tippins and Wittman 2005; Yeamans 2010). In addition, there have been court challenges to them on the grounds that they violate Constitutional guarantees, such as the guarantees of Due Process of Law and Equal Protection. Mothers and their attorneys should carefully weigh the pros and cons before asking for or agreeing to custody evaluations in their cases.

Although custody evaluations should not hinge on surface factors, just as for any interview, first impressions are important. Parents who are undergoing custody evaluations should remember some important things about being interviewed by anyone: be on time; be polite; dress conservatively; speak at a normal speed and normal tone (not pressured or anxious or angry). Parents should also be prepared to discuss their good parenting qualities, giving examples. If a mother has a mental illness, she should be prepared to discuss her treatment and emphasize her current lack of any symptoms that would adversely affect parenting and the support resources that she has put in place. Preparing for questions that might be asked will help the mother feel more relaxed about the interview as well.

Research on the Effects of Mental Illness on Parenting

All custody evaluators should be knowledgeable about the possible effects of mental illness on parenting, but the focus should be on the particular parent (s) involved, not the effects of a certain mental disorder on the "average" or "typical" patient (Herman 1999; Jenuwine and Cohler 2009). If there is no custody evaluator in a case, or if the custody evaluator's assessment is inaccurate, the attorney for either parent may engage the assistance of a mental health professional with expertise in that area to educate the judge on the particular mental disorder

(s) the parent(s) may have, the wide range of effects (from zero to many) those disorders could have on parenting, and the actual effects (if any) on the parent.

Research on serious mental illness in parents is almost exclusively done on mothers; there is very little research on fathers (Jenuwine and Cohler 2009). The mental illnesses on which the most research relating to parenting has been done are schizophrenia, major depression, and bipolar disorder (formerly known as manic depression).

Relatively little research has been done on the effects of parental personality disorders on parenting, although there is some. Again, those studies more often are on mothers rather than on fathers. Antisocial Personality Disorder and Borderline and Narcissistic personality disorders in parents seem related to both parental behavior and later childhood problems. However, a child's behavior problems are not necessarily caused by parental behavior. Genetics or some other factor other than parental behavior could result in childhood behavior problems (Dutton et al. 2011).

The Mother's Approach to Court Proceedings

The most important fact to keep in mind when a mother has a mental disorder of any kind and the mother is faced with a custody case (usually against the father but sometimes against another family member) is that the attention of the court (and a custody evaluator if any) should always be directed away from the diagnosis to the actual parental functioning of each parent.

If the mother can show, for example, that by taking the medications prescribed to her and/or by engaging in therapy she has divested herself of the symptoms of her disorder that may, in the past, have interfered with her parenting, such proof should go a long way toward overcoming any misguided assumption that just the presence of a mental disorder precludes appropriate parenting.

The existence of medications that are assumed to be able to treat a particular disorder can be a double-edged sword, however, because if medications exist for a condition, many people who lack sufficient knowledge may incorrectly believe that every person with that condition should take that medication. In fact, everyone is unique. What might work with one person might not with another. Medications that can be tolerated by one person may not be able to be tolerated by another. One person might be able to deal with the side effects of the medications while another might not. Additionally, an individual could be incorrectly diagnosed, so that the medications prescribed could be entirely inappropriate or even harmful. For example, PTSD is sometimes misdiagnosed as ADHD. These issues arise in custody cases involving parents with mental disorders.

However, if the medications that are prescribed do in fact lessen the symptoms of the mother's mental disorder, then the mother would be well advised to continue to take them (Benjet et al. 2003). Studies tend to show that when symptoms decline, parenting improves (Kahng et al. 2008). Even more importantly for purposes of a court case, judges usually are not favorably disposed to parents who refuse to follow doctors' orders or otherwise refuse to do what they have been advised to do to improve their parenting.

A mother who has been diagnosed with a mental disorder, or who has simply been in therapy at any time, may fear she may be at a disadvantage against a father who has had no contact with the mental health system. She and her attorney should keep in mind that just because a father has never been treated for a mental disorder does not mean he does not have one and does not mean he is a better parent. If the mother's mental health is being investigated, the father's also should be.

This is particularly the case if he has perpetrated any type of domestic abuse. Domestic abuse is marked by a perpetrator's attempt to exert power and control over his partner, whether that is exerted by physical abuse or, more subtly, by mental, emotional, social, or financial abuse. Domestic violence is a behavior, not a mental illness. Thus, abusers are often psychologically "normal" individuals, in terms of mental disorders. However, they can also have various mental disorders, diagnosed or undiagnosed, such as depression, Borderline Personality Disorder, or various types of Antisocial Personality Disorder, especially psychopathy. One study has suggested that about 25 % of domestic violence perpetrators can be classified as generally violent/antisocial (Holtzworth-Munroe and Stuart 1994).

A psychopath has no conscience or empathy for others (Hare 2003). Consequently, a parent who is a psychopath should clearly be viewed as presenting an especially high risk for danger to children. Custody evaluators virtually never test for psychopathy using the PCL-R (Hare 2003) or any other recognized instrument (Bow et al. 2005). Therefore, it is quite possible for a custody evaluator (or judge) not even to be aware that the father is a psychopath while that same evaluator or judge might be overly concerned about a relatively minor mental disorder in a mother (Leedom et al. 2013).

Clearly, more attention should be directed by custody evaluators and judges to those traits and disorders that are more detrimental—even dangerous—to children. After a proper evaluation/assessment, it is quite possible that an evaluator may conclude that a mother, despite her mental disability, may be a better parent than a father who has never been diagnosed with any disorder prior to the assessment.

Situational Disorders

Judges should also be made aware that certain conditions very well may be situational—often related to the circumstances of the separation of the parents. For example, PTSD or depression in an abused (or formerly abused) woman is likely to be affecting her during a custody battle with her abuser (Seighman et al. 2011). Laws in most states do require judges to take domestic violence into account in custody cases. In fact, in many states, a finding that a parent has abused the other parent gives rise to a presumption that custody to the abuser is not in the best interests of the child (Family Law Quarterly 2012). However, the courts are often still resistant to finding abuse. Judges sometimes still say things such as "Well, he only hit the mother, not the children," regardless of research that shows that parents who abuse their spouses are at great risk of abusing their children too (Bancroft and Silverman 2002; Edleson 1999).

Judges still often fail to recognize that an abused mother with PTSD or another mental disorder caused by the abuse probably is only temporarily in a weakened state and can recover and parent as well as before she was abused if the court will help her to get safe and to keep her children safe (Erickson 2005; Sullivan 2000; Levendosky and Graham-Berman 2000).

Thankfully, some courts have recognized that an "abuser cannot take advantage of his acts of abuse in a custody battle with the abused...." (*Lewelling v. Lewelling* 1999). In that case, the father had abused the mother, and she was taking medications for her "nerves." She had also been in the state mental hospital on one occasion. However, the court did not find any evidence that custody to the mother would be detrimental to the child and refused to "remov[e] a child from a parent simply because she has suffered physical abuse at the hands of her spouse."

Involvement of a Treating Mental Health Professional in a Custody Case

If a custody evaluation is performed, the custody evaluator may or may not have the authority to speak with a parent's treating mental health professional or to obtain that professional's records regarding the treatment of a patient. The law differs from state to state.

The patient's records regarding treatment by the patient's treating mental health professional may, depending on the state law, be subpoenaed by the attorney for the other party even if there is no custody evaluator.

Some state laws hold that when a parent engages in a custody case, that parent automatically places his/her physical and mental health at issue; therefore, no confidentiality or privileges apply to records of medical doctors or mental health providers (*Rosenblitt v. Rosenblitt Anonymous v. Anonymous*). Other states take the position that the judge must balance the need for the records or for the testimony of treating mental health providers against the need for confidentiality and privilege (Comment 2001). Sometimes the attorney for the client whose records are sought to be produced may ask the judge to allow certain redactions from the records before the other side may see them or may ask the judge to review the records in chambers ("in camera") to determine which portions of the records, if any, are relevant to the case and therefore may need to be revealed to the other side. The records are likely to contain many entries that are irrelevant to custody.

A father usually would want to subpoena the wife's therapy records if he believed that the records would be detrimental to the mother's bid for custody or visitation. Normally the mother would want her records to be kept confidential and therefore would not want her records to be subpoenaed. On the other hand, the mother might want her treating physician to testify in order to demonstrate to the court that any symptoms of her illness that could possibly be problematic with regard to her parenting are absent. If so, at least some of her records might need to be provided to the judge for determination of their relevancy to the case and their need to be shown to the other parent for cross-examination of the treating physician. State laws differ on this issue as well as on many other issues.

False Allegations of Mental Illness and Undiagnosed Mental Illness

Many people believe the myth that mothers make many false allegations of abuse against fathers (Dallam and Silberg 2006). However, studies tend to show that fathers more often make false allegations of abuse against mothers rather than vice versa (Trocme and Bala 2005). Often if a mother claims the child's father abused her, the father will claim that she is "crazy." In a study of mothers who alleged the fathers abused their children, but where the fathers alleged the mothers were "crazy," investigation revealed that all the fathers were abusive to the mothers (Ayoub et al. 1991).

The attorney of a parent against whom false allegations of mental illness are lodged should strenuously object to a mental health evaluation of that parent, especially without a mental health evaluation of the other parent. Such an evaluation would be a mere "fishing expedition." Typical allegations of mental illness lodged against mothers are allegations of borderline personality disorder, hysteria, paranoia, and bipolar disorder. A parent who alleges that the other parent has a mental disorder should be required to provide evidence of specific behaviors of the parent that are symptoms of such disorders. Even if the accusing parent lies and falsely describes behaviors that appear to be symptoms of these disorders, a competent mental health expert should be able to provide evidence that the mother is not mentally ill.

Other typical allegations are so-called "parental alienation syndrome"/"parental alienation," "enmeshment" or "folie a deux," and Munchausen's Syndrome by Proxy. These require more discussion, because they are either nonexistent or extremely rare.

"Parental Alienation Syndrome" (PAS) is not a valid mental health diagnosis. It is a false diagnosis made up by the late Richard Gardner, who claimed that parents (especially mothers) going through divorce often brainwash their children against the other parent (Gardner 1992). Advocates of PAS attempted to have it included in the DSM-5 (Bernet 2010). They renamed it "parental alienation disorder" (PAD), defined as follows: "a mental condition in which a child, usually one whose parents are engaged in a high conflict divorce, allies himself or herself strongly with one parent, and rejects a relationship with the other parent, without legitimate justification." (Bernet 2010). The PAS advocates were not successful. The American Psychiatric Association announced in 2012 that four alleged disorders—including PAS—were not accepted for inclusion in either the section of the DSM-5 dealing with conditions that are accepted as categorical diagnoses or the section of the DSM-5 dealing with "conditions that require further research before their consideration as formal disorders" (American Psychiatric Association 2012). In other words, PAS/PAD is not even worth further discussion.

Notwithstanding this clear rejection of PAS/PAD, many mental health professionals have become enamored of the concept of PAS, and those PAS advocates who conduct custody evaluations tend to claim it exists in many of their assigned cases. An opponent of including PAS (or PAD) into the DSM-5 states:

> At its best, adopting PAS or PAD as a formal diagnosis in the DSM-5 serves only to further confuse mental health practitioners and the courts. At its worst, it lines the pockets of both attorneys and expert witnesses by increasing the number of billable hours in a given case. It creates an entirely new level of debate, in which only qualified experts can engage, adding to the already murky waters of divorce testimony. We believe PAS(D) has neither the empirical support nor the clinical relevance to justify its adoption as a mental illness. By all means, each side should be allowed to present a robust argument to gain custody in court, but these conflicted children, caught in the middle, should not be labeled as mentally ill (Houchin et al. 2012).

Although there are certainly parents who badmouth the other parents during custody battles, there are few who actually try to "alienate" the children against the other parent (the so-called "target parent") and fewer who succeed. If a child does not want to have a relationship with one parent or does not want to spend much time with that parent, usually such a child is motivated not by any "alienation" perpetrated by the other parent but by fear of the less favored parent or anger against that parent for something the parent has done or has failed to do (Kelly and Johnston 2001; Herman 1999).

PAS is often automatically alleged by a domestic violence perpetrator against the other parent when the other parent is simply trying to protect herself and/or the children by reporting the perpetrator's domestic violence or child abuse (or both) (Erickson 2013, 2010; Meier 2009a, b; Dalton et al. 2004, 2006).

"Enmeshment" and "Folie a deux" are also sometimes alleged against battered women by their abusers in a manner similar to "parental alienation." "Enmeshment" is not in the DSM. It is a term used by Salvador Minuchin and others to describe a situation where the boundary between a parent and child is so unclear and the two are so close that the child is unable to appropriately individuate from the parent. The current use of the term "enmeshment" to approximate the concept of "parental alienation" seems to stem from the fact that the term "parental alienation" has gotten bad press, so those who would previously have alleged "parental alienation" feel they may have better success if they substitute a different term.

"Folie a deux" appears to have been taken up by "parental alienation" advocates for the same reason. "Folie a deux" is in the DSM-IV under the name "Shared Delusional Disorder." It is an attempt to describe another very rare condition in which one person has a delusional disorder (often a paranoid delusion) and another person close to that individual (e.g., spouse or child) takes on the symptoms of having that same delusion. It is therefore obvious that if an alleged alienating parent does not have a delusional disorder, no "shared delusional disorder" with the child can occur.

In the DSM-5, "shared delusional disorder" has been eliminated (American Psychiatric Association 2013a). The American Psychiatric Association states: "DSM-5 no longer separates delusional disorder from shared delusional disorder. If criteria are met for delusional disorder then that diagnosis is made. If the diagnosis cannot be made but shared beliefs are present, then the diagnosis 'other specified schizophrenia spectrum and other psychotic disorder' is used" (American Psychiatric Association 2013b).

Munchausen's Syndrome by Proxy (MBP) was in the DSM-IV in the chapter entitled "Other Conditions That May Be a Focus of Clinical Attention." It was defined in the DSM-IV as "The intentional production or feigning of physical or psychological symptoms in another person who is under the individual's care for the purpose of indirectly assuming a sick role." In other words, one person (usually a parent) makes another (usually a child) sick or exaggerates the child's symptoms. It is considered a form of child abuse. Most commonly mothers, not fathers, are accused of MBP. In the DSM-5 it has been placed "among the somatic symptom and related disorders because somatic symptoms are predominant in both disorders, and both are most often encountered in medical settings" (American Psychiatric Association 2013b). It is exceedingly rare.

In the 1990s it became very fashionable for mental health professionals to claim that they found MBP in many custody litigants, especially mothers. Now, it is clear that some, if not many, of those "diagnoses" were false. Often the mother is concerned about real symptoms displayed by the child that doctors have not been able to explain with any diagnosis. For example, a mother was accused of MBP when it later turned out that the child had lupus disease. Before the lupus disease was diagnosed, however, she lost custody because of the false accusation of MBP.

The issue of false allegations of mental illness is made more complicated by the fact that women tend to seek assistance from mental health providers (and medical doctors) when a similarly situated man would not—possibly as a result of a "macho" attitude that going to a mental health provider shows weakness (Tony Soprano in "The Sopranos" being a notable exception).

Consequently, it is common that when parents are contesting custody, the mother is, or has been, in therapy, but the father is not. This could make her appear to have serious mental issues when she does not and could make the father appear free of any mental health issues when he is not. Her attorney may need to demonstrate that her therapy is not directed toward a serious mental illness but is being sought by the mother so that she can better cope with what she is going through and better care for the children. In that same vein, it can be pointed out that most parents would benefit from therapy at such times and that when a parent tries to tough it through difficult situations, this may be detrimental to his or her functioning as a parent. One court has held that receipt of mental health treatment often enables a parent to provide "a more stable, nurturing, and healthy home for the child" (*Peisach v. Antuna* 1989).

Undiagnosed mental illness is also an area of concern in custody cases, especially in cases where the father has perpetrated domestic violence against the mother. A custody evaluator may not be equipped to ferret out such conditions.

The mother's attorney may need to have her/his client testify in court or report to the custody evaluator regarding the allegedly ill father's behavior in order to show the father's symptoms of possible mental health problems. However, even that information may not be enough to get the attention of the evaluator or the court. For example, in one case handled by this author, the mother/client told the custody evaluator that the father suffered from panic attacks and ran to the hospital claiming he was having a heart attack. Additionally, for months at a time during the ongoing marriage the father had hardly moved from the couch—a common sign of depression. She also reported to the evaluator that he had put a gun to his head and that she had had to talk him out of killing himself. Inexplicably, the evaluator never even mentioned these things in his report to the court. It should always be remembered, however, that many abusers have no diagnosable mental disorders.

Legal Protection for Parents With Mental Disorders

The Americans with Disabilities Act (ADA) and the ADA Amendments Act of 2008 (ADAAA) are federal laws that may help to protect persons with disabilities (PWDs) against discrimination in the courts as well as in other areas. The ADA and the ADAAA prohibit discrimination based on disability in employment, housing, and public accommodations. Courts are places of public accommodation, so court personnel are prohibited from discriminating against PWD and must make reasonable accommodations for PWD, so that PWD will be able to participate in court proceedings on an equal footing with nondisabled litigants (*Tennessee v. Lane 2004*; ADA; ADAAA; LaFortune and DiCristina 2012; Huffer 2012; Seighman et al. 2011).

Originally, under the ADA, physically disabled individuals, not mentally disabled individuals, more often sought protection under that statute. Now, after the passage of the ADA Amendments Act of 2008, more mentally disabled individuals will be able to be protected. In 2009, the EEOC issued proposed regulations to implement the ADAAA, which include "Examples of Impairments that Will Consistently Meet the Definition of Disability":

> Major depression, bipolar disorder, post-traumatic stress disorder, obsessive compulsive disorder, or schizophrenia, which substantially limit major life activities including [but not limited to] functions of the brain, thinking, concentrating, interacting with others, sleeping, or caring for oneself (Regulations to Implement the Equal Employment Provisions of the ADA 2009, p. 48441, emphasis added).

This change in the regulations will make it easier for persons with mental disabilities to qualify for accommodations under the ADA, especially when read together with other parts of the regulations and of the ADAAA that lessen the burden of proving that a disability "substantially limits major life activities" (Regulations to Implement the Equal Employment Provisions of the ADA 2009, p. 48441).

Additionally, custody statutes in some states specifically caution against discrimination based on disability, which would include psychiatric disability (Callow et al. 2011; National Council on Disability 2012). A prohibition on discrimination does not mean that the effects of a disability on the children must be ignored, but it does certainly mean that myths and assumptions about the abilities of disabled parents to effectively parent their children must not be tolerated.

Conclusion

Mothers with mental illness are sometimes threatened with loss of custody of the children to the father or another relative. The mother and her attorney must direct the court's attention to her actual good parenting skills and behavior. By doing so they can wear down the walls of bias that may affect custody evaluators and judges.

Acknowledgments The author gratefully acknowledges the excellent research assistance of Chelsea Dale, currently a senior at Colgate University, and James Jackson, currently a second-year law student at the Benjamin N. Cardozo School of Law.

References

Books and Articles

American Academy of Child and Adolescent Psychiatry (1997) Practice parameters for child custody evaluation. J Am Acad Child Adolesc Psychiatry 36(10 Supplement):57S–68S, Washington, D.C.: Author
American Psychiatric Association (2012) APA board of trustees approves DSM-5. Psychiatric News, December 1, 2012. http://alert.psychiatricnews.org/2012/12/apa-board-of-trustees-approves-dsm-5.html
American Psychiatric Association (2013a) Diagnostic and statistical manual of mental disorders (5th ed). American Psychiatric Association, Washington, D.C.
American Psychiatric Association (2013b) Highlights of changes from DSM-IV-TR to DSM-5. http://www.dsm5.org/Documents/changes%20from%20dsm-iv-tr%20to%20dsm-5.pdf
American Psychological Association (1994) Guidelines for child custody evaluations in divorce proceedings. Am Psychol 49:677–680 [see APA 2009 for current version]
American Psychological Association (2010) Guidelines for child custody evaluations in family law proceedings. http://www.apa.org/practice/guidelines-evaluation-child-custody-family-law.pdf
American Psychological Association (2012) Guidelines for assessment of and intervention with persons with disabilities. Am Psychol 67(1):43–62, https://www.apa.org/pi/disability/resources/assessment-disabilities.aspx
American Psychological Association Committee on Ethical Guidelines for Forensic Psychology (2013) Specialty guidelines for forensic psychology. Am Psychol 68(1):7–19, available at https://www.apa.org/pi/disability/resources/assessment-disabilities.aspx
Annotation (2013) Mental health of contesting parent as factor in award of child custody. 53 A.L.R. 5th 375
Ayoub C, Grace P, Paradise J, Newberger E (1991) Alleging psychological impairment of the accuser to defend oneself against a child abuse allegation: a manifestation of wife battering and

false accusations. In Robin M (ed) Assessing child maltreatment reports: The problem of false allegations 191–207

Bancroft L, Silverman J (2002) The batterer as parent. Sage, Thousand Oaks, CA

Benjet C, Azar S, Kuersten-Hogan R (2003) Evaluating the parental fitness of psychiatrically diagnosed individuals: advocating a functional-contextual analysis of parenting. J Fam Psychol 17(2):238–251

Bernet W (2010) Parental alienation, DSM-5 and ICD-11. Charles C. Thomas, Springfield, IL

Bow J, Gould J, Flens J, Greenhut D (2005) Testing in child custody evaluations Selection, usage, and Daubert admissibility: a survey of psychologists. J Foren Psychol Pract 6(2):17–38

Brown L (1992) A feminist critique of the personality disorders. In: Brown L, Ballou M (eds) Personality and psychopathology: feminist reappraisals. Guilford, New York, 206–228

Busch A, Redlich A (2007) Patients' perception of possible child custody or visitation loss for nonadherence to psychiatric treatment. Psychiatr Serv 58(7):999–102

Callow E, Buckland K, Jones S (2011) Parents with disabilities in the United States: prevalence, perspectives, and a proposal for legislative change to protect the right to family in the disability community: Jacobus tenBroek, Disability Law Symposium. Texas J Civil Liberties Civil Rights 17:9–41

Chesler P (2005) Women and madness. Macmillan, New York

Comment (2001) The use of mental health records in child custody proceedings. J Am Acad Matrimonial Lawyers 17:159–181

Dallam SJ, Silberg JL (2006) Myths that place children at risk during custody disputes. Sexual Assault Report 9(3):33–34, 42–47. Available at http://www.leadershipcouncil.org/1/res/cust_myths.html

Dalton C, Drozd L, Wong F (2004) (rev'd 2006) Navigating custody and visitation evaluations in cases with domestic violence: a judge's guide. Reno, NV: Nat'l Council of Juvenile & Family Court Judges. Available at http://www.ncjfcj.org/images/stories/dept/fvd/pdf/navigating_cust.pdf

Dutton D, Denny-Keys M, Sells J (2011) Parental personality disorder and its effects on children: a review of current literature. J Child Custody 8(4):268–283

Edleson J (1999) The overlap between child maltreatment and woman battering. Violence Against Women 5(2):134–154

Elrod L, Spector RG (2011) A review of the year in family law: working toward more uniformity in laws related to families. Fam Law Quart 44(4):469–518

Erickson N (2005) Use of the MMPI-2 in custody evaluations involving domestic violence. Family Law Quarterly 39:87–108

Erickson N (2010) Fighting false allegations of parental alienation raised as defenses to valid claims of abuse. In: Hannah M, Goldstein B (eds) Domestic violence, abuse and child custody: legal strategies and policy issues. Kingston, NJ: Civic Research Institute, updated and reprinted in Erickson N (2013). Fighting false allegations of parental alienation raised as defenses to valid claims of abuse. Family and Intimate Partner Violence Quarterly 6(1):35–78

Gardner RA (1992) The parental alienation syndrome: a guide for mental health and legal professionals. Creative Therapeutics Inc, New Jersey

Gilman CP (1892) The yellow wallpaper. The New England Magazine (reprinted and currently available in various forms, including free e-books)

Greenberg SA, Shuman DW (1997) Irreconcilable conflict between therapeutic and forensic roles. Professional Psychol Res Pract 28:50–57

Hare RD (2003) The hare psychopathy checklist—revised, 2nd edn. Multi-Health Systems, Toronto, ON, Canada

Herman S (1999) Child custody evaluations and the need for standards of care and peer review. J Center Children Courts 1:139–150

Holtzworth-Munroe A, Stuart G (1994) Typologies of male batterers: Three subtypes and the differences among them. Psychol Bull 116:476–497

Houchin T, Ranseen J, Hash P, Bartnicki D (2012) The parental alienation debate belongs in the courtroom, not in DSM-5. J Am Acad Psychiatry Law 40:127–31

Huffer K (2012) Unlocking justice: the Americans with disabilities act and its amendments act protecting persons with disabilities in court. Fulkort Press, Las Vegas

Hurder A (2002) ABA urges equal access to courts for individuals with disabilities. Mental Phys Disabil Law Reporter 26(5):772–774

Jenuwine M, Cohler B (2009) Child custody evaluations of parents with major psychiatric disorders. In Galatzer-Levy R, Krause L, Galatzer-Levy J, Scientific Basis of Child Custody Decisions (2d ed). Wiley, New York

Kahng SK, Oyserman D, Bybee D, Mowbray C (2008) Mothers with serious mental illness: when symptoms decline does parenting improve? J Fam Psychol 22(1):162–166

Kelly JB, Johnston JR (2001) The alienated child: a reformulation of parental alienation syndrome. Fam Court Rev 39(3):249–266

Kelly R, Ramsey S (2009) Child custody evaluations: the need for systems-level outcome assessments. Fam Court Rev 47(2):286–303

Krause D, Sales B (2000) Legal standards, expertise, and experts in the resolution of contested child custody cases. Psychol Public Pol Law 6:843–879

LaFortune K, DiCristina W (2012) Representing clients with mental disabilities in custody hearings: using the ADA to help in a best-interests-of-the child determination. ABA Fam Law Quart 46(2):223–246

Leedom L, Bass A, Almas L (2013) The problem of parental psychopathy. J Child Custody 20: 154–184

Levendosky A, Graham-Berman S (2000) Behavioral observations of parenting in battered women. J Fam Psychol 14:80–94

Mason MA (1994) From father's rights to children's rights – the history of child custody in the United States. Columbia University Press, New York

Meier J (2009a) A historical perspective on parental alienation syndrome and parental alienation. J Child Custody Symp Domestic Violence Custody 6(3–4):232–257

Meier J (2009b) Parental alienation syndrome and parental alienation: research reviews, published by VAWnet, a project of the National Resource Center on Domestic Violence/Pennsylvania Coalition Against Domestic Violence, http://new.vawnet.org/Assoc_Files_VAWnet/AR_PAS.pdf

Melton G, Petrila J, Poythress N, Slobogin C (eds) (2007) Psychological evaluations for the courts: a handbook for mental health professionals and lawyers, 3rd edn. Guilford Press, New York

Morrell J, Rubin L (2001) The Minnesota multiphasic personality inventory-2, posttraumatic stress disorder, and women domestic violence survivors. Prof Psychol Res Pract 32:151–156

National Council on Disability (2012) Rocking the cradle: ensuring the rights of parents with disabilities and their children. National Council on Disability, Washington, DC

O'Connell M (2009) Mandated custody evaluations and the limits of judicial power. Fam Court Rev 47(2):304–320

Family Law Quarterly (2012) Charts [on family law in the fifty states] – Chart 2: custody criteria. Fam Law Quarter 45(4):494–95

Raub J, Carlson N, Cook B, Wyshak G, Hauser B (2013) Predictors of custody and visitation decisions by a family court clinic. J Am Acad Psychiatry Law 41:206–18

Rosewater LB (1988) Battered or schizophrenic? Psychological tests can't tell. In: Yllo K, Bograd M (eds) Feminist perspectives on wife abuse. Sage, Newbury Park, CA

Seighman M, Sussman E, Trujillo O (2011) Representing domestic violence survivors who are experiencing trauma and other mental health challenges: a handbook for attorneys. National Center on Domestic Violence, Trauma, and Mental Health. Available at http://www.nationalcenterdvtraumamh.org/wp-content/uploads/2012/01/AttorneyHandbookMay282012.pdf

Sullivan C (2000) Beyond searching for deficits: evidence that physically and emotionally abused women are nurturing parents. J Emotional Abuse 2(1):51–71

Tippins T, Wittman JP (2005) Empirical and ethical problems with custody recommendations: a call for clinical humility and judicial vigilance. Fam Court Rev 43:193–222

Trocme N, Bala N (2005) False allegations of abuse and neglect when parents separate. Child Abuse Negl 29(12):1333–1345

Yeamans R (2010) Urgent need for quality control in child custody psychological evaluations. In: Mo H, Barry G (eds) Domestic violence, abuse and child custody: legal strategies and policy issues. Civic Research Institute, Kingston, NJ

Cases

Anonymous v. Anonymous, 5 AD3d 516, 772 NYS3d 866 (2d Dept., 2004)
Lewelling v. Lewelling, 796 S.W.2d 164 (Texas 1999)
Rosenblitt v. Rosenblitt, 107 AD2d 292, 294, 486 NYS2d 741 (2d Dept., 1985)
Peisach v. Antuna, 539 A.2d 544, 545 (Dist. Ct. App. Fla. 1989)
Tennessee v. Lane, 541 U.S. 509 (2004)
Troxel v. Granville, 530 U.S. 57 (2000)

Statutes and Rules

Americans with Disabilities Act, 42 U.S.C. Sections 12101 *et. seq*

Americans with Disabilities Amendments Act, P.L. 110-325, eff. January 1, 2009. For the current text of the ADA of 1990 incorporating the changes made by the ADA Amendments Act of 2008, see http://www.ada.gov/pubs/ada.htm

California Rules of Court, Title 5, Special Rules for Trial Courts, Rules 5.220 (court-ordered child custody evaluations), 5.225 (training for evaluators), 5.230 (domestic violence training for evaluators)

New York State Education Department, Office of the Professions (2009) Guidelines for child custody evaluations. Available at http://www.op.nysed.gov/prof/psych/psychcustodyguide. htm

Resources

Barrier Free Living, P.O.Box 20799, NY, NY 10009-9991; http://www.bflnyc.org

The Leadership Council on Child Abuse and Interpersonal Violence website is a good source for materials ondomestic violence, child abuse, sex-based discrimination in family law, so-called Parental Alienation Syndrome, and many other issues. http://www.leadershipcouncil.org

National Center for Parents with Disabilities and Their Families, Berkeley, CA. https://lookingglass.org/services/national-services/71-ncpd

The National Council on Disability. http://www.ncd.gov

National Center on Domestic Violence, Trauma, and Mental Health. http://www.nationalcenterdvtraumamh.org

LGBT Mothers

8

Mary E. Barber and Eric Yarbrough

Abstract

LGBT women become mothers in different ways, both before and after coming out. LGBT mothers are still subject to bias and discrimination on the basis of their sexual and gender identities, and LGBT mothers with mental health diagnoses may face added burden of stigma related to mental illness. This chapter describes several case examples of issues that may arise for these mothers. Both LGBT mothers and their children can benefit from affirming treatment services and peer supports.

Introduction

Marcia is a 28 year old Latina parenting 10-year old Sofia, her daughter from a brief relationship. Sofia's father has never been involved with her care or support. Marcia has bipolar disorder for which she gets treatment at a local mental health clinic and for which she is on Supplemental Security Income (SSI). She sometimes struggles financially and emotionally as a single parent, but is fiercely proud of Sofia, who is happy and doing well in school. For the past year, Marcia has been in a relationship with Jess, a woman she met in the neighborhood. It is not Marcia's first sexual experience with a woman, but it is her first serious relationship. A tension between them in the past few months has been Jess' wish for Marcia and Sofia to move in with her. Marcia is worried that if Social Services found out about her lesbian relationship in addition to her treatment for mental illness, they might try to take Sofia away.

M.E. Barber, M.D. (✉)
Rockland Psychiatric Center, Orangeburg, NY, USA
e-mail: mary.barber@omh.ny.gov

E. Yarbrough
Callen – Lorde Community Health Center, New York, NY, USA
e-mail: eyarbrough@callen-lorde.org

N. Benders-Hadi and M.E. Barber (eds.), *Motherhood, Mental Illness and Recovery*, 109
DOI 10.1007/978-3-319-01318-3_8, © Springer International Publishing Switzerland 2014

Little has been written about sexual and gender minority mothers with mental illness. Although lesbian, bisexual, and transgender women have been parenting children for a long time, LGBT parenting has only recently come into public consciousness. This invisibility was due to stereotypes of LGBT people not having children and real fears of custody loss for LGBT parents who had children in the context of a heterosexual relationship that ended.

Yet we know despite the paucity of literature that lesbians, gay-identified women, bi women, and trans women have been parenting long before gay parenting was depicted on "Modern Family" (Barber 2012). We also know (and this book makes abundantly clear) that women with serious mental illness have managed to parent, often without a lot of supports, in great numbers as well. This chapter is an attempt to begin a dialogue about the issues, challenges, and strengths of sexual and gender minority moms with mental illness.

Terms

This chapter uses the terms lesbian and gay in describing sexual minority women, because some women with same-gender orientation may self-label as gay women, some may describe themselves as lesbians, and some may use either label interchangeably. Sexual minority is a term that describes people with a minority sexual identity—gay, lesbian, or bisexual. Transgender is a term that encompasses a range of gender identity that does not match a person's birth gender, from feeling like the other gender inside, to living as the other gender, to going through a medical transition with hormones and surgery. Gender minority is another way of expressing this transgender spectrum—having a minority gender identity. Sexual and gender minorities can use other labels to describe themselves as well—for example, queer, gender-queer, pansexual.

Data

As many as one in five Americans will have a mental health diagnosis in a lifetime, a figure which includes mild phobias and short-lived adjustment disorders along with more significant problems. An estimated 6 % (Kessler et al. 2005) have a serious mental illness such as major depression, bipolar disorder, schizophrenia, PTSD, or a personality disorder. Population surveys, although likely to be undercounting, have estimated that 3.5 % of adults in the USA identify as lesbian, gay, or bisexual, and 0.3 % identify as transgender (Gates 2011). A larger group of Americans report same-sex sexual activity (8.2 %) and at least some same-sex attraction (11 %; Gates 2011).

Better population-based data on LGBT parents has become available in recent years, from the US Census and other large surveys. The most recent data shows that about 37 % of LGBT adults have had a child at some time in their lives (Gates 2013). Among LGBT women under 50 who are living alone or with a partner, nearly half (48 %) are raising a child under 18 (Gates 2013). Same-sex couples are four times more likely than opposite-sex couples to adopt a child, and six times more likely to raise foster children. There are an estimated 22,000 adopted children and 3,400 foster children in the USA being raised by LGBT parents (Gates 2013). Thus LGBT parenting is common, and LGBT mothers are an especially significant group.

When the public considers LGBT people in general, and LGBT parents specifically, the image usually brought forth is that of an affluent white male couple in the Northeast or San Francisco. National survey data does not support this generalization. The states found to have the highest proportions of LGBT's raising children in the most recent data were Mississippi (26 %), Wyoming(25 %), Idaho (23 %), Alaska (22 %), and Montana (22 %, Gates 2013). Census data showed that two cities where gay couples are found to be raising children in great numbers are San Antonio, Texas (34 % of gay couples have children), and Jacksonville, Florida (32 %; Krivickas and Lofquist 2011; Tavernise 2011). Same-sex couples and their children are more likely to be ethnic minorities than are parents and children in opposite-sex couple households. Nor does the affluent stereotype hold when compared to national statistics—LGBT singles and couples raising children are more likely than non-LGBT's to report incomes near the poverty level, and the median annual income for same-sex couples with children is lower than that of comparable different-sex couples with children (Gates 2013).

We have no data on how many LGBT mothers have mental health problems. We do know that LGB people in general (transgender people are not included in these data) may be at increased risk for depression, anxiety, suicidal thoughts, and substance use disorders than the general public (SAMHSA 2012; Institute of Medicine 2011). These risks are thought to be due to minority stress (IOM 2011). Convenience-sample data show correlations between being transgender and having an increased risk of depression, suicidal thoughts and behavior, being the victim of violence, and homelessness (IOM 2011). The literature on LGBT people with serious mental illness (SMI) is small (Hellman 1996; Hellman and Drescher 2004; Barber 2009), but professionals who work in community settings where people with SMI are seen can all expect to treat LGBT patients.

Becoming a Mother

LGBT mothers become parents in different ways, just as heterosexual mothers do. In the past, gay and transgender mothers usually came to have children in the context of a heterosexual marriage that happened before they came out as gay or trans. Becoming a parent in the context of a same-sex relationship did happen long before the 1990s and advent of the "gay baby boom." However, gay parenting by intention has become much more common with increased access to reproductive technologies such as donor insemination and in vitro fertilization, more open adoption rules and procedures allowing gay couples to adopt, and better legal protections such as second parent adoption and marriage for same-sex couples.

Having role models in the media and in communities is probably also a factor in LGBT people considering parenthood as a possibility. LGBT parents still have children in the context of heterosexual relationships, and form families in other ways, such as adopting as a single parent, taking in a sibling's child, or starting a relationship with a partner who is a parent. Some lesbian couples conceive and co-parent children with gay or straight male friends, where the man (or one of the men in a gay couple) is the biological father.

Issues for Moms and Their Children

Juliet is a 55 year old white lesbian-identified artist who had longstanding mild anxiety for which she was never treated. She was in a monogamous relationship with her partner Terry for thirty years, and they raised their daughter Megan together. Megan was conceived by anonymous donor insemination with Terry as the birth mother. During her teenage years, Megan developed an addiction to cocaine and pain pills. The substance abuse of their daughter led to fights in the relationship and eventually a separation. Terry blamed Juliet for Megan's addiction and the relationship falling apart. Legal custody of Megan and the family's assets were all in Terry's name, and Juliet lost her retirement savings and was cut off from her daughter with no legal recourse. She fell into a depression and started to have severe panic attacks which led to treatment. She is now trying to resolve feelings about her daughter, who is in recovery, and start over with her savings to create a plan for her retirement.

LGBT parents have many of the same stressors as straight parents, but they also have the burden of dealing with bias and discrimination from family, friends, and society. Like Juliet, parents may be faced with the reality of losing access to a child due to the lack of legal protections in many states, despite the parent having raised the child and provided financially for them. The strains of a relationship have extra weight when the loss of a partner is coupled with the risk of losing a child. While many LGBT parents resolve these issues around a breakup on their own, there may be no legal supports for the parent involved in a stormy relationship. The stress of having no supports led to Juliet's worsening anxiety, panic attacks, and need for mental health treatment.

Olivia is a 63yo lesbian-identified professionally educated woman. She has suffered for many years with Major Depression and was previously mis-diagnosed as having Border-line Personality Disorder. At the age of 42 she was raising a 12yo son with her husband at the time. The relationship was tumultuous and physically abusive. When her husband filed for divorce, Olivia was confronted with both living as a single mother and facing her repressed sexual orientation. She took an overdose of medication and was admitted to the hospital for treatment of severe depression. Her suicidal behavior led to the incorrect personality disorder diagnosis. While in the hospital, her ex-husband was awarded full-custody of her son and Olivia was denied visitation rights. She is now still dealing with depression over loss of her son who refuses to speak with her because of her mental illness and sexual identity.

Olivia experienced discrimination because of both her sexual orientation and her mental health problems. When people come out as gay, lesbian, or transgender, they often go through such symptoms as mood lability, impulsivity, and potential for suicidal ideation. These are similar to the highs and lows of adolescence, but when they occur in an adult such as Olivia who was in her early 40s, they may be mislabeled as a personality disorder by the inexperienced clinician. Clinicians who don't take a complete sexual history may miss the connection between a patient's acute symptoms and stressors involving sexual orientation. If a patient has lack of access to an affirming support system, she may attempt suicide as Olivia did. Her family, unhappy with her coming out, punished her by taking custody of her daughter away.

Numerous studies of gay mothers and their children find that the children show no more depression, adjustment problems, or school problems than the children of heterosexual parents (Stacey and Biblarz 2001; Perrin et al. 2004; Biblarz and Stacey 2010; Gartrell and Bos 2010). The studies have some limitations, as they use convenience samples and mostly represent white, middle- and upper-class lesbian-headed families. This literature has been used to counter custody decisions based on biased views of gay parents as less capable or a bad influence on children, so the main aim of the studies was to show that gay parents were "good enough" parents. This was a necessary aim, as can be seen from all the cases described above. For Marcia, fears of her child being taken away were enough to make her reluctant to move in with her partner. For Juliet, lack of legal recognition of her parent status led to the loss of her child. And for Olivia, discrimination on the basis of both her sexual identity and psychiatric history led to the loss of her parental rights.

Hopefully, these tragic stories will become less common as more states recognize the rights of gay and lesbian couples and their children, and particularly as more states allow gay and lesbian couples to marry. However, LGBT parents with mental illness will continue to face the stigma and bias associated with their mental health diagnosis. In states where marriage is not available, or where the couple's relationship and children preceded the availability of marriage, protections for both parents often require the assistance of an attorney, and LGBT parents with mental health diagnoses may have fewer economic resources available for obtaining legal protections for their family.

A new generation of literature on gay parents is beginning to clarify some of the unique issues the parents and children face and the needs of both. Both the parents and children may feel enormous pressure to be role models, in essence to prove that LGBT families are okay. For the parents, this may mean that when their child is acting out in public, they may have heightened feelings of embarrassment and concern—not only feeling "What will everyone think of my son?" but "What will they think of gay parents?" (Fitzgerald 2010) Children may feel this pressure also. Children of LGBT parents may even feel pressure to be heterosexual and may paradoxically have a hard time coming out if they realize they are LGBT themselves.

"Mother" is a title and role that is very meaningful and emotionally laden. Where there are two mothers, there may be a subtle competition or concern about who is the "real" mother. In a society that favors biology, where one mother is the birth mother, the non-birth mother may feel a sense of being left out, or lacking a defined role. One preliminary study of non-birth lesbian mothers revealed concerns about lack of social recognition for their role during the pregnancy of their partner (Abelsohn et al. 2013).

For LGBT families created after the breakup of a heterosexual relationship, the parents will have the added tasks of managing a blended family, relating to an ex or exes, and coming out to the children. A parent who goes through gender transition after having children will similarly have to come out as transgender to the children. For an LGBT mother with a mental health diagnosis, coping with and explaining her illness to her children is a further task she must determine how to handle.

Harper is a 45yo bisexual-identified transgender woman with depression and complex PTSD. She previously served in the military and fathered a son before transitioning to female at the age of 38. Her friends from the military have been supportive of her transition as well as her son, but she continues to be criticized and rejected by her parents and ex-wife. Building a social support system with accepting friends from her past has been difficult for her because of an inability to feel comfortable around past friends in her new body. She described herself as a "man's man" in the past and displayed many traditional masculine behaviors, and she reverts back to stereotypical masculine mannerisms when she is depressed. She is dealing with her new identity as female but also negotiating her previous relationship as a father to her 17 year-old son. Because of her ambivalent feelings, she has yet to go through changing her identification to female. This creates on-going tension because of her divorce, military benefits, and how her parents refer to her when she sees them.

Harper's case displays a number of tensions present for a trans-identified individual. Her transition later in life sparked controversy in the family and her core support system has been unsupportive of her new identity. Her son and military counterparts are accepting but relate more to her previous masculine self. While this masculine identity may have been a false-self, Harper reverts back to it when she needs support because she has been unable to develop those skills as her female self. This creates complications in addition to the stress she receives from her parents and ex-wife, because she also has ambivalence about changing her identification and other documents. She believes once she makes these concrete changes, her primary support system will disconnect from her.

Treatment and Support

LGBT parents with serious mental illness are likely to get treatment in the public mental health system, a system that sometimes treats patients as children, and may not be supportive of their sexual identity or role as a parent. Gay people have reported not feeling welcomed in mainstream public mental health settings (Willging et al. 2006; Avery et al. 2001). With new guidance and education on how hospitals and clinics can become more open and accepting of LGBT patients (The Joint Commission 2011), this is hopefully beginning to change.

Some mental health treatment settings specific to LGBT's now exist, either run by LGBT Community Centers or as part of general psychiatry clinics. In these settings, sexual and gender minority parents can be open, get support from professionals, and support each other.

Outside of formal treatment, LGBT parents can get support from each other, through local playgroups, web communities or email lists, or through national organizations (Family Equality, see resources). The children of LGBT parents have their own unique issues and their own coming out process and can benefit from support from their own peer group (COLAGE, see resources). They can share feelings about their parents, advice on how to talk to peers, and how to reply to ignorant or offensive questions they may get from peers or adults. Often, children will have different levels of openness and different responses at various developmental stages. Young children may feel comfortable answering "Where is your father?" with a matter-of-fact, "I don't have a father; I have two moms." Teenagers may be more protective of their personal information, choosing when and how to come out about their families to peers or adults.

> Marcia speaks with her therapist about her fears of losing her child Sofia if Social Services found out she was in a lesbian relationship. Her therapist tells Marcia she doubts that they would know or care about this and points to state sexual orientation nondiscrimination laws that would protect Marcia's parental rights. Marcia's therapist refers her to the local LGBT Community Center, which has a parents and kids social group. There Marcia is able to connect with other lesbian mothers, and Sofia has a playgroup with children her age who have gay and lesbian parents. Marcia's therapist also meets with Marcia and Jess as a couple to discuss the possibility of the two of them moving in together and to work through issues they have around their relationship and Jess' relationship to Sofia.

This chapter has emphasized the fact that LGBT women with mental illness have managed to raise children for some time, often through significant obstacles and without a lot of supports. Raising awareness of LGBT mothers and their challenges, needs, and strengths can help clinicians better address those needs and connect LGBT mothers to supports.

Resources

These are not exhaustive lists, but will give the reader a start on resources for LGBT families.

Organizations

- COLAGE—a national group of children, youth, and adults with one or more LGBTQ parents, http://www.colage.org
- Family Equality Council advocates on behalf of LGBT families, http://www. familyequality.org

Affirmative Treatment

- Callen-Lorde Community Health Center, NYC—offers health and mental health treatment, http://callen-lorde.org/
- Fenway Health, Boston—offers health and mental health treatment, http://www. fenwayhealth.org/site/PageServer

Books for Professionals

- D'Ercole A, Drescher J (eds) (2004) Uncoupling convention: psychoanalytic approaches to same-sex couples and families. The Analytic Press, Hillsdale, NJ
- Glazer DF, Drescher J (eds) (2001) Gay and lesbian parenting. The Haworth Press, New York

Books for Parents

- Green J (1999) The velveteen father: an unexpected journey to parenthood. Ballantine, New York
- Martin A (1993) The lesbian and gay parenting handbook: creating and raising our families. Perennial, New York
- Savage D (1999) The kid: what happened after my boyfriend and I decided to go get pregnant. Dutton, New York

Children's and Teens' Books

- Newman L, Souza D (1994) Heather has two mommies. Alyson Books, New York
- Newman L (2009) Mommy, mama and me. Tricycle Press, Berkeley, CA,
- deHaan L, Nijland S (2004) King and king and family. Tricycle Press, Berkeley, CA
- Parnell P, Richardson J (2005) And tango makes three. Simon and Schuster, New York
- Fakhrid-Deen T (2010) COLAGE: let's get this straight: the ultimate handbook for youth with LGBTQ parents. Seal Press, Berkeley, CA
- Garner A (2004) Families like mine: children of gay parents tell it like it is. Harper Collins, New York

Movies/TV

- Cholodenko L (2010) The kids are all right. Universal Studios
- Wade S, director (2008) Tru Loved. Brownbag productions
- Modern Family, TV Series, ABC Studios
- The Fosters, TV Series, ABC Family

References

Abelsohn KA, Epstein R, Ross LE (2013) Celebrating the "other" parent: mental health and wellness of expecting lesbian, bisexual and queer non-birth parents. J Gay Lesbian Mental Health 17(4): 387–405

Avery AM, Hellman RE, Sudderth LK (2001) Satisfaction with mental health services among sexual minorities with major mental illness. Am J Public Health 91(6):990–991

Barber ME (2009) Lesbian, gay, and bisexual people with severe mental illness. J Gay Lesbian Mental Health 13(2):133–142

Barber ME (2012) LGBT parenting. In: Levounis P, Drescher J, Barber ME (eds) The LGBT casebook. American Psychiatric Publishing, Washington, DC

Biblarz TJ, Stacey J (2010) How does the gender of parents matter? J Marriage Fam 72:3–22

Fitzgerald TJ (2010) Queerspawn and their families: psychotherapy with LGBTQ families. J Gay Lesbian Mental Health 14(2):155–162

Gartrell N, Bos HMW (2010) US national longitudinal lesbian family study: psychological adjustment of 17-year-old adolescents. Pediatrics. doi:10.1542/peds. p 2009-3153

Gates GJ (2011) How many people are lesbian, gay, bisexual, and transgender? The Williams Institute, April 2011, http://williamsinstitute.law.ucla.edu/wp-content/uploads/Gates-How-Many-People-LGBT-Apr-2011.pdf. Retrieved July 31 2013

Gates GJ (2013) LGBT parenting in the United States. The Williams Institute, Feb 2013, http://williamsinstitute.law.ucla.edu/wp-content/uploads/LGBT-Parenting.pdf. Retrieved July 31, 2013

Hellman RE (1996) Issues in the treatment of lesbian women and gay men with chronic mental illness. Psych Serv 47(10):1093–1098

Hellman RE, Drescher J (eds) (2004) Handbook of LGBT issues in community mental health. Haworth Press, New York, NY

Institute of Medicine (2011) The health of lesbian, gay, bisexual, and transgender people: building a foundation for better understanding. The National Academies Press, Washington, DC

Kessler RC, Chiu WT, Demler O, Walters EE (2005) Prevalence, severity and comorbidity of twelve-month DSM-IV disorders in the National Comorbidity Survey Replication (NCS-R). Arch Gen Psychiatry 62(6):617–627

Krivickas KM, Lofquist D (2011) Demographics of same-sex couple households with Children. U.S. census bureau fertility & family statistics branch, SEHSD Working Paper Number 2011-11, http://www.census.gov/population/www/socdemo/Krivickas-Lofquist%20PAA%202011.pdf. Retrieved August 14, 2013

Perrin EC, Cohen KM, Gold M, Ryan C, Savin-Williams RC & Schorzman CM (2004) Gay and lesbian issues in pediatric health care. Current problems in pediatric adolescent health care, November/December, pp 355–398

Stacey J, Biblarz T (2001) (How) does the sexual orientation of the parent matter? Am Soc Rev 65:159–183

Substance Abuse and Mental Health Services Administration (2012) Top health issues for LGBT populations information and resource kit. SAMHSA, Rockville, MD

Tavernise S (2011) Parenting by gays more common in the south, census shows. http://www.nytimes.com/2011/01/19/us/19gays.html. The New York Times, Jan 18, 2011. Retrieved August 15, 2013

The Joint Commission (2011) Advancing effective communication, cultural competence, and patient- and family-centered care for the lesbian, gay, bisexual, and transgender (LGBT) community: a field guide. Oak Brook, IL, LGBTFieldGuide.pdf

Willging CE, Salvador M, Kano M (2006) Unequal treatment: mental health care for sexual and gender minority groups in a rural state. Psychiatr Serv 57(6):867–870

Part II

Voices of Mothers: The Journey

Once Upon A Time I Was Silent

9

Anita Thomas

Anita is a 35-year-old mother of three from California. She carries a diagnosis of bipolar disorder and in this chapter discusses learning to take her own mental health recovery seriously after struggling with her symptoms, her family, and becoming homeless. She now works as a peer specialist supporting others in their recovery journey.

I never found it easy to talk about myself before, but I always liked to talk about where I grew up, because it's such a fantastic place. I grew up in Laguna Niguel. If you're not familiar it's a beautiful city located in Orange County, California, near the beach. My parents moved us there when I was 3 years old. I was born in Los Angeles, California, and I am the oldest of three children. I have two brothers Ben and Wesley.

When I was 21 years old I attempted suicide. I was at my wits end with being teased by my mother and brothers, along with other life stressors. I had also ended a serious relationship, but believe it or not, it was the family stress that was the first and foremost reason I attempted tried to take my life. After that I was diagnosed with bipolar disorder, and I was in and out of treatment (hospitals, therapy, etc.) with local mental health providers. I didn't take recovery seriously. In fact, back then there was no such thing as mental health recovery. At the age of 23 I met my now ex-husband where I worked as an exotic dancer. During that time it was easy to ignore my symptoms because I had no parental responsibilities. I was only responsible for myself. Luis (a tall and extremely handsome Cuban man) and I met in October of 2006. By November that same year we were dating. In December 2006 we got engaged and by April 2007 we were married and expecting our first child.

Our son Marshall was born to us on November 8, 2007 weighing seven pounds. I couldn't believe I gave birth to a child. It was a scary thought for me, because I had given up my life as a topless dancer, I got married, and I knew that I would have to face my symptoms of bipolar disorder. Plus, I wasn't sure I married the right man.

Motherhood, Mental Illness and Recovery, DOI 10.1007/978-3-319-01318-3_9,
© Springer International Publishing Switzerland 2014

He was jealous and aggressive in behavior. I also learned after marrying him that he started to use methamphetamines. He actually had the nerve to get high on meth the day Marshall was born when he had to leave the hospital to get a change of clothes. I was devastated. I asked myself, how am I going to take care of myself and *two* children?

The first few months after Marshall was born we resided at my mother's house in Moreno Valley, California, in transition from moving from Orange County to the Inland Empire. Luis and I figured it would be easier if we stayed with my mom for the end of my pregnancy. A few months after Marshall was born we moved to our own place. Luis was the breadwinner. He worked two jobs while I stayed at home with Marshall and went to school online to obtain my associate's degree. This type of situation may sound ideal for some people, but not for me. I was very depressed. Sometimes I didn't know why. I often wondered if I had this thing people called Postpartum Depression, but I didn't have any information on it. I didn't want to harm my son, but sometimes I just didn't feel like being bothered. I was also having problems with Luis. He was still using meth, and his behavior was aggressive. In March 2008 he was arrested for violating his parole after a domestic dispute we had.

I was left alone with my mental health challenges and our child. That's when I sought services with the Riverside County GAIN (Greater Avenues for Independence) department, a welfare-to-work program. I received welfare and mental health services. I got hooked up with a therapist, who after the first meeting I had no intentions of ever seeing again. She actually had the nerve to tell me to stop blaming others for my past and take personal responsibility. How dare she? Didn't she know what I had been through? For some reason I stuck with her. Looking back, it was one of the best decisions I have ever made for my recovery.

Since I wasn't working I had to leave my apartment and moved back in with my mother. Even though I had started to receive mental health services, I was still very depressed. I tried to hide how bad things were and never told anyone because I was afraid of losing my son. I was so depressed that I would just sit in my room for hours, sometimes days, and wouldn't get up. My brother Wesley and my mom (mainly my brother) would have to take care of my son for me. They would yell at me and tell me I was a piece of sh*t mom. I'd cry. They didn't understand. They never did. All I could think about was back to that first time when I tried to commit suicide and I ended up in the hospital, being pumped with charcoal with a tube up my nose. I often think about when I woke up with my mom over my hospital bed. Her eyes were full of tears and her mascara was smeared all around her eyes, but she still (as always) looked so beautiful. I remember her apologizing to me. I remember her asking me why? I remember telling her, and I remember her telling me (and even after I left the hospital) that they'd never tease me, or talk bad about me again, that they'd support me.

I wasn't a piece of sh*t mom. I love my son. I have mental health challenges and that didn't mean that I couldn't be a good parent. Because I wanted to be a good parent and because I wanted to feel well, I kept going to my appointments even though I hated my psychiatrist at the time. He was very non-recovery. When I was breastfeeding Marshall he told me I should stop and take medication. He would not offer me any medication compatible with breastfeeding. I was passionate about breastfeeding and I wasn't going to stop, so I went off my meds, but still kept going to parenting groups on my own will. I wanted to learn the temperaments of my child to be the best parent possible. I was also going to therapy.

Ten months after his incarceration Luis returned; however, he was arrested a few more times between January 2009 and the year 2010 for everything from being under the influence of drugs, to domestic disputes between the two of us, to him threatening me and my family. Between that time we decided to have another child. Elon was born on August 30, 2010 weighing seven pounds. Luis was not there for the birth of his daughter. He was arrested in June 2010. He was finally released on November 20, 2013. During my pregnancy with our daughter, I was the most depressed and symptomatic I had ever been. I didn't think that was possible knowing how horrible I felt prior to her birth. During my first pregnancy I opted to stay medication free, but for a couple of months while pregnant with Elon I opted to take Zoloft which was recommended to me by my psychiatrist at the time. I ended up relinquishing services with this doctor after he suggested I get an abortion. He said I was "so mentally ill that I need medications that are not safe with pregnancy." He also recommended that I "not breastfeed Marshall because I needed to be on medications that weren't compatible with breastfeeding." In fact he was resistant to prescribe medications that were compatible with breastfeeding. I thank the Lord that I was connected with a local social services program because they were very knowledgeable with this type of information, were pro-breast-feeding, and they supported me tremendously through this time. They understood me and what I was going though. I started to see a glimmer of hope.

Even though I was deep in my challenges during this time, I managed to get Marshall and myself in PCIT (Parent Child Interaction Therapy), which we successfully graduated from. PCIT is designed to improve the parent–child relationship and change parent–child interaction patterns. I would engage Marshall in a play situation with the goal of strengthening our relationship. Because my brother was taking care of him so much and because I was consumed by my symptoms, I felt Marshall didn't respect me as much and he only wanted to be with my brother. It crushed me. This is my first time speaking out about how I felt about that situation. I also felt that my brother and mom helped to foster that type of behavior in my son. While living at moms house one of my aunts and two of her sons came to stay there too. There was a lot of arguing and with everyone getting on everyone's nerves I knew if I was every going to get better I had to remove myself and my kids from that environment. When I took Peer Employment Training (P.E.T.) in 2010 through Jefferson Transitional Programs (now Recovery Innovations) one of the lessons that were facilitated to me was the recovery pathways. One of those pathways is recovery environment.

In January 2011 I became homeless with my two children. We ended up in a shelter. It wasn't what I thought when I think of the word shelter. We had our own little room with a closet, couch, TV, and two beds. Our room was located in the back away from the single men and women. I finally had some piece of mind, but my symptoms of paranoia and anxiety increased due to the fear of having my children taken away. While I was at the shelter I worked on a few things. I was trying to become a volunteer as a Mental Health Peer Specialist and I was trying to relocate into a transitional living shelter. Before I became pregnant with Elon, one of the journeys in my recovery had led me to a peer run center and I went through Peer Employment Training (PET) and graduated gaining a certificate as a certified Peer Support Specialist—a person with the unique perspective of having "lived experience" in mental health. We soon moved into the transitional living shelter and I also started to volunteer as a Mental Health Peer Specialist in April 2011. I started to feel a sense of self-worth. One of my impairments due to my mental health symptoms was not being able to maintain long-term employment. At that point in my life I had never kept a job or volunteer position over 9 months.

I don't want to convey that the start of my parenting was all challenging and dark because it wasn't. I had a lot of happy days and times too. Having my kids helped bring so much joy to my life and I was so proud to have them. Words cannot describe how beautiful they are inside and out. I would always get compliments (still do) when I took Marshall out and then when Elon was born here too. Even though I felt weak on so many days, today I know I was strong and still am. I have been through so much. My position as a Peer Support Specialist is one of my proudest achievements. It felt right. I wanted to make a career of this, so I could support myself and my children. Every day I was getting better. I was taking what I learned from the PET training as well as what I learned from the Wellness Recovery Action Plan (W.R.A.P.) designed by Mary Ellen Copeland. I was utilizing my wellness tools and daily maintenance plan to obtain and maintain a life of wellness from my mental health symptoms. During my volunteer time I applied for an internship as a Peer Support Specialist and was approved. During my internship I met a man named Jack. We entered into a relationship quickly and I became pregnant with my third child.

After my internship, I applied for a permanent position with the county as a Mental Health Peer Specialist. I kept my pregnancy a secret because of fear I wouldn't be hired. After I started, I finally I opened up to one of my coworkers because the anxiety was killing me. She encouraged me to speak to my Mental Health Services Supervisor. I was afraid of so many things including being a new hire on 6 months probation and having to leave already. My supervisor and program manager were both very understanding. They granted me an extended probation when I came back. I didn't have enough time off saved up when I left, so I was only gone 6 weeks. My daughter Danielle was born on July 5, 2012 (just guess) ... yes, weighing seven pounds. Six weeks was the shortest amount of time spent with my newborn. It was depressing, but this time I was stronger in my mind. I was better! I had tools! I had recovery! I knew my strengths and I had supports! Support is one of the five key concepts of recovery.

I am not recovered. I still have a diagnosis and I still experience symptoms. The difference is that now I know how to address them and I have the tools to assist myself to reduce them. I have not been in Emergency Treatment Services or an inpatient hospital since 2002. I have not tried to commit suicide since that same time either and I wouldn't. I cannot stop the thoughts however. I don't know why.

I can tell you though that when they come I feel ashamed. The thoughts are things like, "If only I didn't have to live to endure this pain." Things like that. One of my wellness tools to assist myself when I have negative thoughts is to redirect them with positive ones. It works.

From all I have learned with my recovery journey and especially because I am well now, I am not afraid to say I am a parent with a mental health diagnosis. I encourage any parent to reach out for help if they are challenged by their symptoms. If I could do anything different I would have opened up more about my challenges and what I was going through. There is a saying, "Closed mouths don't get fed." There are so many resources out there now and maybe I could have gotten help and helped myself sooner had I been a little more honest about what I was going through. Mental illness is so common and people like me (now that I am in my position as a Peer Specialist) are trying to assist, guide, and support other people challenged by their mental health symptoms. Not to take away their rights or their children. In recovery we have choices. Choice is one of the recovery pathways. The other recovery pathways are hope, empowerment, environment, and spirituality. The Recovery Innovations definition of Recovery is "Remembering who you are and using your strengths to become all you were meant to be." With help and support I remembered who I was and I was able to use my strengths to be the person I am, the mother I am. My children are now 6, 3, and almost 17 months. I have support from my boyfriend Jack. He is a wonderful father to our daughter Danielle and a father figure to Marshall and Elon.

Just because I am in recovery, doesn't mean I am cured. As far as I can see it I am always going to have a diagnosis and symptoms. That's why I am a strong advocate for asking for help and learning all you can about yourself, your symptoms, and the services in your area that can support and guide you to your wellness, especially as a parent. Now that I have gone through my journey (and still going), I have realized that being a parent with a mental illness does not mean someone has the right to take my children away from me. The only reason someone could have taken my children away from me is if I was a danger to them or neglecting them or causing them harm. Looking back I did neglect them by not asking for help and by being so consumed with my symptoms that I didn't pay enough attention to them, so I am thankful that my brother Wesley was there to pick up the pieces. If I could give any advice to parents is that it would be to get help early! I feel like I wasted so much time that could have been spent with my kids. That's not something I can change, so I feel blessed for my future and what is to come. My children deserve the best. I deserve the best!

Moving Out of Darkness

10

Angela D. Burling

Angela is a 58-year-old mother from northern California. In this chapter she discusses her experience with postpartum psychosis that resulted in the drowning of her infant son at 9 months. She was tried and found not guilty to charges of manslaughter and felony child endangerment, and since then has engaged in outreach efforts to educate others of the dangers of postpartum mental illness. Angela has two adult children, a daughter, 34, and a son, 26.

The Tragedy

"Mother Charged in Death." These words headlined a prominent story in local newspapers on September 2nd, 1983. Was that really me? I certainly didn't fit the profile of the monster described in the article. But it *was* me. In the eyes of Northern California, I was a monster. The District Attorney charged me with murder and felony child abuse. Later articles citing my son's death seemed to highlight the words "child abuse."

My mother had raised me Catholic, and I was a practicing Christian. I worked part-time as a registered nurse at a local hospital until shortly before Michael died. Every available afternoon, I spent swimming at the local pool acclimating Michael to the water. My hope was that he would become the same promising swimmer as his older sister, Allyson. I loved my life. I loved being a mom more than anything and I adored my children.

When Michael was 9 months old, after he had mastered the art of eating solid foods and could hold a bottle by himself, I stopped nursing him. My breasts had become so engorged that I bound them with ace bandages. Two of my friends told me that they had done the same thing, so I did not anticipate the peril in which I had placed myself. The hormonal upheaval created by abruptly stopping nursing made

Motherhood, Mental Illness and Recovery, DOI 10.1007/978-3-319-01318-3_10,
© Springer International Publishing Switzerland 2014

me go insane. Within a few days, I began having strange thoughts. The radio was sending me messages. I believed my 9-month-old son was the devil. My husband Jeff was Jesus.

The chemical imbalance I was experiencing completely affected my perception of reality. Then the unimaginable happened. I drowned my beloved Michael in the bathtub. I reasoned that Jeff, through his "divine power," would raise Michael from the dead 3 days later, confirming to the world that Jeff, indeed, was Jesus. I was firmly in the grip of an illness, the very nature of which prevented me from recognizing its existence. I had no idea that my mind was being twisted by postpartum psychosis.

I was an unsuspecting victim of a horrible tragedy and a travesty of misguided medical care. Losing a baby is not all that uncommon. Sadly, every year 25,000 infants die within the first year of life in the United States. Having lost an infant, I know what an emotionally gut-wrenching experience it is under any circumstance. It is something one hopes would never happen. However, losing an infant at her own hands is unthinkable for any loving mother. I could never have thought myself capable of taking the life of anyone, especially my own infant.

During my initial prenatal visit to a local and respected OB/GYN, my nurse midwife had reassured me that all would be okay with my second pregnancy. I had told her of my earlier hospitalization in a psychiatric unit and that I had done some really crazy things following the birth of my daughter 2 years before. Her advice, or lack of advice, set my family, myself, and especially Michael up for a tragic loss.

Although my midwife's reassurance was welcomed at the time, it reflected a system-wide failure of the medical profession. In 1983, the medical establishment did not recognize the severity of perinatal mood and anxiety disorders.

A Normal Childhood

Growing up in a typical home in Salinas, California, I considered myself as normal as anyone else. My parents were loving and active in the community. My father worked as a pharmaceutical salesman for the same company until he retired. He was involved with the Optimist and Sierra Clubs and was a bell ringer for the Salvation Army at Christmas time. My mother worked part-time as a registered nurse and retired from the Visiting Nurses' Association, after a long and satisfying career. Even though both my mother and father were busy, I felt loved and nurtured by them. Our close relationship continued as I became an adult.

My three sisters, my brother, and I got along well. My mother prepared nutritious and delicious dinners every evening that we enjoyed while gathered around the table watching Walter Cronkite on the evening news. There wasn't a lot of shouting, aside from my father's occasional outbursts. After work, Dad enjoyed his daily rum and Coke.

For recreation, our family liked to camp and backpack. Big Sur and Los Padres State Parks were nearby, and we hiked there often. We learned to appreciate nature and hot chocolate on crisp mornings. We logged many miles hiking in the spectacular Yosemite National Park. Dad was an avid photographer and took some amazing shots of the highlights of our trips. One of my fondest memories was the view from the top of Half Dome in Yosemite. On those weekends not spent on organized trips, we all piled into my father's car and went picnicking. As I reflect back on my home life, I think it was a good one.

Academically, I did well in school and had no behavior problems. As children, my sisters and I were involved in ballet and we swam for the YMCA. I continued swimming in high school. Besides swimming, I was active in the Spanish Club in high school and was elected senior class president and graduated with honors.

I had not been exposed to the mentally ill until a brief clinical rotation on a psychiatric unit during nursing school. At that point in my life, in my early twenties, I was judgmental towards the psychiatric patients assigned to me. I hate to admit it now, but I was not very empathetic. I remember thinking to myself at the time, "I am glad I don't have to worry about a mental illness happening to me." I felt I was insulated from mental illness because nothing traumatic had ever happened to me. I was hard working, had goals, and came from a loving family. Yet despite the absolute "normality" of my childhood and early adulthood, I later became the "poster child" of abnormality and postpartum psychosis.

The Aftermath

When my husband, Jeff, arrived home on that horrible day and found Michael's lifeless body, he called 911. He pleaded with the officers who arrived at our home to hospitalize me instead of taking me to jail. He told the evaluating police officers that I had been hospitalized after the birth of my first child, and he believed that Michael's death had psychiatric causes. Graciously, the police gave me the benefit of the doubt and took me to the hospital, which was where I belonged.

When I "came to" and realized that Michael had actually died, I became hysterical and the doctors heavily medicated me. Nevertheless, I had to make court appearances. Even with the medication, I was at times inconsolable. Jeff scrambled to put my legal defense together. He retained an aggressive defense attorney who was very sympathetic. In fact, when Jeff relayed to the lawyer that I admitted to drowning Michael, both men cried in the office. Our lawyer told Jeff, "Angela could have been *my* wife."

The chief defense witness in my case was the director of the county Mental Health Department. He was of the opinion that I was clearly psychotic at the time of Michael's death. Jeff also hired a prominent forensic psychiatrist in the Sacramento region who validated those findings. The D.A., on the other hand, was unsympathetic and prosecuted me with full force. Remarkably, we were able to post bail of $50,000 after the judge reduced it from $250,000. I was allowed to return home under the 24 hour supervision of my retired parents who were responsible for making sure I took my prescribed medications and was supervised when I was with Allyson. She was 4 at the time and her precious smile and joyful presence helped me heal. When she asked me if I had drowned Michael, I told her I had, trying as best as I could to help her understand how sick I had been at the time. She never seemed afraid of me.

My lawyer believed we would have a better outcome with a trial presided over by a judge as opposed to a jury trial. His instincts proved to be right. On July 31, 1984, I was declared not guilty by reason of insanity to charges of manslaughter and felony child endangerment. Although the judgment validated my illness before the law, I still had to cope with being seen as a mentally disordered offender outside the courtroom. I was placed in a local halfway house for 90 days and then released to the outpatient Conditional Release Program. This allowed me to live on my own with frequent monitoring and meetings with the county mental health professionals as well as medical management by a private psychiatrist. I remained under the conditional release program until I was discharged some 20 years later.

From the Ashes: Healing and Working Towards Understanding and Knowledge

When I was in the hospital after losing Michael, I asked God "Why?" I did not get an answer. However, what gave me solace was repeating over and over to myself a verse from the *Bible*, Romans verse 8:28: "God works together for good to those who love Him and are called according to His purposes."

During the month that I was in the hospital, a tall attractive female patient approached me and asked me if I was Angela Thompson. I hesitantly replied, "Yes." She said, "Thank you for saving my life. Following the birth of my child, I had locked myself in my room and was depressed to the point of considering suicide. My friends read about your story in the newspaper and believed I was suffering from postpartum depression. They encouraged me to be evaluated and here I am, thanks to you!"

I came to realize that my plight was not as unique as I thought and that I needed to do something to prevent similar tragedies in the future. Jeff was a lobbyist for the California Correctional Peace Officers Association and was well acquainted with State Senator Robert Presley, who became interested in my case. Senator Presley created a task force to evaluate what could be done to improve medical as well as the peace officer training to include more rigorous education on postpartum psychosis. The task force worked hard and ultimately had Senate Concurrent Resolutions 23 and 39 adopted in the spring of 1989.

Senate Concurrent Resolution 23 set forth various declarations regarding postpartum psychosis. It requested that the Board of Corrections adopt regulations to include a protocol to be used when assessing the mental status of women who have recently given birth and who are charged with serious crimes, especially infanticide. It recommended that a woman be referred to a mental health facility when an assessment indicated a need. In addition, Senate Concurrent Resolution 23 requested that the University of California conduct research to define the illness more fully and to facilitate an understanding of the phenomena: its causes, effects, and treatments.

Senate Concurrent Resolution 39 called for the improvement of the protocols for peace officer training and education so that officers can conduct a mental health assessment of women and availability of community resources, other than jail, for women accused of a crime and who are exhibiting symptoms of postpartum psychosis.

When I look back, I realize just how fortunate I have been. Had Jeff not believed in me, I don't know if I would have recovered. The judge who tried me was compassionate and the community where I lived had a halfway house where I could serve my time. Jeff and Allyson visited me every evening and on weekends, which gave my life hope and meaning.

My testimony proved helpful in the 1987 case of an Orange County, California, woman who, suffering from postpartum psychosis, killed her 6-week-old infant. A jury found the young woman guilty of second-degree murder. Dr. James Hamilton, psychiatrist and pioneer in the field, and I were called to give testimony following the verdict. At the sentencing hearing, the judge, known as a law and order judge, reversed the jury's decision and reduced the charge to manslaughter. This was a bold and gutsy decision. The defendant's attorney and another expert witness credited my testimony as being "particularly persuasive." (Criminal Practice Manual 1989)

During the late 1980s and early 1990s, I was interviewed on over a dozen talk shows in the United States and one in Canada, including *Oprah* and *Larry King Live*. Winfrey and King were skeptical of my defense, but I felt well received by most of the other hosts. The *Los Angeles Times* featured us in "*The View*" in 1987, and we were the subjects of an article in the behavior section of the June 20, 1988, edition of *Time* magazine. Patty Duke even narrated a documentary on my story. My motive for going so public was to educate others about my illness, which had so blind-sided me. I was hoping to prevent others from experiencing the same horror I did.

Prior to our involvement with the Task Force, Jeff and I were faced with the ultimate test of our faith. I became unexpectedly pregnant. It was the fall of 1986 and I had just been accepted into a Masters of Nursing program. I hoped to learn more about postpartum psychosis, the illness that robbed me of my motherhood to Michael and Michael of his life. By this time, I was knowledgeable of the hormonal changes that had made me go insane. I had read British physician Katharina Dalton's book, *Depression after Childbirth,* in which she described a patient's psychosis of a twisted reality that I also suffered. While reading the chapter on postpartum psychosis, I felt as if I was reading thoughts scripted from my own thinking during the acute phase of my illness. It was as if she threw me a life jacket: I no longer felt alone and singled out.

Later on in 1990, I had the privilege of meeting Dr. Dalton in York, England, at the prestigious Marcé Society meeting, which I attended with Jane Honikman who founded Postpartum Support, International. I was happy that I could thank her in person for her work that had played such a significant role in managing my third pregnancy.

When I first learned of my pregnancy, I contacted Dr. Hamilton who developed a postpartum treatment plan and advised my psychiatrist and obstetrician about how to best prevent a recurrence of my illness. He prescribed an estrogen injection immediately after delivery and insisted that not breast-feeding was "a small price to pay to prevent another psychosis." In addition, I was also taking psychotropic medications. Yolo County also required around the clock supervision of my infant and me for 8 weeks. There was social pressure put on me to abort. Not only would that have gone against my values, but also I was confident that the treatment plan in place would avert the disaster that I faced following Michael's birth.

Tommy's arrival gave me a new lease on life. The unhappiness that had plagued me since Michael's death seemed to vanish when I held my newborn infant on May 14, 1987.

I continued my studies and earned my Master's degree in 1991, writing my thesis on the *"Screening Practices of Health Care Practitioners for Postpartum Mental Illness."* My findings were that healthcare practitioners did not adequately discuss postpartum mental illness prenatally or postpartum with their clients. I found that more than half of medical professionals I surveyed lacked sufficient knowledge of the syndrome. I also discovered how behind the American medical and legal systems were by comparison to those in the United Kingdom.

The British medical model includes inpatient Mother Baby Units for women needing hospitalization and regularly scheduled visits by a health visitor (specially trained British in-home visiting nurse) for every postpartum woman.

Under British law, according to the 1938 Infanticide Act, a mother who has given birth within the previous 12 months cannot be sentenced for murder in the death of her infant. However, she can be tried for the lesser offense of manslaughter. This law presumes that the woman was incapable of rational judgment at the time of the offence, due to the fact that the "balance of her mind was disturbed by reason of her not having fully recovered from the effects of giving birth to the child or by reason of the effect of lactation consequent upon the birth of the child." (British Law Reports 1938) This British law was the basis of the Senate Concurrent Resolutions referred to earlier.

Unfortunately, the death of Michael and my unexpected pregnancy strained my marriage to Jeff to the point of separation and finally divorce in 1992. This was an especially dark time for me.

During my separation from Jeff, I began swimming in an adult masters program. By the goodness of God, I met a wonderful man, Jim Burling, who became my best friend. We married in March of 1995 and recently celebrated our 19th anniversary.

My postpartum psychosis triggered a lifelong battle with mental illness, which has required several hospitalizations. I must take medication daily and see a psychiatrist regularly. Jim has remained steady and committed. He is a remarkable husband and parent to my children.

Shortly after I remarried, I received a call from a woman who said she wanted to meet me. She had been involved with the prison outreach for Postpartum Support, International. While sitting in my family room, she recalled an incident after giving birth to her first child. She told me that one morning while standing over the crib of her infant, she had the impulse to drown him. She remembered seeing me tell my story on the *Phil Donahue Show* and ran into her husband's home office, begging him to take her to the nearest psychiatric hospital. She feared for her son's life. She told me she wanted to meet me in person and to thank me for going public with my story.

During the Andrea Yates trial, I was petrified that my new friends in our neighborhood, Jim's colleagues or Tommy's friends would find out about my past. Tommy was in high school, and, since marrying Jim, I had taken a low profile regarding my past. When a local television station called me and asked for an interview, I declined. The producer insisted, "But you are the poster child of postpartum psychosis." I firmly told him this was not something I had aspired to be in life.

However, in January 2008, a local newspaper reported a story about a mother who drowned her baby in the sink when the baby was 8 days old. She was 27, the same age I was when I lost Michael, and she lived only 5 miles from my home. Since Tommy was grown and out of the house, I believed I could help and got involved again. I met her family at a local postpartum conference that was precipitated by her case. While she was a patient in the hospital, I visited her on several occasions.

Currently, I am on the Maternal Depression Task Force of Placer County. I served in the planning committee of the California maternal wellness summit which was held May 2014. I work part-time as a community health educator and enjoy my Spanish study groups.

My greatest joys continue to be Jim and my children. Allyson and Tommy are well into adulthood and are accomplished in their own right. As Jim reminds me, "Your children love you, are best of friends, and love their dad and me. No mother could want more."

The overriding redemptive side to this tragedy is that I have been able to offer both hope and help to others in order to prevent similar tragedies. My story illuminates the strength of the human spirit to move beyond the darkness. It is my ardent desire that my story may continue to serve as a beacon of hope. As the Dalai Lama states: Tragedy should be utilized as a source of strength. No matter what sort of difficulties, how painful the experience is, if we lose our hope, that's our real disaster."

References

BRN Criminal Practice Manual (1989) Trial practice series, Current reports, vol 3, No. 1 January 11, 1989
British Law Reports Statutes (1938) p 329

As My Heart Beats

11

Suzanne DuBois

Suzanne is a 49-year-old mother of two from Massachusetts. She is diagnosed with schizophrenia and bipolar disorder, and in this chapter she discusses the impact of her mental illness, being separated from her daughters, and what she's learned in over 22 years of mental health treatment. She credits her community support counselor, Nicole Caplin, for her support and assistance in putting this story together.

My name is Suzanne; I was born in the year 1964. I live in Norwood, Massachusetts, where I was born and raised. My parents had four daughters and I am the youngest. All through my childhood I enjoyed playing with my baby dolls. But when I started kindergarten things really changed for me. I became more sensitive to how I relate to others. To me, other kids seemed different in their sense of awareness and their self-esteem. They seemed great, and my feelings were at a low. I was hurting at that time in my life. I knew something was not right, and from then on my journey in life was difficult. When I was alone I would ask the Lord questions and pray. I had such a wonderful spiritual experience with my higher power. I felt my family did not spend any time with me as a child, doing things like teaching me, so I would have temper tantrums. Something was wrong with me; I had no interest to learn or remember ordinary things like poems, names of writers, etc. But now I realize what life is about: to have some interests and knowledge. For instance, my favorite song, "My Heart Belongs to Me," by Barbara Streisand, symbolizes some of the struggles I had when I was growing up.

My mental illness diagnoses are paranoid schizophrenia and bipolar disorder. I feel blessed to finally be diagnosed after I had so much trouble growing up. Sometimes I would ask myself why I had to deal with life's problems, and then I was told it's not my fault. For a long time I blamed myself, and I looked at life with a lot of sadness. I feel that my mental illness caused other people to judge me and they didn't think I had the capability to be a mother. I felt like people wanted to see me fail. I never had any help from anyone, no matter how much I reached out. This made me feel very alone, vulnerable, and unsupported. Most of my life I would feel like I was being held against my will because of my mental illness, and sometimes this made me feel like I was being discriminated against. I learned that things weren't in my control, so I was being told what to do for so long. Not only with my mental health but I was being pushed around and I felt like a door mat. I felt trapped and that no one cared about me. I had a lot of unanswered questions about my mental illness, and absolutely no one paid attention to me.

One day I gave up, and I tried to end my life. I was so very close but then my dog licked my face, and then I woke up and rushed myself to the hospital. I had my stomach pumped, and they said I had an acute overdose. From that day on, I wanted to live and to get the help I needed to be healthier. I stood my ground and said I've had enough. I learned there is a greater world out there. I took full control of my life and gained it back in a very positive way. I realize others may or may not have gotten the correct help or the right medications to share their story with us now, so that's why I am blessed to share my story today. Now I hope people recognize me for who I am and not by my mental illness.

When I was in my early 20s I met a gentleman from Pittsburgh, Pennsylvania. At the age of 23, I became a mother of a baby girl. Then 14 months later I gave birth to a second baby girl. Today I am a grandmother of five; four grandsons, and one granddaughter. I am also an aunt to four nephews and five nieces and a great-aunt. As I saw my family grow I realized how precious life really is, and it was very enjoyable to watch my daughters grow into motherhood. Now I see my grandchildren and love them all so much.

Being a mother, I had a greater responsibility than when I was a teenager. As a mother, life's challenges were upon me and there was a time when I could not provide a home for my daughters and myself. I went to a shelter and the state took my two daughters away from me and told me to seek psychiatric help. I know they said I needed psychiatric help because I was unstable, but I never understood why that made them take my daughters away from me. It still remains unknown to me. It was like anything I did in life was against me. I did not have the answers. Then after going to court, I got full custody of my children. And then again, soon after that, I separated from their father and completely lost guardianship of my daughters again. I lost everything and was out in the street with nowhere to live, until I went to get help through a local mental health clinic. Since then I have been prescribed to the right medications and I learned about my depression and my schizophrenia, and how it affects me.

I have a better understanding about my mental illness after being in treatment for over 22 years. Throughout my treatment, I was very worried about my daughters but I knew I needed to help myself. Others agree that I am now in my recovery. Through treatment, I have learned the valuable qualities of life are to set limits and to stay on my medications. The hardest step was when I finally admitted I have a mental illness and need to take my medication as prescribed.

My treatment setting was mainly a day treatment program. The day treatment program helped me a lot as an individual, but as a parent it did not serve me well.

When I was admitted into day treatment, it led the state system to work against me as a parent. The system failed me as well as my daughters. I say this because when I was in a shelter, the state took away my rights as a parent, and then I was not allowed to see my kids. I had no idea why the state separated me from my daughters, and I feel I did not get any answers. From that point on it was a vicious cycle for the rest of my life.

Despite my mental illness, I did the best I could with my daughters and now they both have children of their own. My oldest daughter works with autistic people, and my youngest daughter works at a daycare. Talking to both of my daughters about my mental illness is challenging because they do not understand; they just know I cannot handle too much stress. My relationship with my daughters is limited because we cannot share each other's life stories and experiences. I felt incapable of teaching them about me, and my kids were in denial about my mental illness. They always tell me I'll be ok. It scares my youngest daughter that I am on medication because she is used to seeing pharmaceuticals in the streets where she lives. As my daughters grew up and went to school, my oldest daughter studied mental illness and today she has somewhat of an understanding about my mental health history. She understands that I need to take medications. As for my youngest daughter, she has a different understanding. She says I do not need medications to help me and thinks I am dangerous. She does not understand that when I take my medication I am better and that I am now on the road to recovery. I gave up and prayed that my daughters would be safe and have a little bit of an understanding as to the world of mental health. Deep down inside they do know but it hurts them, as it hurts me, to say I have an illness. My youngest daughter has seen people on drugs and is totally afraid because of that. I think that is why she is in denial about me being on medications. But she wants the best for me as I do with all my grandchildren, as well as my daughters. My two daughters taught me to get better as they learned from me about how much I cared about them and loved them.

I would appreciate if people would not to judge me because of my mental illness, but instead give me respect as I would like to love and respect them. Mental illness was pointed out to me by others. If you notice mental illness in someone and the person does not see it, please help them as soon as possible and get them into treatment. My sister had problems like that when she was 51 years old. If my sister was not in denial about her life problems, she might have got the help she needed and lived a better life. My sister was angry at my family because she had a rough childhood. My sister did not have a mental health diagnosis to my knowledge, but I do think she had some mental health problems. Because of this, my sister also had issues with parenting as a mother herself. I think it was because of her trauma history as a child. My sister gave up hope and was separated from her children just like me.

I know a lot of men as well as women who chose not to become parents because of their mental illness. If I could tell anything to parents with a mental illness, it would be this: Being a mother changed my world. It helped me as a person to face responsibility and to give and have love. In today's society, mental health treatment has a greater role, which is different from earlier times, like the 1930s when it was not spoken of. I would like to say to mothers who face similar challenges that it is one's decision to become a parent. Personally, I wanted to become a mother no matter what, and I was blessed to be able to give birth. It's all how you feel about it. You could be a mother without mental illness but may face similar challenges, due to let's say, alcohol or drug addictions, or even diabetes. Everyone has their problems, and no one is perfect. But you can make the choice not to be a victim and to live in a positive way. I know no matter what, I did a great job as a parent with mental illness. I am proud of the achievements that I have made as a mother and as a person who is recovering from mental illness.

Don't Give Up

12

Taressa Ingle

Taressa is a 33-year-old mother from Ohio. In this chapter she discusses her struggles with suicide and multiple hospitalizations following the birth of her son. After once being so overwhelmed with symptoms she was unable to parent her son, she now treasures her motherhood role, and proudly shares her recovery journey with others.

My name is Taressa. I grew up in a middle class family in Withamsville, Ohio. I lived with my father, mother, and two younger brothers. My dad worked full time and my mother stayed home with my brothers and I while we were younger. When we got older mom worked part time but was always home before we got off the bus. Both of my younger brothers joined the United States Air Force and became Staff Sergeants. My youngest brother, Danny, had two overseas deployments. He passed away in May 2013 from suicide.

I did very well in school and graduated high school in 1998 before going off to college to study business. After attending school for a year, I decided I wanted to work part time and go to college at night. I started working at a bank as a full time teller and went to night school still studying business. At this time I met my future husband, Curry. We decided to get married in February 2001 and I quit school and advanced at the bank to an Assistant Manager. I loved my job and husband. We bought a house in Ohio and decided to start a family. We wanted lots of children.

I got pregnant at 21 years old and had many complications. I had severe hyperemesis, a condition where I dehydrated because of vomiting, and had to have IV fluids at home. At 3 months into my pregnancy I had to have my appendix removed. At 7 months I started having contractions and went on bed rest for preterm labor. I had my son, my only child, in January of 2002. I always wanted lots of children but had to have a hysterectomy after my son. It was hard facing the fact that I would only have one child.

Motherhood, Mental Illness and Recovery, DOI 10.1007/978-3-319-01318-3_12,
© Springer International Publishing Switzerland 2014

When my son was 6 months old I got diagnosed with bipolar disorder. I thought I was struggling with Postpartum Blues that never went away. Never being depressed before or having suicidal thoughts, this was very scary. I remember one August day in 2002 like it was yesterday. I went to work at my job at the bank, and left my husband home that day with our son. I woke up feeling a little down and depressed and I felt guilty leaving my husband and son at home while I worked. I didn't want to go to work and as the day went by I felt like crap. I started having feelings like I would be better off dead and my family would be better off without me. I had been crying more those couple of weeks before, but nothing was unusual until that August day. I called my husband from work and told him I wanted to kill myself.

I wanted to die. I came home from work that day early and my husband talked me into going to the nearest emergency room. I was admitted that night to the behavioral health unit, for observation. A doctor came in the next day and asked if I was still suicidal I told him NO. I wanted to go home; the patients there weren't like me. I had never been to a psych ward before and I was frightened. I was discharged after spending one night and was told I needed to see a therapist. There was a three-week wait. The time didn't go by quick enough for me and I had my first suicide attempt.

After that, I didn't parent. I couldn't quit crying or having suicide thoughts or attempts. I wasn't a parent to my son. My husband and his family took care of my son. I missed out on his first 3 years of life. I missed his first steps, when he quit drinking from a bottle, his first words, when he slept thru the night for the first time. I missed his first and second Christmas. I barely changed his diaper or fed him. I was a horrible parent. I let everyone step in and take care of his needs. I just sat back or slept while he was being taken care of by others. It has caused a lot of guilt in my life. I feel very bad that I didn't take care of him or remember all those special moments of his life. Thank goodness he was young and doesn't remember me taking the back seat and dad and grandma taking care of him. Something that has helped is being very open and honest with my son about my past and mental health diseases. It also has taught me to teach my son not to discriminate against anyone, whether because of race, physical, or mental issues.

When Jarrett was about a year and half, I had my first homicidal thought. My husband was at work and his mom was due to our house within an hour. At that point, I was able to be left alone with my son for an hour or two at a time. I called my husband and told him what I was thinking and that I needed help. I put my crying son in his crib and sat on the porch until my husband's aunt got there about 5 min later. I went to the hospital that day and was admitted. I told the charge nurse what was going on and they contacted Children's Services. When I was discharged we met with them at their local office. I had to speak to a case manager in one room while my husband was being interviewed in another room. They were going to make a follow-up house visit the next week. My husband and I were very open with them about my mental illness and my past. After that my husband and I decided that it was best I wouldn't be alone with my son at all, we stayed with my in-laws while my husband worked. Someone was always with my son and me for about

10 months. That was the only time I was scared I would lose my child, and thankfully never had another homicidal thought again.

I have had three suicide attempts, one of them leaving me in critical condition. I have been hospitalized over ten times. The last time I was hospitalized was April of 2005. I see my psychiatrist every 6 months. I take medication for my bipolar disorder. I now only see a grief therapist. I am at the stage of recovery of giving back. I do a lot of volunteering in the mental health field. I want to help give back to those who have helped me and also show others there is hope and light at the end of the tunnel. I volunteer with Crisis Intervention Trainings, informing police officers about life for an individual living with a mental illness. My husband is a police officer also. I share my story in trainings, and I volunteer with the National Alliance for the Mentally Ill as a peer instructor and teaching a peer-to-peer class. I also now volunteer with American Foundation of Suicide Prevention by sharing both my brother's and my struggles with suicide. In the near future I will be working on a documentary about suicide. I am involved in a program called Celebrate Recovery at my church. Soon I will be a certified peer specialist in my county. Sharing my story helps others but mostly it helps me in my recovery. I still have my down days but nothing like before.

Treatment has taught me not to be ashamed or hide my illness from others. Treatment has not really helped me as a parent though. During therapy we never really discussed my parenting. My psychiatrist and I always discussed my family life or home life though. He always knew I tried to put my son first and consider his best interests when I was able. Today I remain very open. I state I have an illness just like someone living with diabetes; you have to take your medicine, see your doctor, and stay healthy to do well.

Today, my son is almost 12 years old and we are still all together as a family. My husband, son, and I get a long pretty well. We all are happy and want to be together. I have been there for my son since he was 3, I have helped him learn his numbers, ABC's, and manners, and helped him with potty training, writing his name, reading, and learning to be himself. I have watched him grow into a mature pre-teenager. Challenges that have stood out are my guilt about the first 3 years of his life. I wasn't involved. I have issues with stress. Being a parent is stressful, but I have to take a minute some times and sit back, take a deep breath, and say this is just life. I also struggle with perfection. I want everything to be perfect. That's not going to happen. My son is going to be messy, his room won't always be clean, he might not get straight A's on all his report cards, he will get mad at me and not like me from time to time, and I have to realize that's normal. Nothing is ever perfect.

I love being a parent. I try to be the best parent I can be and we have a very close relationship. I have had many open conversations with my son about mental illness. He used to remind me take my medicine at 9 pm every night. He knew what medicine I took. He knows what to look for when I am having a down day, when to call dad, or someone for help. It's hard to be so vulnerable to your child but on the other hand it is nice to know that he doesn't judge me or think I am nuts or crazy. He understands I have a brain disease and need to take medicine and see the doctor. He has gone to my appointments with me in the past. He is one of my support team members. I worry it's a lot on him and has made him grow up too quickly but I am very glad we are an open, honest, and responsible family.

One thing I would like to tell other mothers is, don't give up. There is hope and light at the end of the tunnel. Fight hard to do well in your recovery for your children. They deserve you as much as you deserve them. Children are wonderful. I couldn't imagine my life without my son. I wake up every day for him. I keep working my recovery for him also. Get help right away when you see the first sign of trouble and don't ever give up.

Pregnant on the Psychiatric Unit: One Woman's Journey Through the State Mental Health System and into Motherhood

13

Amanda Standridge and Ellen Darling

Amanda is a 26-year-old mother from northern California diagnosed with bipolar disorder. In this chapter she discusses learning she was pregnant while in jail, going into labor while at a state psychiatric hospital, and early bonding with her son while in and out of different institutions. She also talks about the importance of hope and faith in her mental health recovery. The chapter was written by Ellen Darling following an interview with Amanda.

Mental illness is a really horrific experience. It's like the most intense storm that slams you down, hard. You feel like you're drowning and you have to fight and have a lot of faith to swim back out. Faith is what got me through. Faith and some really good people who were there for me. There's a line from the Bible, Psalm 23 from the Scriptures, that I would think of again and again when things were really bad, and that I still remind myself of now. "He leadeth you to still waters." I grew up in a small town in northern California and my parents divorced when I was 8. I went to live with my brother and saw my dad, who's a handyman, regularly. He raised me really well. He taught me good morals and values, and I grew up with this faith. When I turned 16 though, I had a nervous breakdown. It was my first bout of illness. I dropped out junior year of high school and stopped eating. I dropped down to 89 lb and was having severe panic attacks. They were so bad I didn't leave the house and was lying in bed all the time. I remember around Christmas that year, my sister asked if I was going to go to the annual Christmas parade. I wanted to, but I was too terrified to leave the house so she went with my dad.

I was all alone in the house and I remember thinking that I was doomed. I was so sick. I was so in my head. I wasn't making sense of anything. There's a big tree in our backyard, and I took all my bed sheets and made a noose. I jumped from the tree and hung there. I must have blacked out, because I remember walking down a tunnel, doors were opening and closing. And then I fell to the ground. I cried and

Motherhood, Mental Illness and Recovery, DOI 10.1007/978-3-319-01318-3_13,
© Springer International Publishing Switzerland 2014

cried and cried. When my dad and sister came home, I went and told on myself. That was my worst suicide attempt.

I was in the hospital after that, my first time, for 2 weeks. I saw a children's psychiatrist, and he put me on meds. They gave me lots of diagnoses there. I can't even remember them all—posttraumatic stress disorder, generalized anxiety disorder, schizoaffective disorder. I was good for 2 years after I got out. My dad got me into all kinds of home schools, and I worked hard to try and catch up. I was doing pretty well. I had a job working at the local movie theater, but I was also being a wild child. I had started doing drugs—I was doing Ecstasy, and I ran amuck. Ecstasy is a sex drug, and I was sleeping around. I'd met this guy who was selling drugs and we used to sneak into pools in apartment buildings and go swimming. We'd break into places and steal stuff. We all did it. Everyone I used to run with. We were into stupid shit. They all went to jail, but I went an even worse route.

I was 18 when it all came to a head. My mom's boyfriend had molested me, and I decided to tell her what happened. Only I was high when I told her. Anyway, she called me a liar. I got really mad and broke some windows. She started hitting me and I ran into the kitchen and grabbed a knife. I told her I was going to stab her, and then she called the cops.

I found out I was pregnant in jail. They ran a pregnancy test along with all the other testing they do, I guess. A lot of it was blurry. After I got out of jail, I was homeless. My dad's new wife didn't want to deal with me. My mom kicked me out of the house, and I didn't want to be there anyway, so I slept outside. I slept in cars or on school playgrounds. I didn't have any money so I stole pregnancy tests from stores to see if I really was pregnant. I was.

Eventually, I went through the mental health court system and had a good public defender. Basically, the state became my mom and dad and they put me in lockdown for three and a half years under the state's care. I bounced around to about four different hospitals and have PTSD from the abuse that went on in some of them. They held you down hard and things like that. They were definitely not good to me. Some of the staff were good to me though, but I always got transferred to other places. It was really scary. I got really sick. I was at Crestwood Redding Hospital when I finally got on the right meds. I prayed a lot during this time, slept with a Bible under my pillow, and started getting better and better. I went from lockdown to boarding care homes that are like residential homes in a hospital-like setting, to finally half way homes. I pretty much worked with the system and got out of it and then moved back to Auburn, where I am now. It was such a hard and treacherous journey.

My son Dustin is 7 now. I was 19 when he was born and they took me in an ambulance from the psych hospital to the regular hospital when I started going into labor. They gave me a day pass to give birth. At first no one was going to take him and he was going to go into state care too, but then my mom and dad fought for him and they ended up getting custody. After he was born, I spent one day with him in the hospital before I went back to Rosewood, where I'd been.

My mom brought him to see me when I was in different institutions, but my bonding time with him really got better once I got out of the hospital. Dustin has been the miracle of my life and he's what kept me going for the three and a half years I was institutionalized. I was just pushing through for him—to be with him someday. I really believe God put Dustin in my life for this reason. To keep me going. I live for him.

We have a really great relationship now. We just went to this Halloween festival together, and I bought him these cool skeletons that had these lights on them that he loved. We play videogames and goof around. I help him with his homework, all that kind of stuff, too. We're two peas in a pod when we're together. He's really smart and fun to be around. He loves me too and tells me that he misses me. He's my best friend—he's a total little me. Everybody tells me that I'm a really great mom.

I've tried to keep the dysfunction of our family away from my son. I don't talk too much about my mental health history because he's young, but my mom has told him that I was sick and he remembers visiting me in different places. He knows that I'm taking medicine. He asks about it and says, "Mommy, what are you taking?" I explain, "They're like my vitamins. They help me feel better." Even if I'm really sad, I try not to let him know it because I don't want to worry him. I miss him a lot and wish that I could see him every day. My mom still has guardianship of him and I'm only allowed supervised visits. She's still with the guy that molested me so it's pretty hard to be at her house. That's why I'm trying so hard right now to get into a stable environment.

I'm doing really well now. I'm 26 and live in an apartment with a roommate. I've had a boyfriend for over 2 years and I think we're going to get married eventually. He really loves Dustin, too, and is great with him. I work two jobs during the day and go to school at night. I'm going for an associate's degree in business entrepreneurship and during the day I work at Victoria's Secret at the mall and I also work part time at Turning Point, a mental health counseling center where I did lots of groups and classes.

Turning Point taught me how my behavior is part of my illness and that helped calmed me down a lot. I run a peer-mentoring group there now that's about community building to support each other and fight the stigma and discrimination of mental illness. We do a lot of fun things too. I have a karaoke group, a movie group, and a writing group. I also run a Facebook page for our groups and put lots of inspirational quotes and stuff on there. I've really love this job, and it also reminds me of how important it is to keep taking care of myself. I see a therapist weekly and I still see a psychiatrist on a monthly basis. I take all the meds religiously. Lithium is a new one and it's been really good for me. My current diagnosis is bipolar disorder.

I guess the main thing that I'd tell others is to never give up. For me, it was my faith in the Lord, but however you get your faith, that's what you need. You have to be strong in your faith. I just put this verse up on our group's Facebook page:

I say to you, if you have faith like a grain of mustard seed, you will say to this mountain, 'Move from here to there,' and it will move, and nothing will be impossible for you." (Matthew 17:20)

Even if you only have the tiniest bit of hope, a mustard seed, hold onto it. It will grow. And nothing will be impossible for you.

There and Back Again

14

Maura K.

Maura is a 51-year-old mother of three living in Georgia. She is an LPC and CPS/WHAM certified. In this chapter she discusses how her periods of depression and mania impacted her parenting, as well as coping skills she found most helpful in her personal recovery journey.

My name is Maura. I was born in Iowa and relocated to Florida when I was 6. There were five children in my family; I have three brothers and a sister. We are a total of 14 years of age apart from oldest to youngest. I am the youngest. Our family was marked by the effects of alcoholism, and there was perhaps some mental illness in past generations. There was also abuse by those outside of our immediate family.

I married Mike on July 13, 1991; he was 30 and I was 28. We became parents in January, 1995. In the three and a half years between marriage and children, our marriage was affected by my mental illness. Periods of depression were interrupted by manic spending and occasional anger outbursts. I was hospitalized twice and spent time in a day program, as I tried to balance my career (teaching, at the time) with the effects of having a mental illness. We didn't have any idea the influence that mental illness would have on pregnancy and motherhood.

My first pregnancy went well at first; however, my husband has commented on more than one occasion that my mood swings were worse during pregnancy. This was simply something I didn't see in myself. Our first child was born early at 30 weeks. As those familiar with mental illness know, added stressors in life increase the adverse symptoms of disease. Looking back, I can see this. However, at the time, I hopped on the emotional rollercoaster and there I stayed for many years.

I found that, at times, I was calm and able to tackle many tasks in a given day. I was easy to get along with and spent time with other parents through a mom's group at church. I kept lists of all the things I wanted to accomplish in a given day, week, or month, and I was able to tackle these jobs. Then, just as easily, without any warning, I would make excuses to get out of get-togethers. On those days, I couldn't wait for my daughter's nap time because all I wanted to do was sleep, my escape from the world. On those days, I was tearful and would often start arguments with my husband. Two more pregnancies and children later I found myself with two daughters and a son. I was caught on a ride that wouldn't stop.

Parenting while our children were young was tumultuous at best. Some days, I was as rational as the next person and focused on building their self-esteem and loving our children. The next day, week, or month, I found myself losing my temper, raising my voice. There were times when I threatened to leave which only made a bad situation worse. In truth, I did not want to leave; I wanted to be fully accepted where I was and with the family my husband and I had created.

Parenting now, while in recovery, is so very different. I listen better, reassess situations so that I can stay in the rational world, and my children and I have developed close relationships with each other. But the side effects of my medication affect my mood and there are days I still cycle up and down; the ups and downs just aren't as drastic as they once were. When things were not good, I believed that others didn't want me around or that they were only "tolerating" me. This was simply not the case as my husband pointed out; it was merely a flawed perception. Sometimes when I stepped out of the "rational world," I would look for evidence that I was unwanted, unloved, or unsuccessful. There were times when I was self-injurious, which grew out of irrational beliefs about myself and others.

I am currently stable in my recovery. However, between 2010 and 2012 I had four psychiatric hospitalizations and have had to take leaves of absences from work. I am on a therapeutic combination of medications; I get along with family members, go to work daily, and manage irrational thoughts by constantly challenging the negative with the helpful advice and guidance of a skilled therapist. I am a program leader for a Peer Support Program in northwest Georgia. My current professional setting increases the likelihood of continued recovery. I am challenged to face my fears and overcome trepidation when in new situations and completing new tasks. I work with a good team of peer providers who care deeply for the consumers and the program.

My mental health history has affected my parenting in many ways. When my children were younger, I am certain that they needed more consistency from me. I always wanted to be the parent who could manage multiple tasks without losing my patience; I fear I wasn't so successful at this. And then there were the manic phases when I went overboard in my daily living activities, spent too much, and grew irritable too easily. Parenting was marked by an up and down ride. An example that comes to mind is one year when I decided to make bread for our children's teachers for homemade Christmas presents. A reasonable amount would have been one loaf each for the teacher and para-professional. However, I went overboard and was insistent that I must make bread for all of their teachers, e.g. P.E., art, music, and office staff. There were loaves of bread all over our kitchen counters in various degrees of completion. The word chaotic does not even encapsulate the situation. There I stood, sometimes until one or two in the morning, making gifts for those outside our family, while being impossible to live with for members of our family. At first sight, it seems humorous, but at that time, no one was laughing.

I believe that my periods of deep depression have hurt me and my family. There were the 2–3 hour naps, countered by the 2–3 hour long anger outbursts and the incessant worrying that has affected our relationships. My oldest daughter was recently watching the show, The Middle, and stated "I've lived this. I've experienced this" when the mother on the show became melodramatic. While the example she gave was funny at the time, I'm not so sure that it was funny to her when she was going through it the first, second, or even the umpteenth time.

My mental health has gotten in the way of being the type of parent I've wanted to be. I wanted to have endless energy, be engaged in their activities, and easily make friends with my children's friends' parents. This hasn't come as easily as I hoped or expected it to. However, it is becoming easier.

I have been hospitalized eight times in the last 22 years, and I can say that some settings have been helpful, while others have not. When I was placed in an isolation room in Florida 22 years ago, THAT was not helpful. I had always felt like I had no control; what were they gaining by doing that at the time? However, there was a hospital in Chattanooga, Tennessee, that was helpful; there was staff who had lived experience with mental illness in their families and they shared their stories with me. There was also electroconvulsive therapy, which may have contributed to my recovery at the time. The hospital staff in Chattanooga also took the time to meet with me and my husband, and he in turn conveyed what was going on to our children. I am thankful for the fact that I never lost custody of my children due to my mental illness, possibly because we always kept them aware of what was going on with me. I've never been separated from my children for any prolonged period, although once, my son, after learning I was suicidal and self harming, threatened to leave our home and to live with a friend's family. That was heartbreaking.

Parenting successes that stand out for me come in small, daily delights. Just seeing pictures of them on the credenza in my office brings a smile to my face. All three children have participated in hobbies and sports which are a source of joy for them. They are accomplished teenagers who are in college and high school and who excel at their efforts, both academically and with extracurricular activities including cross country, performing in plays, and playing softball.

The challenge I face daily is having to remind myself of the positives in my life. When I fail to do this, negativity slowly trickles down into what I say and how I say it to family members. Sometimes I hear my mother's voice come out of my mouth. . .I guess all daughters do. Other challenges surface when I take things too seriously and worry obsessively about so many things in my life. On the days when my side effects are most evident; it becomes difficult to remain positive and to keep hope going. But, then, I look on my credenza, read their texts, or listen to their voices and laughter; embers of hope become flames of life.

Conversations I've tried to have with my children about my mental illness usually don't go anywhere. It's like the elephant in the room. However, for this story, they contributed the following statements. Our youngest stated that in living with her mom with mental illness, she has found herself "worried, then frustrated, then worried." Our oldest stated that sometimes she doesn't know from day to day what might happen with me. Our son stated, "Family means no one gets left behind, and by God, we have stuck by that for all these years!"

I've learned that if I take my medication and stay out of the hospital, that's half the battle. The other half is daily combating negative thoughts and feelings. For those who have walked in the shoes of having a mental illness, I can say there is hope. That hope comes in many different forms, but the key for me is to focus on the hope and often times, things just fall into place.

Be True to Yourself

15

Amanda Stettenbenz

Amanda is a 31-year-old mother from Colorado. She has been diagnosed with schizoaffective disorder, anxiety, and borderline personality disorder. In this chapter she discusses the successes and challenges of being a mother, as well as her good relationship with her daughter despite living apart from each other.

I became a parent really unexpectedly. I was looking for love and acceptance and thought I could find it by sleeping with my daughter's biological father. I had a one-night stand with him. After I slept with him, he would not leave me alone until I got the police to tell him to stop. After the police got involved, I got rid of all his information. I did try to find him when I found out for sure, even though I knew right away I was pregnant. Being a mom was rough for me from the beginning. I was severely sick the entire pregnancy, losing 30 lb in the first 6 months.

Once my daughter Michaela was born, the first 2 weeks were okay, mostly getting to know her and how to take care of her. Then, postpartum depression kicked in. I was thrown into mixed episodes. I was exhausted but so anxious I could not sit still. I did not want to take care of Michaela. I wanted nothing to do with her. For the next 2 weeks, we had to have someone over to watch her and me while my parents were at work.

When Michaela was a year and a half, the police were called on me because the mental health center was afraid for me. The police took me to the hospital, where I spent the next 4 months. My parents were terrified that Social Services might get involved, so without warning me, I got served with custody papers from them. I was so devastated. I even almost got arrested because I freaked out and started threatening them. Because of that, I did not see my daughter until the last month of the 4-month hospital stay. In some ways, that really devastated me and in others, she was the one that motivated me. After I got home, my parents gave me a few months to adjust and then they gave her back to me. To this day, I do not know what happened with the custody paperwork after the day I got served.

Two years later, I was so depressed I could not get out of bed. Michaela was forced to take care of herself during the day while my ex-husband was at work. When I was up and about, I tended to scream at my ex-husband, beat myself up (literally), cut, or take a handful of pills. Michaela saw me do this several times and she freaked out. I know it scared her. One night, while I was at school, my ex-husband's mom came over to spend time with them and Michaela told her everything. My parents were called and they took Michaela for a week for me to get everything together. Well, towards the end of the week, I did not get any better and I did not want Michaela to come back into the situation she was in. One of those days, I had a really bad day and I panicked. I called social services on myself. Of course, that invited a ton of people into my life and they knew everything about me. My whole life became social services. At this point, I was 25. I decided that suicide was not an option anymore, and I also knew I could not go on the way I was. I checked myself in for another psychiatric hospitalization. I was there for 2 weeks this time, during which I was told what I needed to do if I ever wanted to see my daughter again. I got involved in every program I could to get better. The mental health center figured out at some point I was serious about getting better and offered me more opportunities than I could ever imagine. For the first time in my life, I knew what I needed and how to ask for what I needed.

I remember crying through all of the social services meetings. In the end, the state decided that I would face Allocation of Parental Responsibility, which is basically a fancy way of saying that I pay child support to my parents but I am allowed visitation rights. When Michaela went with my parents, she was very angry and withdrawn. We also decided to hold her back in kindergarten. Our case lasted almost 2 years. At first, I was only allowed supervised visits at the social services building. That was so hard because I knew they were watching us from another room and we could not do anything against the rules in that room. Then, we made an agreement that I could see her out in the community but that certain members of my family had to be there all the time to supervise. Eventually, the supervised part was dropped but because of the medication I was on; my parents were afraid to let me drive her around. Michaela eventually graduated her therapy and we graduated family therapy as well.

These days, Michaela is 10 and she still lives with my parents. Our relationship is actually really good these days. I do not think Michaela remembers a lot from living with me, thankfully. Michaela goes to parties with me, she helped us pick out the cat we have, and she spends the night here and there. Even with my struggles with mental illness, I am proud to say I have only missed chaperoning two of her field trips over her whole life so far. I help out with school parties and different clubs she joins. Michaela has been to events with my job, and she took part in the National Alliance on Mental Illness walk this year. Because I am closer in age than her grandparents, sometimes she asks me the hard questions, like about boys, being a teen, etc. Michaela knows that I have a mental illness but she does not know all the dirty details. She is 10; she does not need to know everything yet. When she is older, we will sit down and I will explain everything. It is hard though because every year, we have to explain to her new set of teachers what our living situation is, and that I'm really her mom. When I show up at her school for events, her peers ask why she does not live with me. I know it is hard for her because she does not really know how to explain it.

I am diagnosed with schizoaffective disorder, anxiety, and borderline personality disorder. It was a long road, and I am constantly seeking ways to improve on my wellness and recovery but I am happy to say that overall, I am pretty stable. I still have bad days sometimes, but my bad days now are like my good days 6 years ago. For the past 2 years, I have worked full time as a Peer Specialist. A Peer Specialist is someone who is in recovery and helps others with mental illness. Before I got heavy duty into being a Peer Specialist, I was a family advocate for my county's social services. I mostly mentored women who either had a mental illness or were thinking about signing custody over to someone else. I also sat on their inclusiveness committee, bringing the family and mental health voices to the table. I also volunteered heavily at the mental health center.

My mental illness has affected my parenting. I have to watch myself a lot more because I can get angry really fast. The obvious way that my mental illness continues to affect my parenting is the fact that my daughter lives with my parents. That being said, I find that it is so important to spend quality time with her, be a good role model, and also to educate her on mental health issues and being accepting of others.

What really helped me was having my own Peer Specialist. It was the first time I did not feel like I was the only one with mental health issues. She understood but she also had held down a job for more than a few months. I decided if she can do it, then so can I. I also took a lot of wellness classes. At one point, I was going to 19 wellness classes at one time! My therapist was really good, although it was hard because she had to report everything to the state. That being said, I decided going into Social Services; I would be completely honest so that I could get all the help I needed.

Michaela and I have talked some about mental health issues. In fact, she knows many of my friends that have mental health issues as well. We have talked about the fact that it makes me not think or sometimes act like a normal person but we have not gotten into any specific details. I am also honest with her about my experiences. One time, we were at a work event and she called someone crazy. My parents and I had a talk with her about how that woman could not help it and that she has a mental illness. When she was little, we told her I was sick and a doctor could help me get better. Michaela has always taken what I tell her about mental illness really well. But she still asks off the wall questions that I do not even know how to answer sometimes.

The biggest successes I have as a parent is going to school field trips and having Michaela confide in me. One time we were talking about how when you are sick, many people only want a few very important people around. Michaela told me that I am one of those important people she would want to be around if she was sick. At this point, it is encouraging that she is doing well in school and has lots of friends.

One of the biggest challenges is when Michaela asks why she is not living with me. It is also hard having to explain our situation to other people who may be new in our life. The biggest challenge I have, though, is I feel so guilty for everything I put her through.

What I would tell other moms with mental illness is to be honest in the beginning. Had I been honest with my struggles, I may not have lost custody of my daughter. But I waited until I was in a crisis to get help. I would also say, have a good support system! My support system has pulled me through a lot and still does to this day.

Second Chance Motherhood

16

Jocelyn O'Connor

Jocelyn is a 24-year-old mother from upstate New York. She has been diagnosed with a mood disorder. In this chapter Jocelyn alternates between the narrative of her story and her prayers, to give readers insight into her unique perspective and path to recovery.

Jesus is near to those that are broken at heart, and to those who are crushed in spirit he saves-Psalm 34-18.

Life is a journey always full of ups and downs, highs and lows. Sometimes it gets brighter; other times it gets really dark and it feels like it will never get better. A friend from high school told me on graduation day to always remember that all things in life are temporary, good or bad. That is the main quote that has stuck in my head to help me get through each day, one day at a time.

Ok pain... I'm ready for you... u are like a black cloud that continuously follows me around...when it starts to get a little brighter... you pour down rain upon me. Right when I'm feeling better/content in my life the sun shines a little brighter...but then u creep up on me, and I almost never am able to beat the rain. I feel like a cloud in the sky just passing by... unnoticed even on a sunny day. Even when all skies are clear...it just gets darker and darker... and then the rain pours harder and harder...once again.

Metaphorically this is how I feel each day. Living with a mental illness and a secondary disability is...hard. One day you're feeling great and on top of everything and then the world starts crashing down. The next day or week can leave you feeling completely different.

Jesus take the wheel, I am spiraling out of control...I feel like giving up...give me strength within to keep going. But I swear lord if they take him from me I will not be here...I will end it just like you did in calvary...

I am so angry with myself sometimes. I feel as if I have failed in some way. Even though I know I did the best I could at the time, I have been battling a depression

Motherhood, Mental Illness and Recovery, DOI 10.1007/978-3-319-01318-3_16,
© Springer International Publishing Switzerland 2014

and mood instability my whole life. In 2012 I gave birth to a beautiful baby boy. One of the best things that ever happened to me in my life. Being a mother with a mental illness changed me for the best in the long run. Even though no one, not even the doctors thought I would be able to handle the responsibility as a mother. They told me the best thing I could do for myself and my health was to abort him. They claimed that my mental health diagnosis was too severe and that it would interfere with my ability to parent a child. I couldn't believe the words I was hearing. I just wanted to live a normal life and all they wanted to do was doubt and focus on the severity of my illness. So what if my developing baby is only the size of a seed; this child growing inside of me is still life. God would not have planted that seed in me if he did not think it was the right time, but God did. Therefore it was his reason and his purpose that only he knew. No one else. I did not want to mess with whatever God's plan was for me or the new life growing inside of me. I felt it would be selfish to consider abortion. So I chose to give my child life, so that someday he could have life too.

> *Be my strength lord, I am hurt. . .I don't feel hurt, I have been hurt. It is that people use my illness to get by their problems, by putting it on me, instead of them, projecting me as the issue, and using insanity, as a method. I will go far, and face my fears. My illness does not limit me. . .*

Right when I made the decision to proceed with my pregnancy, pro-life advocates came to visit me. Complete strangers that I had never known in my life. At the time, I was getting inpatient psychiatric care for a mental breakdown. But then to find out you're pregnant at the same time. . .that was really hard to take in. And these people seemed to be genuine, caring, and understanding.

Little did I know what their main intentions were. They drew a significant red flag not just to me but to all my providers. They wanted to know a lot of my personal information regarding my income, and I came to find out that they were totally opposed to any kind of government aid. . .food stamps, SSI, and any kind of government assistance. They were convinced that all this government assistance people were getting was robbing the working people from their funds. I did not see this coming, even though I was warned from my providers. Due to my poor judgment at the time, I was willing to take their help. Little did I know they were just wolves in sheep's clothing. They took me in to their home to be cared for and told me not to use any of my benefits, EBT, or anything. They ended up taking me into their home, throwing me off to the streets, and then to a community residence out of state, making it seem like that was the best option for me.

> *Lord Jesus, it is March, and it is so hard to find a good friend. I have a lot of good friends, but they do not live around me. Plus, I have lost contact to a lot of my good friends. Where I am now I cannot connect to anyone. . .its really hard. I don't have the same issues as these women, I don't do the things they do, I don't think the way they think. The friends I have are already successful, they have a career and a job and a life. I'm afraid to get in contact with them because I feel that they would not understand. The fact that I am on a lower status and not good with my life they may not want a part of me. I am not the same inspiring person they once knew. I have changed a lot and lost a lot of self respect for myself, and the system has changed me immensely. I feel alone with the battles I'm facing but I know you're always*

there. I don't know if I feel ready to be a mother. . .I know I can be, but I have no one out here. . .no family, no friends, no support I feel I can trust. . . here I am in New York receiving outpatient care voluntarily, and they want to diagnose me with everything in the book without knowing me at all, or my history. . .but you know lord jesus, and your truth will prevail.

They think I have. . .schizophrenia! Yeah right! I know the difference between what's real and what's not. They think I am not sane. I mean, at all period. This community residence is supposed to be through the church. Yet all the people here, except one person are all hypocrites. They don't believe in any morals, and they certainly do not believe in any of the biblical teachings. They have no moral standards, I cannot stay here! I feel like I'm living in hell on earth. I'm delivering my son in a month, and I do not want him in this environment. I want to go back home, but I am so far away. . . .

Dear lord jesus. . .the enemy seems to always set a trap for me. He tries to take away all of my sanity, my happiness, my contentment. But lord in my heart I know you have good things in store for me and blessings that only you can give and never take away. You never give me more than u know I can handle. It's almost April. Lord first they want me to abort my baby, now they want me to surrender my parental rights and give my baby up for adoption. . .

I know there are still a lot of things I want to accomplish in my life. In my mind I am thinking they are right, but in my heart I feel that they got it all wrong. Just because I have a psychiatric illness doesn't mean I can't live a productive life. I have a hard enough time trying to convince the psychiatrist to lower my medication dosage. He's so closed minded, yet he thinks he knows everything. He doesn't even know me. All I'm trying to do is complete these outpatient mental health groups so I can receive official outpatient treatment. It just feels like a game, a run around a trap. It's so frustrating. . .give me strength to proceed.

I was sitting in group one day, and there was a woman there who was very rude and extremely two faced. I was there to learn from the group instructor. She wanted to flaunt all her knowledge and invade my privacy. I simply told her in front of everyone that she is not the group instructor, and that it is not appropriate to intervene and ask people their personal experiences so she could give her input. Don't get me wrong, she was intelligent, but she was mentally sick. She snapped at me in the most profound way. . .she almost made me cry. She called me crazy and paranoid. I talked to the group instructor after group how I felt, but she was not happy with me. Her response to me was, you have a problem with her because she is sane and you are not.

Lord give me patience, they want to stigmatize me. I don't believe what they say. . .yeah, I know I have issues- everyone does. But only you lord can see all things, and you are the only one that is perfect. . .

Seems like this residence just keeps getting crazier and crazier. . .No one wants to attend spirituality groups, they just want the free hand and not work towards anything. I think to myself that these women are very selfish, they do not want to do the work on themselves, they are taking advantage. Especially when there are women like me who really want to help themselves, and receive the help needed. They are really robbing me of that. Wanda works so hard every day without one break, she is always hounded and stuck. When she was finally able to assist me, she was very tired. She told me she was taking sleeping pills just so that she could make it through the day. She never got one break. Because everybody uses up all her time. I'm so sick of it here, I want to go home. Howard who brought me here told me to stay where I am. He told me to lead these women by example. You cannot help someone if they do not want to accept the help or help themselves. He really does not know how bad it

is getting here, and if he does, he just does not give two flying shits. "Don't fly your jets,
before it lands," he said. I knew I was going to hate it here just by the first looks of it. And I
was so frickin right. Lord jesus, I just wish there was some place other than here I could go,
I will never deny you lord jesus.

Its so sad to think and feel like you have no way out, and to have people mocking you, asking without reason where you are going to run to. They don't know where I have been running my whole life. They cannot put themselves in my shoes, they have not walked with me. At times when I was feeling no way out they were not there. There were many times when I felt like giving up completely and ending my life, but Jesus told me to continue to be strong, that he has a purpose for me, an opportunity, and a second chance.

Lord jesus, I know u love all your children the same, but lord I don't want to follow in her
footsteps, my lord my mother, is in denial with herself, she is very ill. She wants to point the
finger at me, and not look at herself but I know lord that u are with me every step of the
way...

I think back to the day my mother took me in to her home. In the beginning it was so beautiful, but things changed immensely. My mother has been in recovery for years, connecting with her at first was great, but my relationship with her stunted my mental health recovery, she became unstable, and could not provide the comfort a mother should for a child. And even if she was able too, it was only temporary. I look in the mirror, and I see myself, yeah I look a lot like her, but I am never going to be her. I know that when I become a mother I will be a good mother. If I become powerless I will not turn to drugs or the street. I will be responsible, loving, and consistent in my child's life. I will not give up.

As I sat in my room at the residence, I got so mad, I broke my cell phone. I cried so hard and I felt so alone. It's clear that my mother is in denial, but to find out too that my grandfather had passed away, it was more than my heart could take. My window shot open from the wind, and it started to down pour. I cried to my lord and asked for an answer from him.

Lord jesus, what is my purpose here, I'm so sad I feel lead astray. I want to go home...I
hate it here...I feel so trapped. Please give me an answer. I'm losing strength within, and
my baby inside of me is feeling everything I am feeling. I need to stay calm, and stop crying
so much...

I had a dream. In the dream I came across people, places, and situations. I didn't want to face them. I ran away and kept sword fighting, but I would always win. The dream took me to another scene. I was trying to find a place where I would feel at peace and not afraid. As the scenery got better and brighter I felt ok, but when it got dark I would run. I ran on a deck and I looked down below and I was about to jump, but a little boy sat on the edge of the deck holding his feet adrift and he told me not to jump. I was about to jump, I didn't know my way out. The little boy's assumption was that "the elephant was mean." I looked down below, I jumped, and I became much smaller than the elephant. For a moment I got scared, because the elephant was bigger than me. I was about to run away. Instead I met the elephant face to face. I couldn't budge. The elephant opened his mouth and said, why do you keep running away, you are going to continue to face people and places that you do not want to face. The elephant continued to say, face your situations, hit the baseball head on even if you strike out three or more times. The elephant said to me, if you face your problems and situations you will find home base.

I woke up that morning and felt a message hit me. Elephants signify wisdom. Symbolically the message was telling me that I have to stay in one place and stop running from my fears. The little boy symbolically was representing my son and the needs of my son. I realized that when I face my trials and tribulations I can have peace of mind. I realized that I am always going to make mistakes, and that I can learn from my mistakes and do things the right way. Symbolically, just as a baseball player strikes out more than one time, there will come a hit and a home base run.

> *Lord jesus they are going to induce my labor...I am not comfortable. Wayne keeps calling me, but I won't answer. I'm in too much pain right now... I'm about to get an epidural...I'm picturing you lord, and I'm praying for everything to be ok...*
> *My cervix did not dilate fully, so now they are going to do a cesarian section. I'm on my meds, and I feel doped out. All I can feel is a tug here and a tug there...then I hear my baby cry for the first time...*

My son was born on Easter morning in April 2012. He is the best thing that ever happened to me. He taught me to be a strong, responsible mother. Although I felt stigmatized from the start of my pregnancy, I proved everyone wrong. I may have a mental illness, but despite that I am a great mother and it does not limit me. Through my colorful past and journey, I can share my story and experiences with others. Let yourselves be inspired, don't ever feel like you can't do something, always believe in yourself and your capabilities even if no one sees it. God sees all things, and he will always provide for you. Live for today and learn from your mistakes, and make positive changes.

> *Lord I never knew that becoming a mother would change me the way that it did. I thought I was all alone, but you were walking with me every step of the way. I am grateful for the support you give me through family and service providers who always bring out the best in me. I am grateful that my housing program gave me a second chance. I guess that's what you meant for me to have all along. My life, my support, and my son, but most importantly being a mother and having a second chance in life and an opportunity.*

After the birth of my son, I moved back home. I have been stable for 2 years. Even living with a mood disorder and brain illness called fetal alcohol syndrome, I am living independently and successfully. I no longer feel the need to run. I share custody of my son with my adopted mother. My son is striving, healthy, happy, and advanced for his age. Because of all the positive support I get, and the work I put into myself each day, I can now live a life of peace, contentment, and happiness. I enjoy being a mother and all the blessings and possibilities that come with it.

Love Endures Time

17

Jessica Melchick

Jessica is a 56-year-old mother of two from upstate New York. She has been diagnosed with bipolar disorder and was hospitalized continuously from 2003 to 2013.

Many seasons have come and gone
However love endures time and distance
I have watched my children grow up
Behind the jagged points of a barb
My heart breaks
Knowing I can't smell their skin
Wipe away their tears
Comfort them in their time of fear
And cheer them in their times of success
I have photos of memories long ago
Before the age of innocence
Was interrupted
Life goes on as it always does
Trial and tribulation will continue
However my test will become my testimony
However I hope I can let go of my young children
And develop a new love and understanding
With a whole new dynamic
Of a young man and young lady on the verge of realizing their full potential
Remember Justin and Brittany
I love you both fully and unconditionally
From the bottom of my heart to the depths of my soul

Motherhood, Mental Illness and Recovery, DOI 10.1007/978-3-319-01318-3_17,
© Springer International Publishing Switzerland 2014

Part III

Voices of Mothers: Getting Help

Postpartum Psychosis Forever Changed My Life

18

Jennifer Hentz Moyer

Jennifer is a 47-year-old mother diagnosed with postpartum psychosis and bipolar disorder. In this chapter she discusses her experiences of being hospitalized nine times after the birth of her son, as well as being separated from her family due to the lack of education about mental illness in her community. She is an author and mental health advocate, and more information about Jennifer can be found at http://www.jennifermoyer.com.

My name is Jennifer. I was born and raised in Pennsylvania. The youngest of eight children, I was shy and well protected by my two brothers and five sisters, even more so after my father left the family when I was just 4 years old. I was too young to understand but as I grew older the lack of a father became more and more difficult. Growing up with divorced parents was very challenging but with the love, encouragement, and support of my mother and siblings, I managed to overcome the stigma that I felt. I would eventually graduate from college and go on to have a career in marketing.

Seven years after dating, my husband and I got married. We decided to wait to have children. I wanted to finish college and work for a few years before having kids. In 1994, 6 years after we got married, I got pregnant. I was so excited but sadly the pregnancy ended in a miscarriage. It was devastating for both of us.

Eventually we became pregnant again, resulting in the birth of our beautiful son. Although my labor and delivery was long and difficult, everything turned out fine. But life was changed forever. Although I was initially exhausted and had to recover, I was much better within 2 weeks. My son and I bonded wonderfully. Being a parent has been challenging, but it is the most rewarding experience I have had.

It was not until my son began sleeping through the night at about 6 weeks that things started to change for me. He was sleeping great but I was not. It all seemed to happen suddenly, but by the time I was 8 weeks postpartum, I had gone without sleep for several nights. I became certain that my son was in danger and I was going to die. I became so protective; I wouldn't even let my husband hold the baby. What was happening? I didn't understand.

I had no prior history of mental illness and was unaware that postpartum psychosis existed. I had to forcibly be hospitalized at 8 weeks postpartum. Initially I was told I had postpartum depression, but it was apparent that it was something different when I had to be hospitalized again 2 weeks later at 10 weeks postpartum. I was losing touch with reality and had actually heard and saw things that seemed very real to me at the time. Thankfully, after the second hospitalization and a second medical opinion, I did get a proper diagnosis of postpartum psychosis. I wasn't prepared that the psychosis would turn into depression. I would later learn this often occurs with postpartum psychosis.

My son and I bonded well during the first 2 months of his life but when I was forcibly hospitalized, the bond broke. I would try to re-bond with him but each time I was hospitalized, the bonding would be hindered. I lost so much during the first 2 years of my son's life but I am forever grateful for the positive experience I had in the first 6 weeks. By the time my son was two and a half, I felt the joy of being a mother return.

When I was hospitalized in the postpartum period, I felt such guilt and isolation. The other patients were experiencing things completely unrelated to childbirth so I could not relate to any of their experiences. It was difficult to overcome.

I struggled with depression and anxiety for many months after my son was born. I was given medication but I still experienced up and down cycles. Over the course of my postpartum onset illness, I was hospitalized nine times. It seemed the anxiety and inability to sleep would become all-consuming prior to each hospitalization. Every time I was hospitalized, a piece of my heart was broken when I had to be separated from my son. One of the hospitalizations occurred when my son was 16 months old. Everything seemed better. I was working full time again. This was extremely stressful. I was still not experiencing natural sleep. One day I had a sudden panic attack. It came out of nowhere. I had gripping fear that I could not control. As a result, I took all of my medicine. It felt like I had no control over my actions; yet my life nearly ended by my own hand.

I eventually overcame postpartum psychosis and depression but during that time, I never got to talk to any other mothers that had experienced postpartum psychosis. Back in the late 1990s, the internet was not what it is today. Although I had people around me, I never felt like they really understood what I was experiencing.

Things got better but I struggled to become as well as I was before postpartum psychosis struck me. Seven years after the onset of postpartum psychosis, I was diagnosed with bipolar disorder. I eventually learned of the correlation between postpartum psychosis and bipolar disorder and over time, I was able to accept that I would now have to live with a lifelong mental illness. I have discovered that with stress management, proper treatment, effective therapy, and spiritual support, I am able to live my life fully despite having a mental illness.

When my son was 8 years old, my husband left for a month on a work-related trip to another country. In the past, the longest my husband had ever been away from our son and I was 2 weeks. All had been going well during the time he was gone but when his trip got extended for two additional weeks, things got stressful. The school district had plans to change the school boundaries, which would force my son to go to a different school. My son, who loved school, began to get upset about having to go to school. Because of the stress I was experiencing, my sleep began to get disrupted.

I had been doing so well that I was seeing my therapist monthly. As a result of the stress, I contacted her for an earlier appointment as well as assistance with a psychiatrist referral. I had to leave the care of the last psychiatrist I saw regularly because of an insurance plan change. The earliest I could get an appointment with the new psychiatrist was in 2 months.

Along with my son's change in attitude about school was the fact that he was telling me about having "lock-down" drills at school. I became concerned for my son so I contacted my son's pediatrician for assistance. I sought help yet somehow it was turned against me and apparently, the Department of Children and Families (DCF) was contacted. The investigator spoke to my son as well as me. Much time passed; then the pediatrician and the investigator came out and told me my son was going to be removed from me. I screamed, "No way, I have done nothing wrong!" My son came running over to me, climbed in my lap and started crying. "No," he cried. The investigator said to me, "when you get to your house, there will be officers there to talk to you and you will most likely be forced to go to a psychiatric hospital." I was in shock.

Yes, I was sleep deprived but I didn't understand what was happening. Why, after seeking help, was everything turning against me? When we returned home there were two police cars there. Two police officers came into my home to question me. One followed me into my bedroom as I was listening to my telephone messages. I did not trust him. Another officer, looking to be a superior, came into my bathroom and searched my medicine cabinet. He found an old prescription and said, "You are not taking your medicine." I told him it was an old prescription. He refused to listen to me. When I went back into the living room, the investigator from DCF said, "Your son is going to be in temporary custody, until you get evaluated." I asked, "Can I say goodbye to my son?" The DCF investigator was going to let me but the police officers refused.

The next thing I know, an officer is handcuffing me despite my request to get voluntarily evaluated at a facility near my therapist. He handcuffed me tightly as I was scared and resistant. I still have a scar on my wrist today from where the handcuff cut my wrist. The officer refused to take me where I requested, instead taking me to a facility in the opposite direction. I was petrified for my life. I didn't understand why this was happening. I live in a small community. It seemed to be assumed that because of my concern for my son, I was completely unstable.

The officers would not let me call anyone prior to putting me in the police car and speeding off to take me away. I continued to request to be voluntarily evaluated. My requests fell on deaf ears. I was in the emergency room for hours without any psychiatric doctor evaluating me. I did not test positive for drugs or alcohol yet I was transferred to a rehab facility. The intake personnel did not understand why I was there. I had insurance so they were even more confused. I was admitted anyway. All this time, my husband was still out of the country.

I was nearly committed to a state hospital after being overmedicated and assaulted in the rehab facility. Thankfully, I got released after about 10 days. Before my release, my husband, who had returned home, was told by the DCF investigator that if he did not sign a restraining order against me, he would also lose our son. My life was no longer the same. I could not see my son. It was the first time I was separated from him for his birthday and for Christmas. I was forced to face the ignorance about mental illness in the community I lived.

I nearly lost my family as a result of the incident with DCF and again when my husband filed for divorce in 2005. Thankfully, the divorce never happened. Now nearly 18 years after the onset of postpartum psychosis, I am thankful that my family and I are happily restored. But the hell that was forced upon us by authorities that seemed uneducated about mental illness has left a scar on us for life. Finding the right care and treatment for postpartum psychosis and the bipolar illness that followed along with lots of prayer and support from family and friends has restored my life once again.

Despite the adversity and difficulties my family faced, my son is a healthy, intelligent, compassionate, and responsible young man. He will soon be graduating high school and starting college. Looking back I would do it all again to have him in my life. My son has lived through my history so he has seen first-hand the difficulties. He has had professional therapy for much of my illness, which has helped him as well as my family deal with the challenges we have faced. I think he is more understanding and accepting of others as a result.

Something I'd like to tell other mothers in similar positions is, do not ever give up. No matter what you may face, you can prevail. With proper care and treatment, therapy, and support, you can overcome adversity. Do not feel guilt or shame. You are not alone.

Shine Your Light into Darkness

19

Sherri White and Laura Downs

Sherri is a 59-year-old mother from California. She is a mother of three diagnosed initially with schizophrenia, later bipolar disorder. In this chapter, written following an interview by Dr. Downs, she discusses her childhood experiences, development of psychosis, and the important lessons her children have learned in the face of mental illness.

When I think about what I want to say about mothering with a mental illness, I draw a blank. I have never really thought of myself as a mother in a different category than all of the other mothers out there. Yes, I have a mental illness, but for me, this fact has not made my mothering challenges any more difficult than they are for other mothers. I want what all mothers want: children reared to feel loved and protected, safe, and cherished, children that develop into adults with admirable qualities.

My mental illness never made me feel that I should not have children or that I was somehow less equipped to deal with children. I have raised three, but would have happily had more if circumstances permitted. The one thing I knew early on is that I wanted to be a mother—that was the most important thing in the world to me. My own childhood was less than storybook, and I always wanted the opportunity to give to my own children the things I missed. I believed I had an acute sense of what a good parent should be based upon what I was deprived of, and craved most, when I, myself, was growing up.

I was born in Martinez, California, in the 1950s. The polite euphemism to describe my family would be "dysfunctional," although that term hardly seems to do the situation justice. I was the second of eight children (I guess "second" is kind of relative, since I am actually a twin—I popped out a few minutes earlier than my partner, making me second in line to an older sister already in the picture). Four of us siblings had the same father. My mother left my father when I was in the fifth grade, and she moved to Reno with her new boyfriend whose baby she was

Motherhood, Mental Illness and Recovery, DOI 10.1007/978-3-319-01318-3_19,   169
© Springer International Publishing Switzerland 2014

carrying. My father fell apart and kind of checked out, drinking himself into oblivion, spending every night in the neighborhood bar until one of us came to claim him. Eventually, the house full of untended children who didn't attend school caught attention, and we were all taken away. My older sister moved in with a friend, my twin and I went with our paternal grandmother, my two brothers went into foster care, and my two younger sisters were sent to Reno to live with mom.

My grandmother was a good woman who took us to church and taught us about faith, about believing in something larger than ourselves. It was then that the seed of realization was planted in me that there are both forces of good and evil at work in this world, and it is our job to persevere through the difficult times and stay on a path toward fulfilling our destinies.

Difficulties there were aplenty, but I think I did persevere in the end. In the tenth grade, my sister and I moved to Reno to spend more time with our mom. We had to work to earn money for everything we needed—clothes, prom tickets, and so forth—and we did. We lived in the 'hood and were subject to all sorts of senseless violence, particularly my sister, who was beaten-up almost every day, leading her to drop out of school in the tenth grade. I, however, managed to graduate from high school and a year early at that, marking me as the only high school graduate among my siblings.

As soon as I graduated, mom had my sister and I move out. So, at 16, we found an apartment on our own. I took a job at a hotel and casino. It was there I met my first husband, a musician who stole my heart at first sight. We were married a month later and I traveled on the road with him and his band. The marriage ended after about 5 years when I became pregnant and he talked me into having an abortion. It was not what I wanted to do, and I could never forgive him for the coercion. Being a mother had always been a part of my plans.

On a brighter, and somewhat ironic, note this marriage left me with a new friend in my husband's sister, a kind and interesting woman who shared stories about life and work and helped me feel anchored and secure even when things about me were tumultuous. The ironic part is that she was a psychiatrist, and those stories she shared about her work were my very first introduction to the world of mental illness. She was the first psychiatrist I had ever met, but fate would not have her be the last. This positive relationship probably made me more receptive to the profession later on when I, myself, needed help.

Years after the end of my first marriage, while tending bar in a rock-n-roll club, I met my second husband. A year after we married, our first beautiful daughter came along. Two years later, a son.

Then the bottom fell out.

I'd been pressuring my husband to "get a real job". I'd been with a musician before and did not want that life again. And now we had children to think about. He had a tough time parting with the music scene, though, and was ultimately busted on a drug charge and sentenced to 3 years in prison.

One week after he shipped off, I jumped out a window.

We were at my mother-in-law's house. I was there with my 3-year-old daughter and 1-year-old son; my husband had just gone to prison, and I was feeling bad.

Really bad. Maybe I had been feeling bad for a while—I don't know—but on that day, I just broke. I felt the world close in on me, and saw evil everywhere. There were demons in the room. Flames were shooting up from the floors. I needed to find a way out, a way to get my children out of there before it was too late. I ran for the window and jumped through, then tried to come back in, ripping apart the tendons in my leg. My object was not to kill myself, but to rescue my family from the demons in the room.

I wound up in the hospital for 3 months. I was diagnosed with schizophrenia and started on Haldol. I was pretty out of it for a long while. I felt turned off, moving from room to room dragging my injured leg behind me in its brace, closed in and paranoid. I didn't feel much and was disconnected from my surroundings. I think it was the Haldol. I hated this medication, and believe to this day that it made me worse.

My children could not visit the mental hospital, as they were too young. My in-laws cared for them. My children had witnessed their mother have a psychotic break and jump out a window. I did not know what this would do to them in the long run. Fortunately, they were very young and had loving support in my in-laws.

One day in the hospital, I was at the crafts table and suddenly the light clicked back on in my brain. I again realized who I was, that I had a life outside of the hospital, children to get back to, a husband suffering through his own ordeal. I convinced the doctors that I was better. They released me into "boarding care," a supervised residential setting. At least here my children could visit. Three months later I was deemed sufficiently stable to be released back home to care for my children. But I was not stable. I was still on Haldol and, although I could put on a good show face when I needed to, I still believed the world was after me and my children. The paranoia led me to keep the curtains drawn, and we rarely left the house. In my sick state of mind, I did not think I was hurting my children, only keeping them safe.

My luck changed when I went for treatment at the county hospital. There I met a wonderful psychiatrist who re-diagnosed me with bipolar disorder, stopped the Haldol, and finally put me on the correct medications. The black cloud I had been living under lifted, and I came back to myself. My husband came out of prison. He found a stable job. I got pregnant again. It was not planned, but welcome news to me all the same. My husband was less sure at first. Given all I'd been through, was it wise to have another baby? Yes, I told my husband. We would be fine. This baby was meant to be part of our family.

But this family was plagued by mental illness. What would the long-term effects of growing up in a house with mental illness be on these children we wanted and cherished so much?

Life went on and years flew by. I remained in treatment with the wonderful psychiatrist from the county. He was my lifesaver. He helped stabilize me on medications and then taught me more and more about my illness. Most importantly, he helped me learn to love myself. Trust thrived in this atmosphere and I was able to open up to him about all I had buried deep inside me—my difficult childhood, parental abandonment, a failed first marriage, an abortion. He helped me to process these experiences and replace what was broken inside with a healthy attitude.

Throughout this time, my children were growing and my husband and I felt blessed, never burdened in the midst of all that was going on. We watched countless football and soccer and softball games, transported the girls to endless dance lessons and cheerleading practices, never losing sight of them as our first priorities. We both strived to give the children a sense of stability and safety, "normalcy" in spite of my illness, which did not change anything in terms of our being a family.

There were bumps along the way. I am talking big bumps, like 911 calls being made to the house to transport the crazy, delusional woman inside to the hospital. These events were part of life in our house. My children came to understand that mommy was ill, that she sometimes needed to go to the hospital, but that she always came back. I like to think that they knew how much I loved, and still do love, them every step of the way as well. In our home, mental illness was simply something that *was*, and there was no shame. My husband was a rock, and when I had to go away, he was home with the children, nurturing and loving them as I would when I was home. My mental illness was a reality. It was part of our family life, and we all worked it out together.

It has been a gift, too. My children learned to be sensitive to nuances of feeling. They learned that it is important to be attuned to others around you, that the greatest source of help comes from those you love. They have learned to be accepting of differences and that education is an important tool in eliciting understanding in others. Most of all, they have learned the value of humor, that it is okay to laugh when something is funny. They have laughed with me as I have shared my stories of hospital stays and people who came and went through my haze of illness and episodes. We have laughed together because some of these experiences *are* funny, and these experiences are woven into our lives.

I believe that all of us have destinies we are fated to fulfill. For me, my destined place is to be a positive role model in mental illness. I have worked as a peer advocate and as a "navigator," an individual who helps others with mental illness find their path toward recovery and health. I have helped found several programs at various facilities in which individuals work together to shed the stigma of their mental illness and celebrate the gifts given to them. I have shared my story with many in hopes of imparting even a small spark of inspiration to someone who is suffering. In so doing, I hope I have also been a positive role model for my children.

No doubt, life isn't always easy. There are forces that rear up every so often— those forces that try to push us from our path in this world and simply crush us. Personally, 2007 was a banner year in this regard. In 2007, my son was hit by a city bus while riding his bike. My daughter was the victim of a hit and run accident. My son's fiancé was killed in yet another motor accident when her car stalled on the side of the road in the night, and she walked for help. My dog was hit by a car and had his rear leg amputated. My husband was laid off from his job, and we lost our home. And there was more—loss of a beloved grandmother, loss of a mother-in-law, loss of two brother-in-laws. We were buried under a giant heap of tragedy and loss that year. I do not think I can be accused of being overly dramatic when I assert that these stressors could be destabilizing to anyone, let alone someone with a mental illness. In 2007, we all suffered. I suffered with my family, my family suffered along with me. Eventually we all made it through. Some reparations were made: my son prevailed in a lawsuit against the city; my husband was reinstated in his job after we sued. I took time off from my work as a navigator, but eventually went back.

There are indeed positive and negative forces at work in this world. My motto is to never succumb to the negative forces. I believe that a life is not defined by experiences, but by what we *do* with our experiences. Darkness will inevitably come at times. We must believe we have the power to shine light into the darkness. Of course, when one is in the grip of serious mental illness, it becomes difficult, even impossible, to believe we have the power to do anything. Getting out of bed may seem like a power outside of human comprehension at that point. I understand this. I have lived it. I believe I have overcome it. I attribute my ability to do this to finding the right doctor, engaging in the right therapy, being surrounded by a loving family, and fighting for my life.

My journey continues as the years sail by. I feel no shame about my illness, but am instead proud of many things including, as hard to believe as it may be, my illness. Yes, this illness is a part of me and makes me who I am, and I am proud of who I am. I am also proud of the family I have, and the mother I have been. I am extremely proud of my children. My children all bear qualities that have been fostered in our family; our family in which mental illness has played its not insignificant role.

Who are my children today? My eldest daughter has worked 10 years for a well-known retail giant where she is the boss. She has a tremendous sense of responsibility and good common sense overall. My son began doing stand-up comedy in his senior year of high school and is genuinely funny and courageous on the stage (hearkening back to the humor that helped my family through so many rough times). He is now teaching English in Vietnam and China. My youngest daughter is a youth pastor in our local church where she counsels young people, a vocation that comes so naturally to her given the circumstances of her own youth.

Responsibility, good sense, humor, courage, compassion. These are the qualities my children escaped their childhoods with. The paths they took through these childhoods were neither easy nor straightforward, watching their mother struggle through episodes of psychosis and hospitalization.

The impact of living in a house with mental illness is undeniably evident.

What more could a mother want?

Finding Hope When There Is None

20

Kathy Goodwin

Kathy is a 33-year-old mother from Texas. In this chapter she discusses her experience with postpartum depression following intrauterine insemination and the birth of her daughter. She emphasizes the importance of being open about one's feelings and seeking help right away when unable to manage on your own.

From the time I was 6 years old, I knew I would one day become a mother. It was Christmas day in 1986. My youngest sister Rachel was brought home in a huge stocking, and from that day on I was certain that I was her second mommy. Being one of five girls in a small, one-bathroom house, I spent much of my time with my sisters, particularly my two younger sisters. I grew up feeling almost like the oldest child, and in this self-fulfilling role I protected my siblings as much as I could.

In 1999, I met my partner CJ at a local coffee shop in Houston, Texas. We fell in love quickly, but weren't on the same page regarding the timing of children until almost a decade later. At that time, we got married in California and went to a fertility doctor in Houston. We chose an open donor through California Cryobank. I remember my mother and youngest sister Rachel were sitting at the table with us looking at donor profiles on the computer. We all agreed on the same donor. Everything seemed to go so smoothly. I started taking fertility medications in preparation for our first intrauterine insemination. I was naively certain that I was pregnant that first time, but I wasn't. The second try worked but I suffered a miscarriage at 9.2 weeks. I was in the middle of a law school semester and I remember walking up to my Constitutional Law Professor in tears. He was the best law Professor I had ever had, and I somehow felt comfortable enough to tell him why I had to leave early the day of my D&C procedure. It was the third try that brought us Grace, our six-pound five-ounce bundle of joy.

Looking back, I have to admit that the last trimester was pretty rough for me. I worked until 2 days before going into labor, but I was emotionally and physically

Motherhood, Mental Illness and Recovery, DOI 10.1007/978-3-319-01318-3_20,
© Springer International Publishing Switzerland 2014

exhausted. I started getting hormone-related migraines, which were debilitating. I had several emotionally charged moments with my partner days before going into labor. Maybe these were signs of what was to come postpartum or maybe these were experiences that affected my emotional state afterwards. Either way, I was extremely naïve about motherhood. I was the person who sat in the front row at all of our parenting classes, sure that I would know exactly what to do when our baby arrived. I was the one who tossed aside all of the literature I received about postpartum depression because there was no way that "someone like me" would be depressed. I had always wanted to be a mother. I was meant to be a mother. Depression was the furthest thing from my mind. I remember telling CJ there was no way I was going to end up dealing with something like that. "Look at what we went through to get pregnant! Why would I be depressed when this is the one thing I've always wanted?" I asked her during one of our many parenting classes. I tuned out the speaker as she briefly discussed postpartum depression and anxiety, and I never once opened up the brochure on postpartum warning signs. Despite family indicators and diagnoses of major depression, I did not understand it on a personal level. For me, I never anticipated suffering with something so mentally disturbing after the birth of my daughter.

Less than a week before I went into active labor, I started having contractions. I was monitored in the hospital for a brief period and told to go home and rest. I was not in labor. A few days later I was vomiting and having diarrhea. The next morning, on March 22, 2010, I started having unmistakable contractions and knew that I was in labor. We went back to the hospital and they actually told me to sit in a wheelchair downstairs while they got a monitoring bed ready because they didn't believe I was in labor. I guess they were going to watch my contractions again and send me home. I told them about the vomiting and the diarrhea and they finally sent me upstairs to Labor and Delivery.

I remember my doctor coming in to measure my cervix and determine how many centimeters I had dilated. She told me I was at 4 cm and congratulated me. She said that my daughter would be born that day. Looking back now, I remember the panic I felt when I heard those words. The word "daughter" was foreign to me. Something had crept inside of me and left me with a feeling of fear. I didn't want anyone looking at me. I didn't want anyone talking to me. I suddenly didn't belong there. Lying there in that hospital bed, deep inside of me, I felt I wasn't good enough to be a mother.

Nine hours into my labor, I was told that Grace's heart rate was dropping and that I would have to have an emergency caesarian. During my pregnancy, I was adamant about having a vaginal birth, but in those scary moments during labor there was no question. They wheeled me into the operating room. After the surgery, I was separated from Grace for several hours and was told that she was given a bottle of formula before I even got a chance to breastfeed her. I started worrying that she wouldn't want to nurse because she was given a bottle. Then I started worrying that something had happened to her. Then I feared that someone would take her. Days after delivery, worry consumed me. I worried about everything and was extremely tearful. My OB-GYN called me on the phone after my discharge and asked me about the crying. I figured that it was a normal reaction to childbirth. My hormones would naturally be all over the map. But she told me to monitor my emotional state. I was a bit confused at that point. Again, I could not anticipate what was about to unfold.

It was the eighth day. I will never forget it. It was the day that everything shut off inside of me. My entire family, including my mom, was sick with a bad cold so they were unable to be around at all when we brought Grace home from the hospital. I was visiting with friends and eating homemade soup they had made us in our living room. For some reason, I couldn't eat the soup that I had once enjoyed so much. I tried to swirl the spoon around in the bowl because I felt bad about not eating it. But suddenly I couldn't stand the smell or sight of it. I put the bowl down on the table and told my family and friends that I needed to go to the bathroom.

Escaping to the back of my house, I crawled in bed and started crying. Everything had changed. I couldn't stand being in my house, in my clothes, in my own body. I hated everything about myself and my life. The scariest part was that I no longer wanted to be a mother. I wanted my old life back and I kept saying it over and over. There is no way that I can adequately describe just how sudden this change occurred. Maybe there were warning signs, but none of them could have prepared me for this. There I was, a stranger to myself. I couldn't logically explain my feelings to anyone, but I knew immediately that something was horribly wrong. I had these overwhelming thoughts and feelings and I could do nothing about it. I couldn't hide them, nor did I want to. I had no capacity to filter through my feelings and words. I was gone and the few people that I allowed into my hell knew I was gone because I told them. Over and over. I remember fixating on certain things. I would never get better. There was no one else who had gone through postpartum depression like this. I was convinced that I was worse than all of the women who had lost themselves before me. In my mind, no one really knew what was happening to me because they weren't inside me. That was one of the scariest things for me. . .there was no way to control it and no way to fix it with a specific formula.

I couldn't eat anything. The only thing I could manage to ingest was chocolate-flavored Ensure. I was certain that there was a medical reason for all this chaos. I went to see my OB-GYN and I told her that I had cancer. "I think I have brain cancer and that is why I am like this. Or maybe I have stomach cancer and that is why I can't eat without gagging." While still certain I had some undetermined terminal illness, I became fixated on various psychological disorders. I started reading through my old Social Work study guides on mental illness. I was sure that I had at least one or two personality disorders and possibly some form of psychosis. I even worried that I heard truck horns in the fan in my room. I worried about everything. I couldn't live like that. I had no hope of getting better. I truly believed that I would never be Kathy Goodwin again. I never thought that I would graduate law school. In fact, I told CJ that I couldn't believe that I was ever in law school. I didn't think I would go back and finish my degree. I didn't think that I would ever be able to be the mother that I was meant to be.

The one thing I barely managed to do was to breastfeed Grace. Though I honestly thought that I was going to die, I was committed to making sure Grace was given breast milk. I actually called breast milk banks in order to buy breast milk, but was told that I needed a prescription. Breastfeeding was the one thing that I held on to, but I did not believe that I would be able to continue to do it because of my condition. At one point I was only getting about 800 calories per day, and that was only with the help of nutritional supplement shakes. One dreadful night, when I was feeling like I couldn't go on anymore, I sent a text message to my sister Rachel, who had just given birth to her son. I asked her to make sure that Grace was breastfed if something happened to me. Honestly, I didn't know whether that "something" would be a natural death or if I would get to the point where I couldn't live with myself and would do something about it. I didn't trust myself. One night, CJ told me to take Benadryl in order to get some sleep. I did, and half an hour later I knew that I was dying. It felt like my heart was barely pumping blood through my body. I listened to my heartbeat in slow motion, sure at any moment that it would stop beating. In my mind, the mix of Benadryl and my other medications (Zoloft, and occasionally Lorazepam and Ambien) was causing my heart to stop working. There was no logic or rationality—none. I remember lying there wanting to die, but at the same time I was so afraid of what would happen to Grace. Who would breastfeed her? What would happen to her? What would she think and feel as an older person? I told CJ that I needed to go to the hospital and that I was dying. She told me that I was not dying and that she was not taking me to the hospital. I felt so alone and so lost. I picked up the phone and dialed 911. As the ambulance sirens blared through my neighborhood, CJ angrily came into the bedroom and asked me if I had called 911. I told her that I had. She made comments about Grace being taken away from me and I remember feeling like such a failure. But I was sure that I was dying. The EMS people checked my airways and vitals and said that everything was normal. CJ told them that I had just had a baby. One young man said, "Oh. I have seen this many times before." Then he looked into my eyes and told me that it would get better and that I would be okay. I cried and cried and asked him if he would hug me.

The only people I truly felt connected to during my depression were CJ and my mother. Unfortunately, my mom wasn't able to be there in the beginning of my depression due to her being sick, but she was able to be there for most of it. My mother spent 2 weeks straight at the house with me and Grace. I really don't know what I would have done without her emotional support and physical presence. In addition, I was grateful that during those first couple of weeks, my mother-in-law was in town to spend time with Grace and stayed longer than planned to help us get through the chaos. Looking back, I remember my therapist telling me how important it was for me to keep my connections to CJ and my mother, especially because I had literally pulled myself away from everyone and everything else I knew. However, even with these two connections, I felt myself detaching from everything and there was nothing I could do about it. I was disconnecting from CJ, and I could tell that even my mother was tired of hearing the same things every day, though she never once said so. I was so scared that I wouldn't make it out of the depression.

One thing I did right during my postpartum depression was to reach out for help immediately. I knew something was very wrong and I knew I couldn't live with the depression. I was very open about the way I felt: "I want to die." "I don't want to be here." "I don't want this life." "I don't want to be a mom." I spoke to a close friend of mine about what was going on. She was able to get me in for an emergency visit with her psychotherapist. Meanwhile, within a day of the onset of my depression, I sat in the corner at a healthy restaurant trying to suck down a blueberry smoothie while CJ ate the food that I once loved. I called several psychiatrists that were recommended by Grace's pediatrician and by one of my sisters. I needed to be seen immediately. One of the psychiatrists referred me to another psychiatrist who specialized in women's health and postpartum recovery. She squeezed me in the next day. I will always be thankful for that. I remember filling out the Beck's Depression Inventory, an instrument I had seen many times before but had never filled out myself. All of my answers were extreme and all of them showed a negative response. My psychiatrist stated that based on my responses she would not suggest alternatives to a medication protocol. Even though I was hesitant to take medications, I couldn't agree with her more. There was no way that I could leave there with a prescription for relaxation exercises, a brochure about support groups, or even a list of postpartum therapists. I was so out of control and there was no way I could manage my own care at that point. Having never learned how to swim, I needed something to push me out of the deep waters that I was drowning in. She prescribed Zoloft for the depression, Lorazepam as needed for the anxiety, and Ambien as needed for the lack of sleep. The first day I took Lorazepam, I actually smiled at CJ. I also started seeing a psychotherapist weekly who specialized in postpartum recovery. I was able to crawl out of the hole I was in through with the help of my psychiatrist and my therapist. Did I trust the process? I don't know if I did, but it was the only hope I had. I surely couldn't trust myself at that point. I don't know what I would have done without my family and friends who tried so hard to be there for me, even though I couldn't even be there for myself.

Today, I feel like the luckiest woman alive because Grace is my daughter. Every day, I get to look into her eyes and tell her how lucky I am to be her mommy—and it is true. I can honestly tell you that I never thought that I would be able to live the life I am living. I thought my life was over and now I know that the fear and isolation I felt couldn't have been further from the truth. Grace and I were safe all along, and we were surrounded by love. Looking back at the darkest period of my life, I am so thankful that I gave myself a chance to be me again. But most importantly, I gave myself a chance to be the mother I was meant to be.

Too Few Memories

21

Shauna Moses

Shauna is a 44-year-old mother from New Jersey. She has been diagnosed with depression and in this chapter talks about the loss of her brother to suicide as well as her own personal experience with depression and suicidal thoughts. She also discusses her work with Attitudes in Reverse®, a nonprofit organization with a mission to educate society about mental health.

My amazing son. My wonderful parents and sister. My lovable dog. My closest friends. My rewarding career.

All of these meant nothing to me.

Even though I literally talked to myself, trying to force a focus on all these positives in my life, it didn't have the impact that I hoped for—that I desperately needed. It was frustrating and frightening. It became much more frightening as thoughts of killing myself took over my mind. Depression is a demon that dominates rational thought. Miraculously, the demon eventually yielded just enough for me to stop hurting myself and seek help.

My depression started on July 13, 2003. The day started out fine. I was actually in a phenomenal mood because my 6-year-old son, Harrison, would be coming home after a 2-week visit with his dad. I blasted the stereo and sang exuberantly along with Madonna as I drove home from the food store with bags filled with Harrison's favorites.

As soon as I walked into the house, the music in my head came to a screeching halt, and ever since then, I can't bear to listen to Madonna. The morose expression on my husband's face instantly stopped me in my tracks. Rob told me to call my dad right away. I immediately thought and feared that something happened to my mom. The literally unthinkable had happened. My brother killed himself. My older brother, Mike, who everyone loved and admired, who seemed to have everything everyone could want out of life, had given up everything.

Motherhood, Mental Illness and Recovery, DOI 10.1007/978-3-319-01318-3_21,
© Springer International Publishing Switzerland 2014

As if Mike's death weren't enough of a shock, I was also astonished to learn that he had bipolar disorder. All of a sudden, my brother's amazing, creative sense of humor, his ability to make me laugh so easily was overshadowed by another demon: mania. Could it be true that every time he was in a great mood and entertained the entire family without any effort, he was actually ill? And, sure, I saw him depressed every once in a while. There was always a real—meaning tangible—reason: marital or business troubles, stress over these problems, or, earlier, exams or overwhelming homework in high school and college. Or *did* he always have a concrete reason? Could it be that it was always caused by his brain chemistry? These questions and the images associated with them swirled in my mind at a dizzying speed, making it difficult to stand or see straight.

How could Mike not cheer up by thinking of his beautiful daughter Hannah, who was only four and a half years old at the time and already demonstrated an outgoing personality and sense of humor like her dad's? How could he not be comforted by having many friends who loved him? And how could he take himself away from us? I thought I would never understand what made him take this horrific action.

I understand now.

I have understood since March 10, 2012, when the demon forced a dark, steel tunnel around my head. Without being able to find comfort in everything I have to live for, I felt hopeless and convinced that ending my life was the only way to escape the misery. I drove to a dark, quiet neighborhood miles away from home and cut my wrists. It was more like scratching; I fortunately wasn't able to cause any major damage. Then, I got frustrated and felt like I was an even bigger failure. I thought of crashing the car, but I didn't think that would work. Finally, that glimmer of rational thought broke through the tunnel. I realized I can't do this to my family, so, I went home and told my parents I needed to go to a psychiatric hospital.

The tunnel analogy came from a therapist my mother convinced me to see soon after Mike died. I initially resisted because it made sense that I was depressed and I was convinced that no amount of talking would ever get me to feel better. However, I did eventually agree, and after a while, my therapist suggested that I take an antidepressant. I initially resisted that, too, because I didn't want anything to make me happy, which I learned was a misunderstanding. I agreed after my parents pointed out that I was not as attentive to Harrison as I should be. Nevertheless, I stopped the medication after a few months and my depression resurfaced only occasionally over the next several years, usually during holidays, my brother's birthday, and the anniversary of his death. This was to be expected, so I still did not think I could have a mental illness.

Even when my depression started occurring more frequently and intensely, I resisted going back into therapy because no explanation of mental illness and the behaviors it causes—either my brother's or mine—would ever be sufficient help. I would never accept that the few memories I have of Mike are all I have left of him and that the best of life will always be bittersweet because Mike isn't here to share in our lives. I also didn't think therapy would help me get over the feeling of failure that crept up and dominated my thinking: two failed marriages, several other failed relationships, and... well, actually, I think that was it—really not enough to classify me as a total failure in life, as I know in my current, rational state of mind. However, the depression made it seem like the failures (never mind the fact that my ex-husbands mistreated me, which wasn't my own failure—objectively speaking, anyway) completely defined me. And, while I was dwelling on these failures, my brain decided to dwell on other miserable aspects of my life: my lack of a social life and, of course, the loss of my brother. I became re-obsessed with his death. The recurring thought that kept me down was the fact that I had few memories of Mike and that my family and I would never be able to create more memories with him.

To me, "few memories" is not an understatement. Throughout childhood, Mike and our older sister, Candy, "ganged up on me," as I perceived it back then, and I kept my distance as much as possible in an effort to keep the peace. I was the surprise child, born on July 23, 1969, in Abington, PA, about two and a half years after my brother and just over 5 years after my sister were born. We lived in a row home in Northeast Philadelphia. I remember one of the rare occasions when Mike and I spent time together in a pleasant way. We played "office" in the basement, pretending to have an intercom between our "desks" that were not even two feet apart and using imagined technology to share our equipment, like a "high tech" ruler, to help each other with our projects.

We moved to Lakewood, New Jersey, in June 1976. My fondest memory involving Mike is from my tenth birthday when I got braces before any of my friends did. I sat on our front porch, brooding and feeling like my teeth stretched out for at least a couple of yards past my face. Mike surprised me by insisting on cheering me up, and of course, he succeeded. He drew caricatures and did impersonations of the Village People, the band who sang "YMCA." Of course, I started laughing almost instantly, as I always did when Mike told jokes, imitated people, or generally acted goofy.

Mike and I did not spend much time together in adulthood, either. We only saw each other at typical family gatherings. During some of these occasions, I could not help but notice when he was moody and withdrawn. It was a stark contrast to his usual boisterousness. I knew Mike had problems in his marriage and with his business, so I was concerned, but not worried about his health.

Mike held my son during the bris, a Jewish ceremony when the circumcision is performed on the child's eighth day of life. One day—I don't remember if it was before or after Harrison was born—he told me I was the only one out of us three kids who studied what I wanted to study in college and he admired me for that. It was either this conversation with Mike or another one that could have been months or years later when he gave me the best advice: "Always do what's best for you." I remember his wedding almost 3 months after my first wedding and how his eyes glowed red in the photo of him doing the chicken dance. I remember being at his Senior Prom, as I grudgingly agreed to go with the brother of a friend of mine, and I just watched Mike and his friends having a good time.

Those are my few scattered memories, other than the typical Chanukahs, Mothers' and Fathers' Days, and birthdays. Nearly 11 years after losing Mike, it still pains me to think that we will never create another memory with him.

One more memory just occurred to me. It was in November 2002 when we had a family reunion in California about a year after Candy, her husband, and their two sons moved out there. At Disneyland, Harrison and I sat behind Mike and Jake, one of our nephews, on Space Mountain—my niece, Hannah, was too small to go on the ride—and we laughed hysterically the whole time, more from my brother's silliness than the ride itself. The sound of Mike's laughter, every bit as youthful and exuberant as Jake's and Harrison's laughter, was the best sound ever.

Less than a year later, that precious sound became a bittersweet echo that makes me smile at the memory just for an instant and then gives me a strong urge to cry about how fleeting the time was that we had to enjoy the many gifts Mike offered.

Mike's creativity in his humor as well as in art is truly a gift that has been passed on to Hannah, Harrison, Jake, and Zack, who is Jake's older brother. I have also noticed that I picked up on Mike's style of humor. Especially during family get-togethers, the jokes I make are reminiscent of Mike: the content and the delivery are like impersonations of the master himself. I don't do this intentionally, and when I realize it, it gives me both comforting and eerie feelings at the same time. Comforting I guess because it's keeping a part of Mike alive—as some people would say, although I'm not spiritual enough to truly believe that—and eerie because Mike is supposed to be here to make those kinds of jokes. I never thought of it before, but now I realize it's like I'm subconsciously trying to fill a gap that, of course, could never be filled. While a joke may be funny at the moment, I kind of regret saying it because it's a cruel reminder of our loss—not that any of us could ever forget.

I wish Harrison and his cousins had the opportunity to enjoy Mike's personality for many more years. Of course, it's most painful concerning Hannah. I recently saw her play the lead role in *The Little Mermaid* and I cried because Mike was missing it. I could picture him singing along during the play and acting out scenes with Hannah for days after the performance. But, we are forced to miss out on such heartwarming entertainment and Mike was destined to miss so much more in her life.

It also saddens me that Mike will miss so much in all of our lives. My son is now 17 years old and already looking forward to starting college next year. Mike missed how Harrison has evolved into an impressive young man with a terrific sense of humor, missed the moves Harrison made in football games, and will miss so much more. It seems Harrison has innately learned Mike's advice—to do what's best for yourself—as he has selected his friends wisely and has always been self-disciplined and respectful. It hurts that Mike will never know the positive influence he has had on Harrison and me, and I'm sure on Hannah and our nephews, as well.

I have also evolved in recent years, developing in my confidence in ways I previously would not have imagined and in ways that I'm sure would have made my brother proud. In fact, many of my achievements became possible because of him—not directly because of how he inspired me when he was alive, but mostly because my goals and achievements are centered on helping others with mental illnesses to receive treatment and avoid the tragedy of suicide. From the day Mike died, I was destined to become an advocate for and educator of mental health, behavioral health care, and suicide prevention. Of course, I did not know this at the time.

In 2006, I was looking for a new writing job. When I found the classified ad for Director of Public Affairs at the New Jersey Association of Mental Health and Addiction Agencies (NJAMHAA), I felt I *had* to have this job. It was a unique opportunity to use my writing skills to support professionals who serve individuals experiencing struggles like what Mike endured. My passion became stronger when I had my suicidal experience: a passion to help people with mental illnesses, not only indirectly by supporting behavioral healthcare providers, but also directly by sharing my story of depression and recovery.

Since I was hired, I knew I wanted to write a powerful op-ed piece about losing my brother and how the services that NJAMHAA members provide help prevent the tragedy of suicide. I finally did this in September 2011 and it was published. A few months later, my depression started hitting me more intensely and more frequently. I spent several entire weekends in bed and told my son each time that I had a bad headache or stomachache. In March 2012, I experienced the deepest depression ever, as I started to write about earlier in this story. I went into an inpatient unit for a few days, started on an antidepressant, which I still take, and I worked with a psychologist for a while. In May 2012, I wrote another op-ed describing how my brief hospitalization helped me immensely and I paid tribute to the hospital staff and all other behavioral healthcare providers.

Getting these articles published certainly boosted my confidence and, even more importantly, fueled my determination to help people. At the time, though, I didn't know how to channel my passion outside of the writing I do for my job. My last psychologist advised me to find something to do on the weekends that was meaningful and had a social component because my depression was related to the absence of a social life and the vast amount of downtime, which naturally led to obsessive brooding about what is missing in my life. The opportunity I needed became known to me in October 2012.

During a NJAMHAA conference, a woman brought to me a flyer promoting an event to be held the following May by Attitudes in Reverse® (AIR). The name of this organization and the picture of an adorable Pomeranian caught my attention, so I asked what the group was all about. The little bit I learned that day intrigued and impressed me, and I said I would not only promote the event to our members, but I would also write a feature article in our publication, which is sent to our 180 member organizations and to individuals we advocate to in our state and federal governments.

Several weeks later, we finally worked out everyone's schedule and I interviewed Tricia and Kurt Baker, the cofounders of AIR; Miki, the Pomeranian, their therapy dog; and others who are involved with AIR, either by fostering dogs and training them to be Emotional Support Animals (AIR Dogs) for individuals with mental illnesses and other types of disabilities, or by experiencing the profound benefits of having AIR Dogs. From that day, I have been devoted to AIR. I write a weekly newsletter, press releases, website copy, and occasional op-ed pieces for them; I'm a member of their Board; and when I can, I join Kurt, Tricia, and Miki to speak with middle and high school students about mental health, related disorders, and suicide prevention. I share my experiences with the students and urge them to have a strong support network, to not be embarrassed if they experience symptoms of mental illness and to get treatment, which is proven to be highly effective—and I offer some of that proof.

These experiences have further reinforced my confidence. I have also been on the radio and have planned, promoted, and spoken at an event that NJAMHAA and AIR cohosted.

My involvement with AIR, the articles I've had published and the radio spots I've recorded—as well as my depression and suicidal experience—have served another very important purpose. They have brought Harrison and me even closer and created opportunities to educate him about mental illness and to ensure that he does not develop a stigmatizing attitude and that he knows how to seek help if he ever needs it. He has said he's proud of me and he helps with AIR activities when he can.

Another major factor in the close relationship that I have with Harrison is, ironically, my two divorces. The first one was his father's idea. Harrison and I were fortunate to be able to live with my parents. A couple of years later, we moved in with Rob, who I married soon after that and divorced just a few years later. Harrison and I moved back in with my parents. I don't recall experiencing any intense or long-term depression after either of these divorces. My first divorce was more of a blow to my already weak confidence. During my second marriage, I became a stronger person: Rob talked down to me as my first husband did and I spoke up about the mistreatment, despite having never defended myself during the first marriage. After four and a half years, I finally had enough of the condescending treatment from my second husband and the fact that he tried to restrict Harrison's and my personalities. For instance, he wouldn't allow conversation during dinner, which created an environment that I thought was not good for Harrison. I finally had enough confidence to believe that I did not deserve to be treated this way and, more importantly, that Harrison needed and deserved to live in a happier home. Aside from getting help for my depression, this was undoubtedly the best decision I ever made because it strengthened my relationship with Harrison and enabled both of us to develop confidence.

I believe that becoming a stronger person before my depression became severe enabled me to seek help when I needed it. I think that if I were still weak, I would have succumbed to the depression much more than I actually did. Considering my ex-husbands' statements that I was being dramatic whenever something bothered me, I know that neither of them would have been sympathetic toward my mental illness and, as a result, both of them would have imposed a barrier to my getting help. Even more significant is that I might not have discussed my depression and my brother's suicide with Harrison, which would mean the loss of a critical opportunity for him to better understand mental illness and know how to handle it if it ever became an issue for him.

My message to every mother, whether or not a mental illness is present, is the following: Communicate with your children and be a strong, positive role model. If you do have a mental illness, share that fact with your children if they are old enough to understand. Explain that it is a real illness and nothing to be embarrassed about and tell them how you are managing it. If you need to occasionally spend a day alone to escape depression through sleep, you will still be a positive role model by having a safe, effective way of getting through the depressive episode. It would be the same as if you needed a day in bed to get over a bad cold or a stomach virus.

If you see your children struggling, express your understanding of what they are experiencing, emphasize that help is available, and seek that help as soon as possible. Above all, don't perpetuate stigma. A negative, non-accepting attitude and lack of understanding could ultimately introduce danger into your children's lives.

Thanks to my medication, my productive endeavors through NJAMHAA and AIR, and especially the loving support of my family and close friends, I rarely feel the need to sleep a day away. When this need does arise, I accept it as necessary treatment for an occasional intensification of my chronic depression. Suicidal thoughts do not enter my mind. What convinces me to take the temporary escape is when I feel not only deeply depressed, but also irritable, impatient with everything and thinking—momentarily—that there is no point to doing anything.

So, after a long, deep nap, I wake up with relief that I can safely and successfully deal with my depression. Even more importantly, I feel gratitude not only that my wonderful family and all the other positives in my life exist, but also that I am able to continue enjoying them and making the most of them in my life. That keeps me going and nearly always keeps my depression at bay, where it belongs.

Until a Better Time Comes

22

Joanna Friend

> *Joanna is a 34-year-old mother of two from southwest England. In this chapter she discusses her struggles with labour complications with her firstborn, postpartum mood symptoms and her decision to use antidepressant medications during pregnancy.*

My name is Jo. I live in a village near Exeter in Devon in southwest England. It is a beautiful place full of green rolling hills, beaches and hedgerows. I moved here from the South East when I was 18 to study English Literature at university. After university I went on to study youth work which is where I met my husband Paul. We got married when I was 24 and he was 22 and then settled down where we live now. We had been married for exactly 5 years when I gave birth to our first son Zachary (meaning 'God has remembered'), who is now 5 years old. We also have a second little boy, Charlie Eron William (meaning 'free man', 'peace' and 'joy'), who is 2 years old. I spend most of my time going to toddler groups, running back and forth to school, zooming about the village with Zach on his scooter and making things out of lovely fabric. I love to run, read and sew as hobbies.

My husband and I decided that we wanted to be married for 5 years before we had our first child. We wanted some time together alone before we started a family, so 4 years after we got married we started to try and get pregnant. My periods had always been irregular so I didn't expect to get pregnant quickly and it took us a year to conceive. I found it hard when others around me got pregnant before we did but I felt it would happen at some point. I knew I was expecting when for the third night in a row I got up to use the toilet; something I had never done before. In the middle of the third night I did a pregnancy test and it was positive! I was so excited I couldn't sleep.

My pregnancy with Zach was very easy and smooth. I was happy and relaxed throughout and did suffer some morning sickness in the first 12 weeks but it was manageable. I was fully expecting to enjoy being a mum and was very confident in my mothering ability as I am the eldest of four siblings and felt experienced at looking after babies. I felt that I instinctively knew what to do when the baby was finally born. I was not worried about anything, even the labour.

I went into labour 8 days late and laboured for 27 h. Zach was in a posterior position and failed to turn, meaning that although I dilated to 10 cm I couldn't push him out. He became stuck, and as I was in a midwife unit I had to travel in the ambulance to the main hospital. My local hospital was closed so I travelled another 45 min to the next nearest one whilst fully dilated, Zach's head stuck in my cervix and with only oxygen.

When I arrived in at the hospital I was examined and told by the obstetrician that there was no way for Zach to be born naturally; he was stuck. I was given a full epidural anaesthetic immediately and taken into operating room. First, the obstetrician gave me an episiotomy and tried to manually turn Zach unsuccessfully. I was then prepped for an emergency c-section. As soon as I had the epidural I was happy again and glad that the decision had been taken out of my hands. Zach was born 9 days late and weighed eight pounds eight ounces. I recovered quickly in hospital and healed brilliantly. I felt a real euphoria throughout the 4 days I stayed in hospital and didn't really sleep the whole time I was there. Looking back, this wasn't normal or healthy, but it seemed fine at the time. I now believe I was experiencing mania.

I left the hospital and then on the fifth day after I had Zach I started feeling strange. I felt increasingly anxious as the days went on and was terrified of doing anything with Zach. I loved him and wanted him, but I was so overwhelmed with the responsibility of a new baby that it was making me completely incapable of touching him and interacting with him. I felt like I had no idea what to do with him and felt I was doing everything wrong and that I had made a terrible mistake that I couldn't take back. Mainly on my mind were fears about what I was going to do with him when he was awake, how I was going to get him to sleep through the night and how I was going to stimulate him enough. Breast-feeding was going well physically and I had enough milk for an army, but as feeding time approached I would get more and more anxious until I sobbed through each feeding experience. I was also obsessively reading parenting books and feeling sick with fear at the fact that Zach wasn't behaving as the books detailed. Above all I felt I never wanted to be left alone with him and I kept telling people that I would never be able to look after him on my own.

About 2 weeks after we got home from hospital things came to a head and I started refusing to get out of bed and spent my time howling and screaming in the bedroom. I would shout over and over again 'I need somebody to help me' and threaten to jump out of the window. I didn't want to die; I just wanted to hurt myself badly enough that they would take me back to the hospital and help me look after Zach. After 24 h of this my husband Paul called a friend over who was a nurse. She immediately saw that I was in a serious condition and called the mental health crisis team. They came straight away and gave me some Lorazepam (a sedative) which transformed me into my old happy self in about 20 min. Unfortunately, the effect only lasted for about 4 h.

The next day I went to see a consultant psychiatrist who prescribed Sertraline, an antidepressant. I was to take the sedative with the antidepressant until they started working. Antidepressants take 2–6 weeks to start having an effect and it was an awful time as my body started to adapt to the drugs. After 6 weeks I felt considerably better but still not well at all. I was also not sleeping so they augmented the Sertraline with Mirtazapine, a different type of antidepressant. This combination worked brilliantly for me, and by the time Zach was 6 months old, I was completely fine, happy and enjoying parenthood, caring for Zach alone and really loving life. All this time my church family and my mum had been with me constantly, giving us regular meals and staying with me so I was never alone with Zach until I felt able to be. When Zach was 18 months old I reduced the medication until I was off of it completely and I felt totally well.

Just before Zach's second birthday we decided we would try and get pregnant again (yes, I actually went for it even after the first trauma!). I fell pregnant straight away this time. The day after had my positive pregnancy test I started feeling very sick, much worse than I had with Zach, and when I woke up the day after that I could feel my mood spiralling out of control again. Once again I was in the depths of despair and misery, this time lying on the cold kitchen floor refusing to move and wailing again. It was a Friday, and the doctor couldn't see me until Monday. These were some of the worst moments of my life. No-one can understand the power of mental suffering and the intensity of it if they have not experienced it for themselves. I literally could not see how I could get through the next minute, let alone the 2 days until the doctor's appointment. I had no medication left from my last episode, and even if I had, I felt like I wouldn't have been able to take it as I was pregnant. It felt like I was being tortured, consumed by utter terror. It was unbearable and I finally understood why someone would want to take their own life.

I arrived at the doctor's office on Monday morning an hour early as I couldn't wait any longer, wailing and screaming like I was in labour. They took me straight in and sedated me. Over the next few days I got worse and worse until they finally admitted me into a psychiatric unit. I was there for 4 days while they worked out what medication they could give me during pregnancy. This was the first time I met the midwife specialist from the perinatal mental health team. She came and visited me at the hospital and made an appointment for me with the consultant psychiatrist for when I left.

The team on the psychiatric unit made the decision that I should leave and go home as they thought it better for me to recover in my home environment than if I recovered in hospital and was released at a later stage. I was so anxious on leaving hospital that I was physically sick and sobbing uncontrollably. I was in a terrible state. Because we wanted to protect Zach he went to stay at Paul's parent's house for 3 weeks so I could get better. I at no point feared he would be taken into child protective care as I have a very supportive family and friendship base. I also knew that Social Services strives to keep family units together as far as possible through my work in schools.

During this time I continued to see my psychiatrist. One day as I waited to see her I was getting more and more anxious to the point that when I finally got into the office I was sick all over the floor. I expressed to her that I felt unable to carry on with the pregnancy (I am not someone who would have ever considered abortion before) and that I felt so terrible I didn't see how I could live any more feeling the way I did. It was at this point that she made the judgement that, on balance, the risk to me and the baby was greater if I didn't take medication than if I did. I started taking the Sertraline and Mirtazapine immediately even though there was hardly any research data on taking Mirtazapine during pregnancy.

By the time Zach returned from my in-laws I was on the mend although I never fully recovered during the pregnancy. I went back to living a normal life and caring for Zach, but I suffered from periods of low mood, intense sickness and severe symphysis pubis dysfunction that prevented me from walking in the last month of the pregnancy. I was supported by a weekly visit from a specialist perinatal mental health nurse and less regular meetings with my midwife and psychiatrist. We put together a care plan for after the birth of Charlie which included raising my medication to the maximum dose after he was born and being moved into a family room after the birth so that Paul could stay with me overnight in the hospital.

Charlie was born vaginally 8 days early. I had a 'sneeze' birth which was recorded as lasting 55 min, a real change from Zach's birth! I enjoyed the experience immensely and it is something I really hold on to as being positive after all the difficulties I had had in my pregnancy. I stayed in the hospital for 5 days so that the paediatrician could monitor Charlie as he had been exposed to 9 months of antidepressants. He was very sleepy and wouldn't wake for feeds, and also didn't cry for the first 10 days of his life which broke my heart. I felt immense guilt that I had done this to him even though I had no choice in the matter; it was a case of just surviving. My church had covered Charlie in prayer for the whole time I was pregnant; one lady had an image that Charlie was like a joey in a kangaroo's pouch and was completely protected from what was going on in the outside world and that he would come to no harm. I held on to this image and to God like a climber clinging by her fingertips on a rock face.

It took me 10 weeks for my mood to stabilise after the birth, during which three dear friends rotated nights looking after and feeding Charlie so I could sleep. I found myself absolutely top notch again which proved to me that it had been the pregnancy hormones that had been triggering my mental health issues. Charlie was, and continues to be, a delight. He is the most joyful and peace-filled little person and is totally unaffected emotionally by my months of mental suffering or physically from the medication. I am so blessed that he was protected the whole time I was pregnant and it desperately pains me to think of how I felt I wanted to die and take him with me. However, I know it was the illness speaking and not me. Zach is a calm and contented child who deeply cares for others and has a great deal of empathy. He remembers absolutely nothing of the 3 weeks he was away and also nothing of my suffering in pregnancy. He remembers nothing but me being a stable, normal, fun and reliable mummy who is always there. My boys are absolutely precious to me. I find love, joy and happiness in mothering them and I never wish I had never had them or feel I made a mistake in getting pregnant.

After I gave birth to Charlie I was taking three different medications. One medication I slowly reduced and stopped taking all together about 2 years ago. Eighteen months ago I stopped the second medication. Now, I have nearly completed my taper of the last medication. I would say that I am completely recovered in every way. I am back to the person I was before I had the children, except with two lovely boys as additions. I still have bouts of mild anxiety related to my menstrual cycle, but I allow them to pass and live through them mindfully, and I am definitely more aware of my mood than before. I have had to go through a grieving process where I have felt robbed of my time with the boys as newborns and the enjoyment of pregnancy. I didn't have the opportunity to breast-feed Charlie even once due to the drugs I was taking and this has been a source of sadness to me. I also have to guard against bitterness when watching women sail through motherhood and enjoy all the things I feel I have missed out on. However, I recognise how fortunate I am to have two healthy, loving, fun-filled children who give me so much joy, and I know that many women don't have that opportunity. I am also aware that each person has things in life that cause them pain; they are just different things for each individual. My attitude towards suffering is now to endure it until a better time comes and focus on the good things I have and be positive. I try to never moan about what has happened but rejoice in the good that has come from it. I feel that I am a 'can do' person now.

A strange positive that has come from my experience is that I seem to accidentally meet people who have past or present mental health problems. Many of my friends have experience with these conditions in different forms and I feel I am able to help and understand in a way I couldn't before. I have been able to assist people when they are in need which has been great. A friend of mine who suffers from bipolar disorder even recently held a 'Glad to be Mad' party that I was invited to!!

I would like to communicate to any person experiencing perinatal mental health issues reading this book that you *will* undoubtedly get better. Either medication or therapy will help, or just time passing. An expert once said to me that *everyone* recovers from postpartum depression and it's true. Everyone I know that has suffered has got better. I was extremely ill and now I am totally fine. If you are thinking that you should never have become a mother and that you made a mistake or that you haven't got postpartum depression and it's just your personality that is causing you to feel this way, these are lies and it is the illness making you feel like that. Don't be afraid to speak out about how you feel to a trusted partner or friend or medical professional, as suffering in silence will only make your suffering last longer. It is nothing to be ashamed of.

Finally, don't worry too much about the effect on your children. They are very unlikely to remember it. When my husband was 8 his mum had to spend a lot of time in bed with a neurological disease. Paul only recently mentioned it and I asked him why he hadn't told me before. He replied that it was because he had forgotten all about it and that he only remembers happy times from being a child. You will get over this, you will go on to be the best mum your children could ever need, and they are likely to forget it ever happened. All the best in your recovery.

Post-Traumatic Mothering

23

Janice and Sarah Noble

Janice is a 44-year-old woman diagnosed with borderline personality disorder and posttraumatic stress disorder. She has two children, an 18-year-old boy and a 16-year-old girl. This chapter, written following an interview with Janice, discusses the impact of trauma on motherhood and the importance of screening for mood disorders in the postpartum period.

Introduction

Janice has a history of physical and emotional trauma from her mother throughout her childhood; they have been estranged since she was 18 years old. Because of this she had no model for mothering when she gave birth to her own two children, nor did she have the built-in support of a mother. She suspects that it was this early, repeated trauma that set her up to be a "victim" and perhaps an easy target for the sexual abuse that happened in her teens. Within the course of a year she was raped at knifepoint, sexually assaulted by a teacher for 6 months, and then raped by three members of the basketball team who were coached by the teacher who had been molesting her.

Like many women with a history of trauma she had a difficult postpartum period. Studies show an association between trauma and postpartum depression, depression during pregnancy, and elevated scores on screening tests for depression (LaCoursiere et al. 2012). Others have shown that there is a higher point prevalence of PTSD in pregnant women (7.9 %) than in the general population (4–5 %) (Seng et al. 2010).

In addition, LaCoursiere showed that social stressors around the time of pregnancy can increase the appearance of depression when there is a history of trauma (LaCoursiere et al. 2012). As you will read in Janice's interview, not only was she dealing with the sequelae of her trauma experiences, but following the birth of her

Motherhood, Mental Illness and Recovery, DOI 10.1007/978-3-319-01318-3_23,   195
© Springer International Publishing Switzerland 2014

children, she was struggling financially and had a stressful work environment as well. Her story shows the importance of screening for depression in the postpartum period, as well as the impact trauma can have on parental functioning. In retrospect it was apparent that she would have benefited from treatment immediately following the birth of her daughter, if not during her pregnancy.

With the help of trauma-informed mental health treatment, Janice has been able to carve out a life for herself despite the challenges she has had. Two of the coping methods she has relied on when her PTSD symptoms flair up are vision boards and writing poetry.

I was nervous. I hate to say this but I had always wanted two boys because I just thought boys have it easier in this culture. When I found out I was having a daughter, I was scared. I was scared for the kind of life she would have so it was a worrisome pregnancy. I had been off of psych meds for so long; I had my son first, and then I was breast-feeding him for almost a year, so I was completely unmedicated. And then it was only a short time before we had Gloria and I was nervous.

I really broke down within the first couple of months after having her. No one diagnosed me with postpartum depression. It never came up. It was always considered part of the problems I was already having. I was already facing depression and suicidal thoughts and it was just one more thing. But I felt I wasn't going to be a good mother. I mean, I really panicked and just didn't believe that I deserved these kids. I thought they would be better off without me and I just kept sinking deeper and deeper.

The job I had when I was pregnant with the kids was really easy and my bosses were very accommodating, but I wasn't getting paid very well. So while I was on maternity leave with Gloria, I got recruited to work in the mall in Lerner's, a big clothing store in the local mall. It was also a vertical management position, and a ton more money. So I went back to the place I had been for 3 years and said, "Guess what, I'm back from maternity leave, here's my 2 week notice, I'm quitting right now and I'm going to go work in the mall."

I went to work in the mall and it was so much harder than I had remembered from my previous years. There were so many more problems with the shoplifters, there was sales pressure, the management pressure, hiring, firing, controlling; it was all very hard for me to do.

Because of my physical pain, I was on a lot of painkillers. I was drugged up to the gills, facing depression, every night I used to cry. . . I mean, our district manager made us all cry. And everybody left. We had such a high turnover in the district, like 50 different managers quit. It was a really stressful job. I was there for a year and I never saw Gloria because I was working 12–14 h a day in the mall with an almost hour-long commute.

After I was at Lerner's for 1 year, I went to Mellon Bank. It was hard to work when Gloria was a baby. I felt very distant from her. One day I won some prize; it was a big stuffed lion because I sold the most investment products at the bank. And I gave that to her and I felt so guilty about it because during that effort of trying to sell those products and win the contest, I was never home and I was never with her. There was guilt involved with the amount of work I was doing outside of the house.

When Gloria was 2 years old, I found out that the teacher who had raped me in high school had raped another girl. I went to the police, but they said they couldn't help me because of the Statute of Limitations. They talked to the other girl and she didn't want to press charges. That's what pushed me over the edge. I had a complete and total separation from reality.

I was ready to kill myself. I mean, I was literally trying to find a way to kill myself. I had it all set up. I was trying to cause an auto accident because I knew I would get double insurance from my employer if I died on the way to or from work. But I didn't want to do it myself, so I thought maybe someone else would end my life for me. I was doing really crazy stuff; picking up hitchhikers, stuff like that.

When my shrink found out he put me on disability. He's like, "You don't work again, you're done working. Go on vacation right now." And I freaked out. I felt like the biggest failure. I had always worked. I worked since I was 16 years old. So I shut down. I didn't want to go on disability, I didn't ask to go on disability, I was shocked when my shrink brought it up, and he'd already done the paperwork. I was floored and it just sent me into this tailspin, and I was down for the count for a couple years.

I went crazy. It triggered a complete dissociative thing and I was gone. I was gone to the point where I laid on the couch for a couple of years. I didn't do anything. My husband had to take care of everything. He had to take care of the kids and me. He had to take care of the food, the groceries, the laundry, and cleaning. I was literally on the couch for 2 years. I just thought I didn't deserve my children and I thought they could do better. And I really thought if I were dead, my husband could remarry and find a good wife, a good mother for the kids. I thought I was a bad mom. We were poor and struggling and trying to keep food on the table and trying to do everything we could for the kids and it was it was very difficult. I was having crazy thoughts. Before I was really medicated, I was having thoughts like I was being tested and I had to feed the kids to pass the test. I thought the TV was talking to me.

I did think I was going to lose my kids, although not that social services would take them. I thought they were lost, and they thought I was lost to them. I got that feedback from my family after I started feeling better. They're like "Janice, we never thought you were going to get better. You were just on the couch for two and half years, like we never thought you were going to get up, we never thought you were going to find a way out of that." I never thought I was going to. I thought I was just done, you know. It was a very horrible time in my life and I don't even really remember it.

It wasn't until September 11, 2001, when the planes hit the towers in New York City that I actually got shaken out of my mental fog, and all of a sudden I realized that other people have way bigger problems than me; that I'm obsessed and controlled by my problems from the past, from my high school, and now America is facing real big problems. The irony is, in the end it was a traumatic event that both triggered my symptoms and then saved me from myself.

And then everything that happened politically after that reminded me that I used to be a political activist before I got married, before I had kids, and I found purpose in political activism. So after my kids got older and I started recovering and going through therapy, I got involved in political activism. That's one of the things I do now to keep myself well.

By 2003 I kept having flashbacks in the middle of the night, I was having bad dreams, I wanted to attack people, I wanted to get vengeance on my school and how they hurt me, and I was calling this rape hotline all the time. I was constantly talking to these women and they helped me get a victim's aid grant to get trauma counseling. That's when I really started down the road to recovery. I had a lot of support on the Internet. I joined message boards. The first thing I joined was a rape survivor's message board and that helped me a lot.

I'm doing better now but for so long the mental health system did not help me. When I was honest about my drug use (which was mostly in the past), that was all they wanted to talk about. And I'm like, "you don't understand, I'm not a druggie, I am just a screwed up person trying to escape these memories and trying to escape the feelings that I'm having." So it was not until I got the trauma counseling that I really got the help I needed.

I've also been declined by psychiatrists who don't want to treat a borderline patient. And finding a psychiatrist in private practice who took my insurance [Medicare] was really difficult; the only way I got in with this guy was because my sister was seeing him and she was leaving as a patient because she moved, so she begged him to let me have her slot.

We've also been through counseling with my son and we have a better relationship now. He's almost 18 and things are better now than they were before. There are still some communication obstacles, but I don't think it's related to our childhood problems. I mean, my daughter, she's almost 16 and is a typical teenager. She tells everybody else's mom she loves them, doesn't tell me she loves me. And then, "Mom you know I love you." I'm like, "You never tell me, though."

So I don't think that there are any real negative results from my kind of absentee parenting during their youth. We have a good relationship now, and we can talk more or less. I mean, I think it's normal for teenagers. I don't have anything out of the ordinary. That's even what my son's counselor said. She's like "The things you guys are arguing about are things like finishing your homework. Every parent is arguing about finishing your homework." So it's nothing out of the ordinary.

My husband's parents never pushed him to do anything. He got accepted to West Point, and they were ambivalent about him going. They didn't say "Hey, this is a great opportunity, you should take it, it's a once in a lifetime chance." They were like "Oh, do what you want." His parents were laid-back hippies and all I had were bad parenting models so I tried to do what was good. And now I'm involved with a women's social group. We're all moms and we all talk to each other about parenting and they all have younger kids mostly. So I can say, "I remember that, oh yeah, they're never going to eat those peas so don't even try. Just give up; it's not worth the fight." Sometimes I'm not sure if I have the right advice or not. I can only talk about my own experience and my own results. But I like to say the proof is in the pudding, I have two well-behaved kids who get good grades and people welcome them in their homes and so I'm proud of my kids.

I just did the opposite of what my mother did. I keep the kids in sports, I try to encourage them to get good grades. They're on honor roll and they do really well. And I try to do all those mom things; they want a ride to the mall, they get a ride to the mall. They want me to bring five of their friends, I bring five of their friends. I'm the taxi mom, that's what I call myself. My parents never drove me anywhere and my husband thinks I spoil the kids by driving them all over, but I'm like "I don't want them walking around crossing big highways when it just takes me five minutes to drive them where they're going." I don't think that's spoiling them, and I want to do that mom stuff. I mean, I'm the mom that has the Kool-Aid on the cabinet for when company comes over. I'm the mom that tries to have snacks on hand.

In the women's group I found a sense of community that I didn't have before. At first I needed them to help me navigate through some of the feelings I was having and now I'm able to relax and enjoy and just have a night where I'm not doing activism, I'm not selling my group, I'm not getting people to sign a petition. So I have more of a well-rounded life now than I've ever had. And I try to keep well-rounded and try to expand my boundaries and make more friends, network with more people, do more things. I don't want to be saddled by my mental illness. I'm still seeking a sense of unity and friendship with other women and especially other parents. And I haven't found that in my town so I found that on the Internet and through this group a couple of towns over.

I still have problems, sometimes I have to stay home and it's hard for me to do some events. I do a big event then I stay home and I'm in my pajamas for 2 days because it takes a lot out of me. If I have to give a speech it takes me a couple of weeks to gear up. I do it and then it takes me a couple of days to calm down from having done that. Sometimes I can get into a conversation with someone that will get emotional and then I'll just get over emotional and I can't regulate my emotions on my own. But I do things now like meditation, which is hard for me, and I've made vision boards, which is where you cut out positive uplifting statements and flowers and stuff. The vision boards help me meditate and focus on my goals. I'm just seeking personal harmony.

I guess if I had one message, it would be that you can recover, depression can be beaten, it's treatable, it's a medical symptom of an underlying problem that is treatable. Borderline personality doesn't go away, but it's still manageable. You can still have a life even if you have the black-and-white thinking and those impulsive behaviors.

"Anniversaries"
12/28/2001
Here we go back in time across that borderline
And everybody knows I can't afford to travel
Now I feel the whole thing wasn't real
But unfortunately I'm still me-
So Uncle Sam pays me Social Security
And I'm in poverty on Disability
Yes I would rather be out in the world working
But I am usually a liability
 'Cause
 All those things that no one wants to talk about

Is all that's on my mind, yeah
And all those things that no one wants to hear about
I'm fearing all the time, yeah
   I'm just a little bit crazy
   You can't change me
So if you talk to me I promise you will see
The reason why they tell me I am crazy
I used to see the man but my insurance plan
Said all I needed was another pill-
I tried art therapy seeking recovery
I drew a calendar for my anniversaries
But all that they could see was my drug history
And they discounted the weight of all those dates
And
   All those things that no one wants to talk about
   Is all that's on my mind, yeah
   And all those things that no one wants to hear about
   I'm fearing all the time, yeah
     I'm just a little bit crazy
     You can't fix me
Forget the counselor I need an editor
A little funding and a major publisher
It sometimes makes me laugh no one will see these drafts
I cannot complete tasks unless you kick my ass-
No nothing's stopping me except reality
The insecurity and my personality
So what gives me the right to bitch and moan and whine
I can express myself ever so eloquently
But
   All those things that no one wants to talk about
   Is all that's on my mind, yeah
   And all those things that no one wants to hear about
   I'm fearing all the time, yeah
     I'm just a little bit crazy
     Just crazy

References

LaCoursiere DY, Hirst KP, Barrett-Connor E (2012) Depression and pregnancy stressors affect the association between abuse and postpartum depression. Matern Child Health J 16:929–935

Seng J, Rauch SAM, Resnick H et al (2010) Exploring posttraumatic stress disorder symptom profile among pregnant women. J Psychosom Obstet Gynaecol 31(3):176–187

Emotional High to Deep Despair

Helen Broome

Helen is a 37-year-old mother from England. She was diagnosed with post-partum depression following the birth of her son and in this chapter she discusses her birthing experience, as well as the treatment and support she received from The Beeches service at Royal Derby Hospital, a national forerunner in the inpatient and outpatient care of mothers with perinatal illness.

My illness began shortly after I found out I was pregnant. It was February 2010 and John, my husband, and I had been trying for a baby for some 15 months when we got a positive pregnancy test. Our initial thoughts were happy ones. I was glad that we had finally conceived but then slowly but surely (after we did the second test just to be sure the next day) my mind went into a total panic and I thought " Oh my gosh"! "I have no idea about how to look after a baby." "What on earth am I going to do"? "How do I make sure that our baby is okay when it is developing inside me"?

These were just some of the questions and thoughts that I had which eventually manifested themselves in severe anxiety. John and I went to see our family doctor who failed to allay my fears about becoming a mum. He confirmed my pregnancy and rather than providing a raft of leaflets, websites, and information he merely told me to think happy thoughts for a happy baby and eat green leafy vegetables!

We decided that we could not keep the pregnancy a secret. I needed to talk to someone and that someone was my mum. I arrived at her house in a flood of tears. She was concerned something had happened to John or our cats and I just blurted out that I was pregnant, I was going to be a mum, and I hadn't a clue what to do. I spent the whole day crying unable to square in my mind why I was like this. I was happy yet incredibly sad at the same time. My emotions were in turmoil.

I worried every minute of every day. I was strict with myself on taking vitamin and mineral supplements and I cut down my caffeine intake from off the scale to

Motherhood, Mental Illness and Recovery, DOI 10.1007/978-3-319-01318-3_24,
© Springer International Publishing Switzerland 2014

two cups of caffeinated drinks per day. I ate a sensible diet and restricted my intake of what I found out were banned foods. I don't smoke and never drank. I didn't want to take any chances.

We got to the 3-month milestone and saw a midwife for the first time. We filled out numerous forms and the conclusion from the meeting was I was fat, old, and with depression in my family I was at risk for all sorts of pregnancy complications. That did nothing to put my fears to the back of my mind. The leaflets and booklets we had were filed straight into the news rack. I couldn't read them. It was like I was in denial that I was pregnant. I was unable to feel happy just in case something awful went wrong or my baby was born less than perfect.

Our association with the first midwife we saw was brief. I made a complaint about her timekeeping and seeming obsession with my weight and her inability to take blood from me forcing a visit to another hospital. At this point I was introduced to another midwife, with whom immediately I felt in safe hands. Our initial meeting was difficult. I explained to her my fears and anxieties and she was empathetic and willing to help me. As I was in tears at every session and continued to struggle with coming to terms with becoming a mum, she referred me to The Beeches, a specialist mother and baby service at the Radbourne Unit, at the Royal Derby Hospital.

In July 2010, some 5 months into my pregnancy, I had my first appointment with a psychiatrist. I had mixed feelings about the appointment as I didn't really know what to expect when visiting a psychiatrist. The appointment was difficult for me. John accompanied me and I spent a sum total of an hour talking about earlier episodes of depression in my life, my fears, my anxiety, and my inability to bond with the baby inside me for fear of something happening: something cruel, which would see my baby being born ill or worse.

My psychiatrist could clearly see that I was struggling. She arranged another appointment to see her in 4 weeks. I continued to see my midwife and then someone new came on the scene, a senior occupational therapist who my psychiatrist recommended. Before I became ill I had no clue that such a service existed for women suffering from perinatal and postnatal illness. Furthermore, I had no clue that occupational therapists worked with people who had mental health issues. I was clearly naïve and I was soon to have my eyes opened to a service which quite literally has turned my life around.

My second meeting with my psychiatrist saw no change in my mental well-being. My sleep was poor from worry and I was tired and exhausted from the burden of carrying a baby and the burden of its care. The doctor explained the options to John and I about medication. After hearing what she had to say I was adamant that I would not medicate myself as no guarantee could be given about the effect on unborn babies. I would never forgive myself had my baby been born with something wrong with him; I would have attributed it to any medication I chose to take. I was reluctant even to take over-the-counter pain medications, let alone an antidepressant. At no point did the psychiatrist try and impose a view on us. She accepted the decision and scheduled further meetings and knew that both my midwife and occupational therapist were monitoring my mood.

My mood continued to plummet. As a teacher, I had a whole summer holiday to dwell on what was going on and the nearer the birth became the more and more anxious I got. I couldn't talk about having a baby. I just ended up in floods of tears.

During the summer of 2010 my midwife arranged a visit to meet the matron of the maternity unit at the hospital we had elected to have our baby. The meeting for me was horrific. The matron's office was next to a delivery room and all I could hear was screaming, shouting, and swearing and it heightened the feelings I was having. John and I, along with my midwife, spoke about my anxiety and my referral to The Beeches. Further visits were arranged and planned including a familiarization visit one evening. We saw the delivery ward and because of my issues surrounding being "clean" during the birth I was shown a side room with its own facilities and this was the room I would be given when the time came to have my baby.

My baby was due on October 8th and sadly this date came and went. Further issues in my antenatal visits leading up to and after my due date served to make matters for me worse. I was booked for an induction on October 19th. The day before my induction I finally plucked up the courage to read a how-to guide about birth, childcare, and the like! I had no sleep all that night. I was nervous, anxious, and tried to persuade John not to make me go to the hospital the next day. John was insistent. The journey to the hospital was awful. I felt sick and worried that something was wrong with me and/or my baby as he hadn't yet arrived.

The induction process was a living hell; not at all like photocopied pamphlets we were handed on the day of the booking. That night I was left in the worst possible pain of my life. I thought something serious had happened. Pain relief was denied as I'd already had the limit of pain medication for that day and I had strict instructions in my birth plan stating a preference for medications that do not cross the placenta.

My occupational therapist had taught me breathing exercises as part of managing my anxiety and panic attacks. I had fortnightly meetings with her in the outset of my pregnancy. I was so thankful to her whilst kneeling on the floor alone in a side room clinging to a chair. The breathing exercises were invaluable to help prevent my blacking out with the pain I was suffering. This ordeal went on for hours and hours. I was not going to have the pain medication that crossed the placenta and whilst some may say that this horrifying experience was of my own doing, I would argue that I had the right to choose.

On October 21, 2010, at 9:37 am an emergency cesarean section was performed. I felt totally calm. All of the stress, panic, and "wrongs" I had suffered whilst in the hospital were put right. I had a beautiful 9-pound, 12-ounce baby boy who was perfect in every way. I dared to believe that I had got over the worst, but little did I know, it was just the beginning.

My baby was ravenously hungry and I opted to feed him myself. At first all seemed okay. I was sore and tired from my sleep deprivation for some 3 days and I was anxious about caring for him on my own when John was forced to leave the ward for the night. The nights were terrible. I continued to go without sleep as George cried and cried as he was hungry. I was trying my best to feed him and fill him up so I could sleep, but it simply didn't happen. I had another sleepless night in hospital and after another night, day five without sleep, I agreed that George could have some formula and I got a whole 3 h rest.

We arrived home as a family and opted to combination feed George. I wanted so much to feed him myself, to develop a bond, and to have that quality time with him but after 8 days I ceased doing so. Mastitis and the fact I spent an hour feeding him myself and then topping him up with three ounces of formula every 3 h took its toll. I had failed again in my eyes. I failed to give birth to him naturally and I failed to feed him.

The cold, dark month of November seemed to linger long. I felt like a bird with my wings clipped. I wasn't allowed to drive myself around owing to my C-Section, I was constantly clock watching so I could feed George on time, and John had to return to work after his paternity leave, one week of which was spent in the hospital. My parents, in-laws, cousin, and friends came to visit and I put on what I call my party face. Happy and smiling and trying to convince the world I was loving being a mum. Inside I was exhausted, tearful, felt sore from my operation, and my anxiety was through the roof.

I had a Health Visitor visit to check myself and George. She made my fears and feeling of inadequacy worse. I did the Edinburgh postnatal test and came out with a score which indicated depression. I laughed it off and tried to say that all mothers feel the way I did; I didn't see the Health Visitor again.

My deception about my coping continued. I saw my clinicians and told them I was fine and that I was wasting their time and that other people should have my appointment space. I guess the occupational therapist had heard it before and saw me a week later to set her own mind straight. She discharged me and I was free of these people who in my opinion were all waiting for me to fail.

January 2011 saw me eating my own words after issues with my husband over him hiding things "to make me go mad" and shouting at my mum, who for some 3 months religiously came down to help me each morning with George. I found myself ringing John (who was trying his best to hold down a very responsible job), constantly in tears and telling him I could cope and couldn't do this and having thoughts of burning my washing as I couldn't cope with getting it washed and dried on a particularly wet day. My mum, dad, and in-laws were already offering daily support, cooking and cleaning. I was unable to do the things I believed I should as a mum and wife. The time had come to acknowledge that I was ill. I couldn't maintain the façade any more. I made the decision to ring my occupational therapist and ask for help.

I wouldn't have blamed her or my psychiatrist for putting me to the back of the queue. My therapist visited and hastily arranged a visit to the Psychiatrist. I was exhausted constantly, couldn't look people in the eye, couldn't remember things, couldn't hold a conversation, and my sleep pattern, despite my exhaustion, was terrible. My brain wouldn't let me rest. I would go over and over things, I clock watched, and I was like a "cat on hot bricks," unable to settle and enjoy normal things. I struggled to be what in my eyes was a "normal" mummy. It was so stressful taking George out, I felt people were looking at me, judging me, waiting for me to fail again.

I opted to take medication. The first medication I had failed to have any impact on my mood. My psychiatrist listened to my ramblings and of course consulted with my therapist at team meetings so that she was informed and able to make further suggestions to me. My psychiatrist always spoke to me politely and courteously. She was respectful that I am a chemistry teacher and as a consequence needed to know everything and how it worked. I felt part of a decision-making process which was aiming to get me well.

My second medication didn't suit me either. Whilst it was lifting my mood the side effects were awful; I developed huge boils under my arms from the severe sweating it caused and that made me even more miserable. My mood plummeted again. All through this time my therapist was there for John and I. I frequently told John that he and George would be better off without me. My meetings with the therapist seemed to start with me in tears and end with me in tears. I was negative and saw no way out of the despair that I was in. The whole time she remained positive. Her weekly visits were invaluable to me and my family. She always told me I would get well. That I needed to be kind to myself. That I needed to have priority A's, B's, and C's. She offered practical advice about taking George out and about. She offered advice that only someone who was a mum herself could. She was a godsend!

It was discussed and agreed that I had a day to myself each week. George went to his grandparents to give me a break. At first I was wracked with guilt. I was his mummy and I should be looking after him. I spent much of the day in bed asleep but that was what I needed. I struggled to balance my unrelenting desire to be a good mum, a good wife, and a good friend with the overwhelming desire to rest. I felt totally wiped out and exhausted after doing very little. My immune system was shot, I seemed to pick up colds, coughs, sinus infections, ear infections, and all sorts and this just dragged me down further.

My third medication and the warmer, brighter days saw my mood slowly start to lift. I kept a diary of my days and wrote two positives and one negative each day. I scored my day out of five and John was overjoyed when I told him I felt like I was "normal" for just one day!

The support continued from The Beeches. I saw the nursery nurse on several occasions and she helped with ideas about weaning George, answering questions I had about his development. I also met a mental health midwife specialist, who went through my maternity notes with me over four long sessions. I had questions I needed answering about my pregnancy, my treatment in hospital, my failure to give birth, and my failure to feed George. Her expertise was invaluable and answered lots of nagging questions I had. The sessions were exhausting. Reliving what was a nightmare time temporarily caused a huge dip in my mood. I summoned up the courage to lodge a complaint about my treatment at the hospital regarding my antenatal care and outpatient appointments.

My psychiatrist and therapist were unwavering with their support. I had a care plan which worked in steps to get me well and back to work. July 2011 was when I should have returned to work. I was in no way fit to teach at that time and I was given a sick note. My employer was fully aware of my issues and following procedure referred me to occupational health. This freaked me out. I was anxious about the interrogation I would suffer. I thought that I would be judged. My therapist attended every single occupational health review meeting with me; I took my letters from my psychiatrist and was fully supported over my inability to work at that time.

In January 2012 I returned to my job. My therapist attended my return to work interview along with my union, head teacher, and local authority personnel advisor. My phased return to work was negotiated over an 8-week period (the longest my head teacher had ever offered). The support from The Beeches team was acknowledged and it was agreed that I should see occupational health twice during my return period to ensure my needs were being met.

Returning to work, albeit part-time, was a major shock. I felt de-skilled, my memory had gone, I couldn't do all of the things I could do so easily when I left to have George. My therapist continued to support me as did my psychiatrist. They helped put strategies in place to help me cope. They stressed the importance of keeping my scales balanced. My therapist was always on the end of the phone when I needed her and for that I am eternally grateful.

In August 2012 I was finally discharged from the care of The Beeches. It was a major milestone for myself and my family. It was a happy day and whilst I acknowledge that I am still taking my medication and probably will forever, I would rather be that than be as low as I was when I was severely ill. No one can appreciate how debilitating this condition is if they have not suffered it.

The Beeches program and its staff are wonderful. It is a program that offers completely tailored care to the whole family as it is not just one person who suffers when someone has postnatal depression. As a "thank you" for everything I have received, I decided, and this bares testament to my recovery, to raise some money to help the program. I organized a grand raffle by writing to local and national firms/organizations telling them about my illness and the help received. I also got funding for the raffle tickets and license from the council and hosted a Pampered Chef evening in September 2012. I estimated I received donations for prizes totalling over £500. Another £834.50 came from my family, friend, and colleagues who were also so generous. I hope I can, even in a small way, help the team who helped me and my family come through a terrible illness.

I always smile when people say "you're a lifesaver"; often this phrase is used too flippantly. I mean it when I say that without the help and support I got from my program, I wouldn't be here today. Yes, I missed milestones in my baby's life such as his Christening and his first Christmas and I have hazy recollection of his first holiday and birthday. At 37 years of age I feel that I now know more about myself that I ever dreamt possible. I have learned to recognize my triggers to low mood and I am aware of my priorities in life. I have a beautiful, bright, and lively little boy and a fabulously supportive and tolerant husband and I am thankful that I have been allowed to experience what being a "proper family" is like after nearly 3 years of battling depression.

On October 21, 2012, George turned two. He had a fabulous party and yes he is spoiled by his parents and his grandparents. I am thankful to have the chance to spend quality time with him as I still work part-time in order to keep myself well. I am looking forward to the future: a future I didn't believe could or would be possible.

It's Okay to Get Help

25

Jennifer Christine Milner

Jennifer is a 31-year-old mother of two from New Jersey, currently living in California. In this chapter she discusses her mental health history including suicide attempts and cutting, as well as parenting in the context of domestic violence.

I am 31 years old. I grew up in Budd Lake, New Jersey, a small town full of farms and woodlands. I have a twin sister and a younger sister. Both my parents were ministers. We all grew up sheltered and very religious. At different times we would have church members living with us in the house and, for a while, we had a live-in nanny. We were not rich but always comfortable, middle to upper-middle class.

I first became a parent at age 24. At the time, I was in a very violent and abusive relationship with my daughter's father. He took me from Jersey to Virginia. He always threatened to have my child taken away if I ever called the cops because of my previous mental health record. Before I met him I had been in and out of inpatient psychiatric wards and two halfway houses for the mentally disabled.

For three years, his threats worked on me and I was scared. When I finally did call the cops, my daughter really was taken away! I was not receiving any mental health services and didn't ask for any which resulted in my losing custody of my daughter. I then married at 28 and had another child at 29. My husband had his own mental health problems and history of being in psych wards and knew about my past history. When I had our son, he used the same domestic violence tactics as the father of my daughter had to make me follow him around the country to keep my child and put up with the abuse. I finally got away from him as well, but he took custody of my son away from me. Child Protective Services took custody of my son away from his father a few months later. CPS gave custody back to me about a month later. I was okay for a while. Then I had some more mental health problems, ended up cutting myself, and lost custody again to CPS. It took a month to get my

Motherhood, Mental Illness and Recovery, DOI 10.1007/978-3-319-01318-3_25,
© Springer International Publishing Switzerland 2014

son back. It's been 6 months and I have retained custody and gotten mental health help.

It took me a long time to realize I needed help. Growing up, my family didn't believe in mental illness. They thought I just needed to be taught how to control my mind and emotions. When I was feeling anxious or upset, they said I was possessed by evil spirits and that my mind was "too weak" for an exorcism to work.

I remember a few times as a young teenager the school requested that I get a psychiatric evaluation. My parents would say it was against our religion and it wouldn't happen. I have had over 20 suicide attempts. I have been a cutter since age 15 or 16. I suffered from anorexia since about the same time. I have been on and off medication and in and out of inpatient and outpatient programs since I was 18. I have tried halfway houses and shelters, been homeless, and used drugs for self-medication. I have been given multiple diagnoses: bipolar, borderline schizophrenic, suicidal/homicidal tendencies, dissociative personality disorder, PMDD, severe anxiety, and PTSD.

When I cut myself and lost my son in December 2012, I have made a serious effort to get better, to keep my son. I have stayed on my medication. Thankfully the mental health program here in Placer county found the right combination of meds that actually work and help me. I half-heartedly tried in other places but never got the kind of help I received here. During my hospitalization in Reno in 2011, they put me on three different medications. They all gave me terrible side effects and made me feel that I would never be awake enough to take care of my son. So I stopped them as soon as I got out of the hospital. It was a combination of treatment that didn't help and not making the best choices on my part. I'm glad now to be in treatment that is working and that I am taking it seriously. Before, I never really made that decision. I was tired of living this chaotic life and really wanted help and to get better. I now have my own apartment, a small studio, but still my own place for the first time where I make my own rules. It is scary and difficult at times. I still get help from counselors, friends come over and help sometimes, and I get checked up on. But, I am doing much better! I have better self-esteem, and feel like a productive part of society again.

My mental health history was of course, used against me as threats from the fathers of my children, unfortunately those threats came true and I lost custody of both of my children. I eventually got my son back but permanently lost parental rights to my first child. My bad relationships and my mental health problems caused quite a bit of extra stress with my children, and I didn't handle situations well. I never injured or seriously endangered my children, but I did make poor choices. I have learned a lot through parenting classes, and my therapists have helped me gain tools for patience and parenting skills with my mental health issues.

Unfortunately with my son, I have seen him copy behavior of mine, I see him lose his temper and experience anxiety. For a while he started eating less because I didn't eat. I would feed him but not myself, and he started not eating unless I sat down to eat with him as well. Losing my first child completely and facing the same possibility with my second is what gave me most of my courage, strength, and resolve to get better.

The challenges for me have always been patience, not getting so frustrated and anxious, and being able to control my outward actions. What helps me keep going are victories like getting custody of my son back, improving manners, and not having temper tantrums—changing bad behavior to positive, both for my son and for me!

My son is only two and a half years old, but he has seen my scars and often asks if I'm ok. I always tell him yes, but he can tell when I start getting upset or scared, and usually tries to hug me. I feel bad about that, (especially when he sees me cry), but his response usually helps me shake it off faster so I can be a good mom.

If I could start to get better and make progress in life at age 30, anyone can. It's never too late. There are always more tools and resources you can get and use. I would tell any other mother out there facing problems, don't feel ashamed to ask for help. Don't feel ashamed to need help. No one is perfect and no one can be Supermom all the time. Use the love for your children as your strength and motivator to get through the hard humps.

Hope Soars

26

Paula Ward

> Paula is a 50-year-old mother from Oklahoma. She was diagnosed with bipolar disorder and posttraumatic stress disorder only a short time ago, and in this chapter she reflects on the impact her childhood physical, sexual, and emotional abuse and subsequent substance abuse has had on parenting her children.

My name is Paula. I grew up in Madill, Oklahoma, approximately 15 miles north of Lake Texoma. My mom was 15 and my dad 16 when they married. They were 21 and 22 they started having children, and ultimately had two daughters and one son. My sister was born in 1961, I was born in 1963, and my brother was born in 1965. My dad was and still is a semi-truck driver following in his father's footsteps, leaving my mom to care for three young children.

Although my mom's parents were always ready and willing to help out in any way possible, my mom still physically, mentally, and emotionally abused us, especially my sister and I. My sister and I have had flashbacks, but my brother remembers nothing at all. My mom would tell dad things that we had supposedly done (things that we never would have dreamed of doing) and dad would go so far as to drag us out of bed in the middle of the night when he got in and spank us with his belt, while getting on to us for whatever mom had told him. We never denied it for fear of getting a worse spanking because he thought we were lying. I can remember one time my mom hit my sister across the back of her knee; it swelled up so big that she could hardly walk, and mom told her: "If you tell your Memaw or Papaw or anyone I will do it again, but worse next time." My sister, brother, and I had to do all the cooking, cleaning, laundry, taking care of all the animals, and taking care of a huge garden, which we had to hoe by hand because we didn't have a tiller. If my mom found the least little thing out of place or "not done right" she would break wooden broom and mop handles across us wherever it happened to hit. I remember being about 6 years old and I didn't hang a long sleeved shirt up "right" so she knocked me to the ground, began kicking me and yelling: "What's wrong

Motherhood, Mental Illness and Recovery, DOI 10.1007/978-3-319-01318-3_26,
© Springer International Publishing Switzerland 2014

with you? Why can't you do anything right? Are you that dumb and stupid?" I heard things like that not only from her, but from my dad also. I remember being 12 or 13 and believing that I was retarded or something. In junior high I stayed grounded all the time because I always seemed to have at least one "D" on my report card. That always started another discussion of my being dumb and stupid; I was even told that I "wasn't coordinated" enough to mow the grass.

I began playing softball, but my parents never drove the three miles to watch me practice or play. Yet, every weekend they would haul my sister and her horse and later on my brother and his horse from Madill, Oklahoma, to Bowie, Texas, to race, getting home anywhere from 4:00 am to 7:00 am Sunday mornings. Since they couldn't support me I quit playing softball.

Our uncle would sexually molest both my sister and I when we were young. Neither one of us understood what was happening neither did we understand that it was wrong. He told us that if we told anyone that we would get into trouble, so once again we were forced to keep silent. My family should have known something was going on because of some of my actions, but no one seemed to be willing to rescue me or my sister.

I didn't realize just how much this had affected my life until I started seeking mental health services approximately a year ago. I didn't realize that most everything I was doing wrong stemmed back to the childhood abuse that I went through, and how the abuse traumatized me to the point that I started using drugs and drinking heavily to numb the pain that I was carrying inside of me. I didn't realize that by doing so I was putting myself at risk of being abused and traumatized even more, which was exactly what was happening.

I got married 2 weeks after I graduated high school to the man who introduced me to both alcohol and drugs and who also turned our marriage into a dictatorship. The alcohol came first: we would go out dancing every weekend and I usually got drunk, but I also realized that it felt good to numb the pain I had carried inside for so long. So began my life as an alcoholic. After we had been married about 6 months I began wanting a baby, but I had trouble conceiving. I went to a gynecologist who after examining me suggested I drink a little wine and relax and that I was too uptight. I started getting very drunk but nothing worked. My husband's brother-in-law was a drug dealer, so they began telling me: "If you will smoke just one joint, it will mellow you out and you will get pregnant." I wanted to get pregnant so desperately that I finally gave in and I tried it, and they were right, I got pregnant. I didn't smoke while I was pregnant with my son, but I did start back up after I had him. So began my drug addiction.

My husband would make sure he had his pot before our bills got paid and we had food. Once I had our son I wasn't allowed to work, as my place was at home. When we would get cutoff notices, he would go to his parents and they would give him however much money he needed with no questions asked. When I got pregnant with our daughter and my son was a toddler, my husband would leave me at home with no phone or vehicle. It just so happened that his mom came and got me to go home with her on a Thursday before I went into labor that Sunday.

Within about 4 years I was smoking a joint every 2 h, from about 2 o'clock in the afternoon until I went to bed—and I also had a whiskey and soda pop mixed in. One day I was watching TV and a commercial using a fried egg to symbolize your brain on drugs came on and I decided right then that I no longer wanted to live like that. So I told my husband it was either the drugs or me and the kids and that I was giving him a month to change. I guess he didn't think I was serious because nothing changed, so after a month I put my kids to bed and then I told him to call his mom because I was divorcing him.

I was single for about a year, and then I married a man who couldn't keep his pants zipped around other women. After I had proof of that I managed to hold the marriage together for a while, and then we divorced. After another 6 or 7 months I remarried a man who always had a beer in his hand, but he treated both my kids and me good, that is, until he beat my son who was 9 years old at the time. I tried to work it out, but he began coming home more and more reeking of whiskey and getting violent with me, so I divorced him too.

I moved back home, and went back to work at a nursing home, and before long I made friends with a girl who I was giving rides to and from work. This girl lived close to a convenience store, and one day I stopped in there and met a guy who seemed nice. Somehow my dad found out that I was seeing the guy, and he came to my house and called me all sorts of names and threatened to take my kids away from me if I kept seeing this man. I arrived home one day when I expected my kids should have gotten home about 5 min before I did, but when I got home no one had seen them. I went to my parents' house and learned they had kidnapped my kids (even though they were on the school's pickup list, they did so without my consent) and it took me an hour to get my kids away from my mom. I decided to leave town after that.

I gave my ex-husband temporary custody of the kids with the agreement that when I got set up in Kentucky that he would send the kids out to me. But when I called for him after I got settled he claimed that he was not sending them to me. So I came back to Madill, got a job in a local nursing home, and moved in with my parents. After a while I rented a house from my parents right across the road. My son decided to live with his dad, and my daughter wanted to live with me. When I moved in across the road from my parents I never thought about how much control I was giving to them. When I was at work my daughter was usually with either my mom or my dad, mostly my dad. They bought her school clothes and her sports equipment because after paying my bills I was lucky to have 50 dollars left to get 2 week's worth of gas. If I made plans on my day off with my daughter that conflicted with something my mom had planned for her it was always a fight. It became easier to just let it be, which I should have been strong enough to never allow. I wasn't emotionally, physically, or financially capable of fighting with my mom. She was and still is a drama queen and if she can keep the pot stirred she will, often using any means to do so, and no matter how much or whom she hurts in the process. If my dad catches wind of something she will lie and turn it around so anyone else is at fault and she's done nothing wrong, and of course he will believe her every time. She has even started a fight with me in front of my daughter and threw in my face all they provided for my daughter and then said; "What do you provide?" as if I didn't appreciate their help, which was not true. Although I didn't appreciate her not allowing me to be a mom to my kids, I had no say over what my daughter did and did not do, my mom did, and I couldn't do anything about it. One day my daughter decided she wanted to move to Lone Grove, Oklahoma, which was closer to where I worked, so I began looking for a house. When my parents saw that we were serious about moving they threatened my daughter that if she moved they would sell all her cattle and her horse and told her that we wouldn't make it. All that did was make her more determined to move, and eventually we did.

Shortly after the move I began to drink again, putting myself at risk of more abuse and trauma. After about 2 years my daughter and I got into an argument and she moved out to live with her father. That was about 10 years ago. I then met my husband that I am married to today; we have been married 8 years now. He has been the only one who has willingly stuck by my side regardless of the circumstances and he is the first person who has been willing to support me even in my worst times. Neither one of my kids has anything to do with me because of my lack of being the parent they desperately needed me to be. I wasn't strong enough to fight my parents. Nor did I have the proper tools to be the parent I should have been. I did try to be the only kind of parent that I could be at the time, sadly it wasn't enough for them.

I can see now after being in counseling, and being diagnosed with bipolar and posttraumatic stress disorder how my childhood abuse and trauma has played a part in ruining my life and my relationships with many people, especially with my kids. Before counseling I was always on edge and always uptight. I was fighting everybody and my life was in constant chaos. I just wanted to die; I even jumped out of a vehicle going down the road, and I even prayed that I would die. I remember telling my husband that I felt like I was a dart board, with everybody throwing darts at me for the fun of it. I felt horrible. I finally walked away from my parents, and today I do not allow drama in my life at all, and if someone wants to create drama, they can stay away from me. I started seeking counseling about a year ago: I am in group and individual counseling, and I visit with a peer supporter. I am now also a member of The Church of Christ. I now for the first time in my life have full control of my life and I no longer drink, do drugs, nor do I smoke cigarettes. For the first time in my life I feel calm inside, and I feel strong; my life in general is a lot calmer. There is no more chaos in my life, and I enjoy being alive today. I am now taking psychology classes online and I believe both my classes and my counseling are the reason why my life so much better today. But I had to make that first step which is the hardest, that is, to seek mental health treatment.

Part IV

Voices of Mothers: Motivation for Healing

Motherhood Saved My Life

27

Patricia Greene

Pat is a 52-year-old mother of three from California. In this chapter she discusses her experience with sleep deprivation leading to postpartum psychosis, suicidality, hospitalizations, and what it took to be correctly diagnosed with bipolar disorder years later.

My name is Pat. I am 52 years old. I have three kids, two of them grown, one almost so. I have a husband who travels a lot and a housemate who doesn't. I am currently underemployed and looking for work. I have an undergraduate and a graduate degree from prestigious institutions that are always ranked within the top ten in the nation in their respective classes, neither of which degree I actually use.

I also have bipolar disorder.

I probably have had bipolar disorder since I was a teenager; I certainly suffered from major depression, but in retrospect some of the symptoms I had were signs of bipolar disorder. There is no way to know—my parents were dealing with another child who was much later diagnosed with schizophrenia and they really did not pay that much attention to whatever much subtler symptoms I was showing.

I managed through college, the years of helping my husband get his Ph.D. and through my own law school experience. I had episodes of what was diagnosed as major depression and was in and out of therapy. I nearly dropped out of law school following a depressive episode after my first year.

Following the birth of my first child, I became psychotic. The hallucinations, suicidality, and delusions I was having made me a danger to my son. It was one of the worst experiences of my life, and it affected the relationship between myself and my eldest son for a long time.

As all babies do, he needed to be fed frequently. I was still exhausted from a twenty-six hour labor, and being woken up every two hours to feed simply deepened that exhaustion. My husband called my sister and a local La Leche League consultant. No, it was important that we never supplement. I was ready to throw in the towel, but he held firm. (In his defense, he didn't know anything more about this than I did.) My exhaustion deepened; I began to feel as though I was completely disconnected from the world. I did not yet know that I suffered from bipolar disorder, and how important it was for me to get sleep.

I have suffered from depression a lot in my life, but nothing was like the pit I descended into then. It was as though the ground had dropped beneath my feet, leaving me in utter blackness. I began to lose contact with my surroundings. My sleep deprivation was becoming severe. And the baby needed to be fed every two hours.

He started to cry all the time. Nothing would soothe him. I would hold him, and he would be okay, but soon he would be crying again. I could not escape the crying. I started being unable to sleep between feedings, because the baby was crying all the time. I would walk into his room, and he would be sleeping, but the moment I stepped out, he would start again.

I began to think that something was wrong with my son, but his well-baby checkups went fine. I began to feel myself closer and closer to the edge, afraid that I would soon snap. I feared going into his room because in the back of my mind I knew there was a strong possibility that I would simply cover his face until he stopped crying—until he stopped breathing.

I still remember the day I went to the store to get a few items. I was on the way back when the baby started crying again. I felt such despair; the baby was crying again—would it never stop? Was there nothing I could do?

The baby was not in the car with me, but at home with my mother.

It says something about my mental state that it was not until several months later that I recognized the fact that I had been hallucinating. And probably not for the first time: about a year ago, my husband and I were talking about when my son was a newborn. "He cried all the time," I said. My husband gave me a strange look," No, he didn't, no more than the other two. He didn't get colicky until he was several months old."

I was in freefall. Things came to a head a week later, when my husband had to go out of town for a business trip, leaving me and the baby alone in the house (my mother had gone back to Florida a day or so before). I looked at him calmly and said "If you leave, one or the other of us won't be here when you get back." What I did not tell him—or anyone—until years later was that I had already known I was going to kill myself. I thought there was a good chance I was going to kill the baby, too, and whatever spark of compassion I had in my soul (not fear of damnation—I was already damned) made me feel that this was grossly unfair to the baby. It wasn't his fault I was his mother; he shouldn't have to die for that. And I knew that if I did not kill him, he would die of dehydration after I died and there was no one to care for him.

My husband got angry, but cancelled his trip and called my obstetrician, who had me hospitalized. The first things the doctor did? Take the baby from my care, have my husband feed the baby formula, and have me sleep for twenty-four hours. When I woke up, I felt far more sane than I had in the previous two weeks. Again, I did not know I was bipolar. I had no idea that sleep was as important as it was in my mood.

There was still a lot to be done—my relationship with my son had been damaged by my psychosis and that needed to be repaired. You may notice above that I refer to "the baby"; that was how I thought of him, as something or someone totally detached from me. The social worker made me start calling him by name, and seeing him as my child rather than an alien being. When I think of those first days, I can't help but think of him as being born during my second hospitalization—that was when I got to know him and see him as my child.

Even after I got better and began to bond with my eldest son, I have always felt slightly differently from him than I have from my other children. I love him dearly, as much as his brothers, but there is also a slight element of detachment. He was always his own separate person in ways that it took me effort to see in my other two. I tended to over-mother my other kids, to only let go of responsibility for them with great reluctance and long after I should have. In the end, my eldest has grown up more responsible and independent at an earlier age than his brothers, and I am pleased about that.

Following my psychotic episode, my husband and I supplemented breast-feeding with formula wherever it was necessary to make sure that I had at least four to six hours of uninterrupted sleep. And we did this with the second and third children as well. In the end, I chalked the entire thing up to simply a combination of very severe sleep deprivation and hormonal influences.

I had a similar—if less severe—episode following the birth of my third son. I was diagnosed as having "postpartum psychosis with delusions"; mainly the grandiose delusion that I knew what would happen in the future. Again there were extenuating circumstances: my father had died a few months before, and other stresses in my life had caused the world to seem upside down. This time, though, I was not faced with the hallucination of the crying baby. I never felt my youngest was a threat to my sanity that my eldest was. The delusions were centered around myself, around who I was and what I could do. This was in spite of the fact that he had been unplanned, at a time when I had already started looking forward to reentering my professional life as a lawyer.

It was after the third child that my mental state took a nosedive. I began to be depressed most of the time. The car accident that nearly took the life of my eldest—and which I blamed myself for, although I was not the driver that hit him—only dragged me further down. I was hospitalized in 1999, when my children were nine, five, and three years old.

The 1999 hospitalization changed my life in one very important way: it reduced my susceptibility to suicide. A psychiatric social worker met with me the third morning of my hospitalization. With no preamble, she asked, "Do you know the suicide rate among the children of maternal suicides?" I did not, so she told me. I cannot remember the number now, but it was horrific. I gasped. "Do you want to do that to you kids?" she asked. "Never," I responded. "You need to find a reason to live for yourself, but in the meantime, I'll take it." Ever since then, suicide has not been an option. The danger has increased as they have gotten to be adults, and I feel they need me less, but I still hold on to the "don't hurt the children" mentality.

It has always been a point of pride for me that in all my episodes, my children have never gone without food or clothing. They have never missed school because I could not get out of bed to take them. I may not have always been the best, most involved mother, but they always had the necessities. Still, the hospitalizations have taken their toll on my kids, even as they are necessary to keep me alive sometimes. They cannot talk to their friends about why their mother is in the hospital. (In fact, when they were very small, they did not have a lot of friends—because of my disorder I was neither willing nor able to take them to playgroups. They developed friends later in life, and now will have them over to the house occasionally.) Twice, I have spent my youngest son's birthday in the hospital. (I tend to have mood episodes in the summer, and his birthday falls in August.) One of these, his twelfth, he identifies as the worst birthday of his entire (admittedly young) life. I am sure his sixteenth, during which I was likewise hospitalized, was no barrel of monkeys, either.

I had gone a long time without being diagnosed in part because I was being asked the wrong questions. I saw residents who often were not experienced enough to describe mania in ways that seem to apply to my situation. "Have you ever felt high or irrationally exuberant?" No. "Have you ever spent money you didn't have?" With credit cards, who doesn't, occasionally? Not anything major. "Have you ever engaged in risky sexual behavior?" Heh. No. And so it would go. The only query I could answer yes to was, "Do your thoughts race?" But on closer questioning I had to say that they didn't do that all that often. I would be diagnosed with major depressive disorder, and given drugs, and the drugs would not work, so I would be given more drugs for a condition that I didn't have, and so forth.

Finally, one young woman resident looked at my chart and said, "I notice that you have had postpartum psychosis. There is a strong correlation between that and bipolar disorder. Have you ever been diagnosed as bipolar?" I sighed inwardly. Here we go again. "No. I haven't." She ran through the list of familiar questions. Like always, I answered in the negative. But then she broke new ground. "Have you ever been told you have an explosive temper? Have you ever felt violently towards someone without being able to explain why? Do you ever have irrational rages?" "Yes! Yes! Exactly! Mostly towards my children." "You are bipolar," she said. "But I'm not manic," I replied. She explained that mania could take different forms sometimes, and the rages were part of my condition. She also said that given my particular set of symptoms I would be classified as bipolar II. Many people would have been depressed by a diagnosis of bipolar disorder. I was not. "I don't care if they diagnose me as a pink-polka dotted penguin, as long as they can treat me," I wrote in my journal.

Finally, I could be given drugs designed to help people who have what I have. Since then, I have had a struggle getting the right medication regimen—for years, actually—but I am more likely to have periods of stability. The drugs have occasionally taken a toll on my family, and not just when they stop working. When I was hospitalized in 2012, I was given meds that, although initially effective, soon affected my personality. I became less interested in what was going on around me and less able to experience the world fully or to engage in the interactions with my children that we had always enjoyed. I became a shell of my former self. When my son came home from college for the summer last year, I was at the height—depth?—of my experience with this drug. He sadly said to his father, "I want Mom back." Trials with other drugs ended up with me back in the hospital, albeit more briefly.

I have always had a love–hate relationship with my medications. One summer a few years ago, I talked to each of my three kids about what effect my bipolar disorder had had on their lives. At that point I was more or less stable, and had been so for several years, although I was to lose that stability a few months later.

It started when my youngest asked me about my medication regimen. He began by asking about my tremor, since he has a slight tremor himself, and I described how my tremor was familial and benign but exacerbated by the meds I was on. He asked what other side effects were from the meds, and I told him: weight gain, memory loss, and occasional cognitive impairments. He was aghast. "Why do you take them, then?" he asked. "Kevin, what was I like before I was on meds?" I replied. "You could be fun, but then you would scream at us for no reason at all. You yelled at all of us, but mostly David, and we could never figure out why. Then you would get depressed and not talk to us." "And that, Kevin, is exactly why I take the meds. So I won't do that."

Later, I asked his older brother David. David has high-functioning autism, so he was less able than his brothers to see storms coming and so ended up getting the brunt of my rage. He said pretty much the same thing, except that he hastened to add that I was "so much better now." That helped ease my feelings of guilt, but not by much.

I finally asked my eldest son, James. He was silent a long time, and then he looked at me with tears in his eyes. "Do you know how I apologize for everything, even when I have done nothing wrong? I started doing that because of you. Because I wanted you to be happy, to feel better." I started crying. Aside from a very occasional spanking (never done when I was extremely angry), I had never hit my children. And yet they had been terrified of me. I struggle with guilt over that. I struggle with guilt over the way my illness has prevented me from being what I see as the best mother that I can be. I struggle with guilt over the anger I sometimes feel towards my children, that somehow this is their fault that I didn't have this disorder before they were born (although I know intellectually I probably did). I struggle with the anger I feel about the years that I was only able to be a mother, because that took all of the emotional energy I could muster aside from dealing with my illness; the years lost that meant that I lost my profession. When you are out of the practice for long enough, it becomes impossible to go back. (Realistically, my disorder was only part of the reasons I was a stay-at-home mother: as I said, my middle son is autistic, and he was less functional as a younger child than he is now, and required more monitoring. I needed to be available at a moment's notice to go to his school to help deal with a crisis.)

I have also struggled with fear.

I fear for my children. Bipolar disorder has a known genetic component. I look on them with dread every time one of them (usually the youngest) appears too revved up: is it his ADD, or is he beginning to manifest bipolar disorder? He asked me the other day where in my family the genetic tendency towards mental illness came from. I said I did not know, although I suspect it was from my father's side. But who knows? We didn't talk about mental illness.

I fear that I will someday, once the kids are all grown, kill myself. I fear that I will hurt them. I fear that that would be too much for them and that one or more of them would follow my example. I fear that if I were to die in an accidental manner, they would forever wonder if it was self-induced. But to tell you the truth, if I did not have a family, I would be long dead, meds or no meds.

My kids love me, even with my disorder. I am more grateful for that than I can express. They are the most important people in my world, and knowing that they are counting on me to take care of my mental health, even now that they do not need me for their direct physical needs, helps keep me safe, and often sane. It means I take my meds, and see my doctors, and check myself into the hospital when I am a danger to myself.

Being a mother has saved my life.

The Darkness Isn't So Dark Anymore

28

Diana Babcock

Diana is a 55-year-old mother from upstate New York. In this chapter she discusses being diagnosed with depression, posttraumatic stress disorder, and anxiety in her 40s, after coping for years with the impact of childhood emotional and sexual abuse while parenting her three children.

Sometimes I like to think that my natural mother named me after Lady Diana Cooper, an English socialite and actress, because she had high hopes for me. I grew up in the Albany, NY area. I have two sisters, two half brothers and a half sister, three adult children, four grandkids with one on the way, and a whole bunch of nieces and nephews with their children. My sisters and I like to say that we are the matriarchs of the family.

I was adopted by my paternal uncle and aunt right before I turned six. The memories I have of my first years with my natural father and mother were filled with fighting, alcohol, and hiding. My sisters and I were born close together, and when I was two and a half our natural mother abandoned us. My father remarried, and then had three more children with my stepmother. The fighting and alcohol didn't stop; there were times I hid my siblings in closets because we were so afraid. My memories of those years are filled with alcoholism, sexual abuse from neighborhood boys and a babysitter, my parents fighting, and beatings. I remember running away to neighbors' houses around 2 or 3 years old, once to play on a swing set and another to ask a lady who answered the door if she would be my mommy.

I start off with this because it's the foundation of my parenting skills and also a mental health diagnosis I would receive in my 40s. There is a one-year period that I don't remember where my sisters and I lived with my grandparents before my natural father remarried. I believe this is where there was some normalcy and a time of steadiness, but by this time, for me, it was about survival and taking care of others. My father remarried and had three more children before my sisters and I

Motherhood, Mental Illness and Recovery, DOI 10.1007/978-3-319-01318-3_28,
© Springer International Publishing Switzerland 2014

were adopted by my aunt and uncle. The next 9 years were filled with the
uncertainty of raging and sexual abuse. I left home right before I turned 16, lived
with a school friend for a bit of time, and started drinking, partying, and doing
drugs. Emancipated when I turned 17, I spent the next 5 years traveling with the
carnival and doing a lot of drugs.

I'm trying to remember a time when I wasn't numb inside, but can't. There was
always a sense of disconnectedness—that I didn't quite belong anywhere. My
daughter was born on the road a month before I turned 22 and enraptured, I
would spend my time singing, laughing, and being with her even though I still
felt disconnected. I had stopped doing hard drugs when I learned I was pregnant and
that was difficult, not because I was addicted, but the drugs helped me feel happy.
Now that feeling came from my daughter and it created a desire to stop the cycle of
abuse, drugging, and drinking that went back at least two generations in my family.
So I went from being a carnie and traveling on the road to coming home, settling
down, and becoming a member of a church. I left my daughter's father when she
was 18 months old and nestled into a wonderful place of support for myself and my
daughter, feeling safe, supported, and loved. But always that numbness stayed with
me, never letting up.

Now because of my upbringing, I don't really have a compass for picking men
who are stable and comfortable with themselves. Eight years later I fell in love with
someone, got married, and had two more children, both boys. I thought this was my
"ever after" love and the things I longed for, a stable home, church home, and love
into my old age had finally arrived. But the cycle of abuse and alcoholism continued
on his part and after 8 years of marriage we divorced and I became a single mother
again. By this point that determination to break the cycle was the most important
thing in my life. My children were going to have good lives and be happy. It didn't
matter if I was happy, as long as they were. I worked three part-time jobs to pay
rent, put food on the table, and make sure they had everything they physically
needed. We laughed, played games, sang, and I loved my kids the best I knew. But
the numbness was always there, lurking around in the background of my heart
and mind.

I tried to see a mental health professional a couple of times while my children
were growing up. It didn't work for me because they wanted me to express deeper
emotions. I couldn't do this. Anger meant rage, sadness meant the dark place, and I
wasn't going there; it was too scary. But gradually the stress of carrying this around
caught up with me. By this time I had an excellent job that I loved, was still part of
the church family, and thought I was on the road to success. My daughter was
grown and had a child of her own and my boys were 9 and 10 years old. But for
2 years one of my boys was struggling and already involved in the judicial system. I
was going to church because I was supposed to, not because I loved it. My job had
become overwhelming. I kept pushing though, making myself work harder, not
going easy on myself, and ended up having to resign from my job.

I became overwhelmed with an emotional darkness that was unrelenting, and
one evening the thought kept crossing my mind that I didn't want my youngest son
to see what I was going to do. I had no plan; I just knew I would do it. The desire to

end my life became so strong I called my pastor who advised me to go to the ER and my pastor's wife would meet me there. I dropped my son off at a church member's house and went to the local emergency room. My memory isn't clear about all that went on that night. I know I spent most of the night in a small room and was admitted to a psychiatric unit. I know that my oldest son was in respite and my youngest son stayed with someone in the church while I was in the hospital. I stayed in the hospital for over a week. By the time I was released I was on seven different psychiatric medications and had received diagnoses of clinical depression, post-traumatic stress disorder, and anxiety disorder. I had never had a diagnosis in my life, although it would have been easy for it to happen. And the funny thing was, I still wanted to end my life but I hid it well from the doctors and staff. I was worried about my boys; they had no idea what was going on.

At this point I was so broken in my spirit and emotions. I had no strength and there was no one to take and care for my boys so the case manager for my older son and the people I was seeing at the hospital recommended foster care for both of them on a voluntary basis. I no longer had my job and had to give up my apartment and began giving and throwing away my belongings. Now I realize that this was because I still wanted to end my life. I moved into a local homeless shelter. I went to the programs and groups and made sure I did everything they said because I wanted my boys home. Then 9/11 happened on the same day I was at my stepmother's funeral. I drove back to the homeless shelter speeding well over 100 miles an hour trying to end my life. Somehow it didn't happen and the next day in the day treatment group I talked about what I had tried to do. I was back in the hospital that afternoon. I don't remember how I got there. All I could think was I couldn't be with my boys. My memory of this time is very foggy. I remember sitting in a little room with my boys once a week and there was a case manager in there with us. I wasn't allowed to be alone with them, there was always someone there. I could see the confusion on their faces and I was so shut down I couldn't comfort or encourage them that it was going to be okay. *I* didn't know if it was going to be okay. Even though when my boys went into foster care and it was supposed to be voluntary, it wound up being 2 years before I could get my youngest son home. It took longer for my older son because he was in residential treatment facilities and having a really difficult time with what was going on with me. I learned there was a law that said I had to make sure I was in family court every 6 months or they could have been taken away from me. And while making sure I was in court I was penalized for not attending groups. I spent the next 8 years in and out of the hospital and going to an intensive day treatment program.

It's still painful when I think about this time of our lives. The separation was devastating and I think this is why I had repeated hospitalizations. I don't know if anyone thought the boys were in danger from me, but looking back now it appears they thought so. I know I would never hurt them. I had no personal experience with having a mental health diagnosis and didn't understand why anyone would think I was a danger to my children. I was scared. I was afraid that my children would carry the mental illness gene. I thought I would spend the rest of my life on medications and in and out of the hospital. I went to the library and researched mental illness, clinical depression, and all the other things I'd been labeled with. All this did was deepen my despair that I would never get well—that there was no recovery.

My support system had fallen apart. I stopped going to church, pushed people away, and fell into the psychiatric system. The medications helped me feel numb and for once in my life other people were taking care of me. I stopped crying and completely shut down. The system calls this a blunt affect. I call it pain, deep heart-wrenching pain. Pain to the point where I couldn't talk to anyone, just take the medications and go to groups. I would visit my boys and go back to my little room at the homeless shelter and sleep. After 10 weeks the program I was attending told me I was done, no more groups, and I was to continue to see a psychiatrist once a month and therapist once a week. There were no expectations of recovery, no hope on their part that I would become well or get my boys back.

This is where I made a decision that probably saved my life. I picked up the phone book and started looking in the yellow pages for something, anything under mental health listings. The first place I called was specifically for drug addiction and the person on the phone thought I should call Turning Point, a local intensive day treatment program. I got an appointment for the next day. I had to take three buses to get there. I'm still amazed I was able to do that. I was so shut down, I don't remember the ride. What I do remember is sitting with the person and all of a sudden the floodgates opened. I couldn't stop crying. It took 2 hours just to get through the paperwork. I started intensive day treatment the following week.

Now it would be all hunky dory to say this was the start of my journey to recovery and everything was smooth sailing. The reality is that it's hard work getting out of the mental health system once you've become a part of it. It can easily become a cycle of programs and medications and for me it was like this for about 8 years. I had to continue dealing with the family court system, traveling to see my boys who by this point had been separated, one in residential treatment facilities and the other in a therapeutic foster home. After 2 years and a long 6-month battle I finally managed to get one of my boys home, but my other son had become a part of the juvenile psychiatric system and it took longer for him. That's a story in and of itself.

I worked hard to recover. For me, it was like an education. I learned about myself. I took what I got in the groups and from my peers and applied it to my life. I did mood and emotion charts, wrote about my feelings, prayed, meditated, and worked like I was studying for an advanced degree. I began to understand the impact the trauma of my childhood had on me and asked questions on how people heal from that. I started using Wellness Recovery Action Plan, which helped me to deal with the dark side of my emotions. It took a while, 8 years, before I felt safe enough to start stepping away from intensive day treatment and become involved in the community again. There were those who thought I wouldn't be able to do it and that I would need the mental health system for the rest of my life. But there were those who did and their voices and support are what helped me as I went through the process of putting myself back together. I learned I needed to go slow and not make any hasty decisions. I used my wellness plan to help me over the next 2 years as I weaned off the psychiatric medications. This wasn't easy for me because the medications served the same purpose as when I was using.

Now I make decisions based on what I feel is best for me, not everybody else. I allow myself to feel. I think this is the most important part of my recovery. My childhood essentially ended at about 3 years old. I had to learn how to feel, what those feelings were, and then how to allow myself to express my feelings. I needed to learn how to set healthy boundaries so I could have healthy relationships. I use breathing techniques to help with anxiety. I started attending church again. I slowly built a support network of people who I trust and who I can go to if I find myself struggling with dark thoughts or melancholy. I walk and listen to music. I enjoy my children and my grandchildren. I've recently started telling myself that I am a good person and today is going to be a good day as soon as I wake up. It's not easy; there are days when I want to climb into bed and stay there. So I schedule what I call grunge weekends where I do absolutely nothing from Friday night until Monday morning. I started working again, first part-time, then full-time, and I made the decision to go back to part-time after having heart surgery. There is still stress and difficulties, but I enjoy my life now. The darkness isn't so dark any more.

An Eccentric Mother

Dorothy Scotten

> Dorothy is a 73-year-old mother of three from Massachusetts. She is a Licensed
> Independent Clinical Social Worker and obtained her Ph.D. in Educational
> Studies. In this chapter she discusses her mothering and the label of 'mental
> illness' which she feels deemphasizes one's personal strengths.

When I initially saw the title of the book that spoke about mothers and mental
illness, I was repelled by the words, *mental illness*. Those words and that label still
bring tears to my eyes even though now I am 73 years of age. I never considered
myself mentally ill; I considered myself a person with extreme perceptions and
feelings about the world around me.

My story coincides in numerous ways with many of the clients I have had the
pleasure of serving over the years. It is a story of feeling strong alienation and
abandonment from very early on. My story was a struggle for finding a God who
would love me and who would protect me. I couldn't find anyone else who would
do—these people walking about in my life were strangers and were a species that
were foreign. I grew up in fear, I married in fear, I raised my children in fear—
always the fear, the underlying feeling that I would be annihilated and I still did not
know what love was.

Yet, when my first child was born, something happened. There was fear, to be
sure, but this little creature needed something from me. Even though I didn't know
what love was, and was not sure I could give it, I tried, and I kept trying with all the
children to make sure they did not grow up feeling unloved. Meanwhile, there was
always this deep feeling of separation, that I was two distinct persons, cut in half,
and the pieces would not fit together.

I have often described myself as a lonely child, a middle child from a middle
class German-American family. I had two brothers, one 5 years my senior and the
other, 7 years younger. I was virtually mute as a child and did not really speak, nor
could I interact socially with others. When alone, oftentimes, I would rock back and

Motherhood, Mental Illness and Recovery, DOI 10.1007/978-3-319-01318-3_29,
© Springer International Publishing Switzerland 2014

forth and have conversations in my head. I was frightened by people and could not make eye contact and would withdraw into a corner, so others could not see me. As I have mentioned in an earlier work (Scotten 2003), my childhood was "bereft of sensory and social stimulation."

My father was an extremely labile person who oftentimes had temper tantrums and raged or withdrew from family activities. My mother, to me, was akin to a martyr, a submissive homemaker who catered to the boys especially and supported my father's whims and extreme emotions. My childhood was traumatic and at times overwhelming, and the memories have followed me throughout the rest of my life.

I always was excessively shy. Somehow I knew something was profoundly wrong with me, but did not know what. I was a good student in school and, in fact, excelled in my studies. However, I did have challenges with reading and concentrating. My teachers sometimes were puzzled that I performed beyond my ability level determined by "normed" test scores. I graduated from college and became an elementary teacher in order to conquer my shyness and learn how to speak. I subsequently married, had three children about a year apart in age, became a homemaker, and also became very involved in civic and church activities.

In my late 30s, I decided to go back to school for a Master's degree in social work, after having had a traumatic experience with a psychotherapist that prompted an internal feeling "to do therapy" better than what I had experienced. I also was determined to learn how to think more clearly and to become more articulate around my peers, which had always been problematic for me.

After graduate school, I made a major move with my family to an island community and started a new job with an agency as a child therapist. This move, combined with a series of losses, ill health, and marital difficulties, seemed to precipitate one crisis after another. After a 25 year marriage, my husband left, just after his mother died and as the children were leaving home.

A few years later, I had lost my home, my mother, and became quite ill, and then left a clinical job as supervisor in a local counseling center to work in an innovative 30-day treatment center overseas, hoping that a change of venue would prompt a healing process. That appeared to backfire when all my childhood and adult traumatic memories surfaced once again as I began to dialogue with a colleague about my life. The colleague suggested I start drawing. I sat down one evening and drew about 20 pictures. It looked as though a child had drawn these, and it opened up a part of my unconscious that I didn't even know existed. The more I drew, and the more I wrote, the more I started to dissociate in ways that were impossible for me to handle. A friend came over to the island where I was working and took me back to the states to a woman's trauma unit in Boston (Scotten 2003) where I stayed for 2–3 weeks.

My life turned around at the hospital. I was fortunate; I found a therapist there who was cued into the transcendental qualities of psychosis. I also found my niche and people who really understood trauma. My therapist accepted and supported my spiritual proclivities and understood just what I needed to do to heal. She never would really discuss my diagnosis nor was I interested in hearing it. My focus was on healing and finding spiritual assonance. The term "mental illness" connoted that something was fundamentally wrong with me as a human being. For me, the problem of my disengagement was a spiritual difficulty, not an organic disease to be "treated." I viewed my therapy as an ongoing spiritual process that has been described in the literature as a Shamanistic process, traveling inward to the disorganized parts of my psyche. My drumming circles were very helpful adjuncts to this process. My healing process has been a long one, but it all began then.

While this was my first hospitalization, it was not my first "episode." There were others and I managed enough to find therapists along the way to "save" me from the system that did not seem to treat me like a human being. I had had years of therapy with different therapists who I could really "con" and I was always fairly clever when it came to hiding feelings.

I also went through the 1970s when popular self-help psychology weekends were abundant and I went to most of them, trying to "discover" myself and find some internal peace. There was the week with the Adlerians, Gestalt workshops, Opening of the Heart, writing workshops, Expressive arts and trainings with Paolo Knill and others, the original *B.R.E.T.H* (Breathing to Release Energy for Transformation and Healing) founded by Kamala Hope Campbell, Psychodrama, Shamanism, Parapsychology, Music, Reiki, Polarity Therapy, Trauma training—and the list goes on. After my divorce, I even went on a 3-week wilderness survival course that combined psychological work with Robert Gass and his wife, Judith. I can't even remember everything I did. All I wanted to be was whole.

My Children

I have three children, two daughters and one son, who are now 47, 46, and 44 years of age, all of whom are married. Sometimes, when I look back, I don't know how I handled being a mother. They were close enough in age that it was like having triplets, and the youngest was very ill and had surgery when he was 9 months old as well as asthma. I carried him around with me and insisted that he not be constrained by his illnesses, even as I battled my own demons. I did not want him or the girls to know how vulnerable I was. I didn't have time. If things were really unsettled for me, I would remove myself, so I would not hurt anyone.

The children were quite active and I was determined that they would not feel as unloved as I had felt. We lived in a small community and that helped. In terms of my own emotional issues, I was nervous and stressed and compartmentalized them. Sometimes, I would go into the bedroom and just literally hang on to the bed in terror. I could not let them nor my husband know how poorly I was feeling.

At one point I remember worrying so much that I went down the street to a local doctor and told him I didn't feel well. He gave me benadryl and valium to take three times a day. I then discovered that he had been trained as a psychiatrist and I felt ashamed. I threw the pills away and kept hiding, putting on this act to cover up the *other* me. I viewed the pills as a message from the doctor that I was crazy. So I had to protect my children from thinking they had a *crazy* mother.

My saving grace was that I was a good cook and I focused on that and making over-sure that the children and my husband were fed. The children were energetic and fairly balanced. They really bonded with each other and we lived in a regular neighborhood with other children who became a part of our everyday life. We had what I thought was a fairly normal family life and did many things as a family with our involvement in church and community activities.

My husband left when the children were almost out of the house. My eldest daughter, then in college, took a leave of absence and came home. My son, I think, was afraid that he would have to take care of me, even though I made it clear that I was independent. Of course, inside I was terrified. I had been a housewife and suddenly at age 50, I had to start over again.

After the divorce, my relationship with my children took on a new dimension. They were adults and they had their own lives. When I became seriously ill and decided to leave my job for another overseas, I left them. I thought I needed to put myself together and they needed to see that happen, so they could go on with their lives. So when I had the major breakdown and had to be taken home a year or so later, I elected not to tell them. They had been through enough. When my son found out, he was disappointed that I had not contacted him. He said he had this dream that I had fallen off a cliff and it frightened him.

I still would not tell them what was really happening and even today I am not as forthcoming about my inner challenges, because even though they are adults, I remain their mother and they don't really want to hear the details. I have spoken to them about our relationship and have continued our conversations over the years. For this chapter, I revisited those early times in their lives with them. I asked each of them if they knew what was going on and how did they feel about living with an "eccentric" mother.

My older daughter told me that she and her sister and brother didn't turn out "so bad," especially compared to some of her friends. She said some of the issues involved simply the times in which we lived where "you and dad weren't around that much." She spoke of how she felt all of her siblings and she had low self-esteem and that she wished that I had been more assertive with her father, and, I think, more assertive in general, because she felt she was told she can do anything she wanted and be a success. The problem was, we gave her no sense of what her possibilities or potentials were. However, she learned a great deal about herself: "I am a good mentor now to students because of my gift. . .I am plain spoken." I said to her: "You lead by example, and I am afraid that I wasn't a good one for you." Other themes arose as a result of our conversation: themes of dissonance and themes of good times: "I learned poetry and music from you and I remember you sitting on your bed, playing the guitar. I started writing poetry for you when I was little also. . .and my favorite memory was you baking bread at night and waking me up to give me the first piece." She shared other thoughts as well: she felt that we could be more affectionate and perhaps I could have been more present. She felt that she never learned how to be angry and always was more passive-aggressive and had to unlearn that in her 20s. She said as she and her siblings got older, we began to show more affection and this disarmed her.

I received similar feedback from the other two children in terms of my apparent lack of "presence," and not being there especially after our move. My son expressed some unsettlement about how he felt that he might never be able to take care of himself. He had to work through that issue and has mainly done so via the novels that he has written. He is a writer and owns his own personal chef business as well as doing small contracting work. He has had some issues and feelings about being heard and I can see how he has been working through those as well. In terms of our relationship, that has matured over the years and he has been able to process many more things with me. One item he shared with me not so long ago was his discomfort about my looking at him. He said I "stared" too much. I really smiled when I heard that. I said, "I will try to stop"...but this is part of my childhood, too. I had to learn how to "stare," to look at people. I would never look them in the eyes. Now, I believe that the eyes are the windows of the soul.

My middle daughter thinks I had a borderline personality...that I was flamboyant all the time, changeable, and everything was "all about me." Interestingly enough, I thought the same about her. We seemed, throughout the years, to mirror each other. I felt she constantly projected her own "stuff" onto me and many times I believed it and tried harder to be a better mother to live according to her "standards" and vision of the perfect mother.

My grandsons are 19, 16, and 7 years old and are quite a wonderful handful. Each of my grandsons is different and has his own issues, but my daughter and her husband are very committed to full-time parenting, certainly on a more conscious level than I had been. And now, the little one is facing issues that warrant more support as his mother (my daughter) is about to undergo a stem cell replacement therapy for t-cell lymphoma. I feel I am being given another "shot" at mothering with these boys and I am learning a great deal about teens and modern technology as a result and more about just plain being present. As I have matured and worked on my own healing, I see the changes in my children and in how I deal with them and with my grandsons. I am a much better grandparent and mother now than I was earlier, I surmise. I keep apologizing to my now grown children and ask them to work on their "mother issues" before I am in the grave.

Have there been issues over multiple generations? Quite possibly. My eldest brother's three children were hospitalized when they were young and my nephew was diagnosed with schizophrenia. He subsequently passed away when he was 38 years old. There is a family history of alcoholism and depression on my maternal side and my younger brother has had his challenges. Perhaps it's in the genes...I don't know. It is not important to me now. I just want a normal life and this "thing" called Mental Illness somehow always kept getting in the way. Who really defines what is normal, anyway? Throughout my professional career, for example, I see many persons who make public policy in the medical and mental health field as true "dissociatives"— very much out of touch with how I would define "normal." Normal is the integration of the heart and head in my opinion. Given that definition, many of our leaders and policy makers could be labeled as "mentally ill"—what do you think?

Advice to Parents

My advice to you parents who have been through the process of so-called mental illness is to really focus on your own mental health. Seek therapy and work on being in relationship with your therapist. Working on that relationship will support the other relationships in your life including the ones with your children. I think in that way you will both protect yourself and your children and grow in ways that will strengthen their sense of self. It's important for them to feel secure, safe, and loved. If you as a mother are experiencing all these emotional challenges and cannot take care of them and to begin to love yourself, it will affect your children. Your children depend on you as the nurturer and protector. Yet children are resilient. They know that you love them, despite your faults.

Be actively engaged with your children. If you haven't learned to play, start now. You have this marvelous opportunity to use your "crazy," witty self to be creative and to laugh along with them. Their innocence and thirst for knowledge is contagious and it helps you to be in the "here and now," marveling at how your world and theirs is in constant flux—that is life-affirming. I am now enjoying this finally with my grandchildren and especially the young one. I have a second chance, and I can go to bug farms and to McDonald's. I can draw with him and do the things unfettered by my childhood terrors. I can even yell at him and we laugh and hug. . .and I run after the older boys as well, bribing the 19-year-old with chocolate brownies, if he would only wash the dishes. Oh, how I missed all those things all those years. . .the joy of being in the "here and now."

You can do this, you can drop the fear in a basket and throw it in the river and let the current take it away. The fear is not you; the You is a moving, dynamic. and creative being. If you can put fear aside, you and your children will grow in very special ways.

Reference

Scotten D (2003) Preverbal trauma, dissociation and the healing process. ProQuest Information and Learning Co. UMI Microfilm 3081620

Together We Are Whole

30

Dena Miller and Harita Raja

Dena is a 48-year-old mother of two from Texas. She was initially diagnosed with depression and then bipolar II disorder, anxiety, attention deficit hyper-activity disorder, and posttraumatic stress disorder. In this chapter she discusses her realization of the importance to take care of her own mental health first, in order to be the best mother to her children.

I was falling apart inside, but I put their needs before mine. I knew that was what was right. I wanted to be a good mother, though deep down I was terrified of losing them. Would they leave me, or worse yet, would they be taken away? These are the thoughts that would repeat themselves in my mind. I had to put in so much effort to ensure that they would remain mine.

I was born and raised by my parents in Texas. Life was pretty good as a child. I had a younger brother and an older brother and we all got along okay. I had everything I wanted. Unfortunately, all the good things were invalidated by my being abused by the neighbor kids. I would rather not talk about that.

I got married in 1987. The first year was pretty good. Unfortunately, I did not see my ex-husband much since he was in the military and very involved in it. I guess it was for the better looking back. He was an alcoholic too. Within our first year of marriage, he was assigned an overseas position in Korea. I thought I would be able to handle it, but his departure was a turning point for me. It threw me over the edge. I had also been dealing with the death of my older brother one year before. I was tired of my life and in a lot of emotional pain. I just did not care anymore and felt that I had no one to live for. I had enough and declared that life was not worth living. I tried to commit suicide.

I used a razor to cut my wrists. I went to the emergency room at the military hospital. They asked me a couple of questions. I told them how I was feeling. Their response was that there was nothing that they could do about it and I should not feel like that. But if I could not feel the way I did, I was not sure how to feel. They did

Motherhood, Mental Illness and Recovery, DOI 10.1007/978-3-319-01318-3_30,
© Springer International Publishing Switzerland 2014

not even try to help me. I was told to get it together. I just left instead. I was too numb to think any more. I can think back on it now though. Thankfully, I survived. Unfortunately, I did not seek help again for a long time.

Years later, I decided that this had to be a turning point for me. I decided if the military would not help me, I would help myself. I started attending more religious services at a local church and enrolled in a medical assistant program at a local school. I sucked it up and pushed through. Although I had friends, I could not face them. I was ashamed; what would they think? Would they treat me differently? Moreover, I needed to help myself first, before I could ask for their help. I could not have done it alone though. I became an avid follower of the National Alliance on Mental Illness (NAMI). If you have not heard of it, I would recommend you look it up. It allowed me to meet people who were suffering like me and make me feel that I was a *part of the whole*. I was not unique in my situation and felt comfort in having support through this difficult time. It felt like a hand on my shoulder guiding me through. NAMI also helped me to find the right therapist. There were so many to choose from, but NAMI was able to help me to sort through them. I began seeing a therapist and I also joined a support group.

My happiness slowly returned. My pregnancy with my first son proceeded great. I was so excited, as was my husband and the rest of our family. We felt so lucky. It was only after he was born that I began experiencing postpartum depression. I felt a lot of emotional pain and felt that life was no longer worth living. I did try to seek some guidance from my obstetrician at the time. He said it was natural to feel a little overwhelmed since it was my first child. I guess I did not know any better and took his words at face value. He told me to take walks and hot baths, which should help relax me and help me feel better. In hindsight, I feel that he never understood the extent of my symptoms.

The second pregnancy was even worse for me. I was depressed even before I knew I was pregnant. I wanted to end my life. I had been thinking about it and was on the verge of suicide. Within a few days of coming up with a plan, I found out that I was pregnant with my second son. I was not sure how to feel at first. Eventually, thinking about my first son and my coming second son, I became happier. This time around, I decided to consult with my psychiatrist before talking to my obstetrician. My psychiatrist wanted to put me on medications, but my obstetrician was against it. The obstetrician told me that I could harm or even kill my baby with medications and I should not take any such medications. A part of me wanted to feel better, but my maternal instinct jumped in and refused any psychiatric medications. Looking back, I wish I had taken something to help me. It was not an easy pregnancy.

I have been blessed with my two sons, now 18 and 21 years old. Unfortunately, having children did not make me immune to further repercussions of my illness. I was diagnosed with depression, then later bipolar II disorder, anxiety, and ADHD in the past 10 years. It really did not matter what they called it; I felt terrible and uncomfortable in my own skin. It was hard for me to get out of bed and take care of myself. I was not sleeping well. I would stay up much of the night. This made me irritable and very moody. I would be happy and then sad within hours of each other. I started thinking that there were people out to get me; I was paranoid. One of my biggest problems was over-shopping. I would go on shopping sprees even if I did not have the money to do so. I would buy shoes, purses, clothes, and other such items. Credit cards were easy to charge and that is what I did: charge. I felt that I was in control most during these moments. Ironic. More recently, I was diagnosed with PTSD. I felt like it was nearly impossible for me to be a parent, much less be a good parent. I was unable to think straight and unable to tell right from wrong. I tried to get involved in my sons' schools when I was not working as idle time was my enemy. When I worked or spent time at my sons' schools, my symptoms would quiet down.

My limits were tested when my eldest son was diagnosed with bipolar II disorder and ADHD. I felt guilty about this. You bring children into this world hoping they will have a better life than yours. I did not want him to hurt or suffer. I wondered what I could have done differently and it was hard not to blame myself. Honestly, I still do. I was constantly taking care of his needs and unable to even see what my needs were at the time. I let myself go and just hoped the medications would work like magic.

I could not get myself together. I basically did not care about myself anymore. I was committing fraud and was put in jail and then on probation. This was a wake-up call for me to have a serious conversation with my ex-husband, whom I divorced in 1998. We decided that my sons would go live with their father in 2008. Initially, I was still falling apart inside and out. I did not want them to leave, but knew it was for the best. I was unemployed and had not held a job in over a year, so I decided to live with my parents. The whole transition was easier than I anticipated. I think I realized that I needed to take this time to take care of me. Medication was not equivalent to magic. I needed to put in my own efforts to get better. The reality is, it became easier and harder after they left. While they were mostly cared for by their father during this time, I remained a significant part of their lives. It was during this time that I decided to tell them about my struggles with depression and anxiety. It was hard at first, but my therapist helped me. Therapy was an important part of my treatment. We role-played what I would say and what they might say. Then, I brought my sons with me to my session with my therapist, as they were familiar with her from past sessions of their own. We had extensive family therapy. Being honest with my sons took a great deal of weight off of my shoulders.

I currently am a Peer Recovery Specialist. I understand the importance of having others who understand your circumstances. It has been a fulfilling role for me. I am in my recovery process now. The key word is process; it's an ongoing challenge. My advice to other women with mental illness is to take care of yourself first. It is not a selfish act. By taking care of yourself, you are indirectly helping your children. My sons were clearly my motivation to get better. They gave me the opportunity to be a better person and I want to strive for the best. I have learned the value of patience. Our love for each other has allowed us to thrive and *together we are whole*.

Worried Sick: Postpartum Obsessive–Compulsive Disorder

Ellen Darling

In this chapter Ellen Darling, a doctoral student in Clinical Psychology, tells the story of a mother's experience with postpartum depression and obsessive–compulsive disorder. Written following an interview with this mother, who is also a psychiatrist, the story emphasizes the importance of access to support and treatment for mental health recovery.

While depression is commonly thought of as the most frequently occurring psychological disorder associated with pregnancy and the postpartum period, recent research has identified anxiety as more prevalent during this time. A meta-analysis of the literature in this area suggests that postpartum women are particularly vulnerable to the onset of obsessive–compulsive disorder (OCD) and are almost twice as likely to develop OCD as their non-childbearing counterparts (Russell, Fawcett, & Mazmanian 2013). While increased anxiety related to a newborn's well-being and subclinical OCD symptoms are relatively common (e.g., over 80 % of postpartum mothers report experiencing intrusive worrisome thoughts at times) for a minority of women these symptoms are severe enough to cause significant personal distress and relationship upset and impair their ability to function (Brockington, Macdonald, & Wainscott 2006). Additionally, researchers have found that postpartum OCD (ppOCD) may present with distinct clinical features from OCD found in community samples. In ppOCD, the obsessional content may be more focused on extreme fears of intentionally or accidentally harming the infant and the compulsions are not solely overt, but often include thought-blocking and excessive reassurance-seeking (Speisman, Storch, & Abramowitz 2011).

In this story, a psychiatrist in her late thirties recalls her experience of post-partum OCD and discusses key factors in her recovery. She wished to remain anonymous, but wanted to share her story in the hopes of dispelling the shame and stigma that can surround mental illness during a time in which the cultural expectation is joy and fulfillment. She also offers her story with the wish that others

Motherhood, Mental Illness and Recovery, DOI 10.1007/978-3-319-01318-3_31,
© Springer International Publishing Switzerland 2014

struggling with similar symptoms find both comfort in knowing they are not alone and hope that with treatment a full recovery is possible. Several details have been changed to protect her anonymity.

When I look back, the truth of it was that I was scared from the beginning. I was worried about whether or not I was really ready to become a parent and I was terrified of giving birth. Would my body really be able to do something as unbelievable as push a seven-pound creature out of an internal cavity? Beyond the fear of birth, I was nervous of how becoming a parent would affect my marriage, impact my career, and what would become of "me"—my sense of self as an independent woman. Despite all these worries, my husband and I did, truly, in our heart of hearts want a baby. We had shared our dreams of having children together just after the first "I love yous" were whispered between us, and in the years before our daughter was born, we had even gone as far as dreaming up a make-believe little girl about whom we'd tell each other stories before we drifted off to sleep at night. We'd planned when we wanted to begin trying years in advance, both saw our doctor for preconception physicals, and had even begun looking through real estate listings for houses with backyards. If any two people were ready, we were ready.

We had the good fortune to conceive after the first month of trying. I was thirty-three, had just finished my psychiatry residency, and was blessed with a textbook healthy pregnancy. The only complicating factor was that I was on antidepressant medication. I had been taking antidepressants for almost 15 years, since my first episode of depression in my early teens. Over the years, I tried numerous times to come off medication, each time unsuccessfully. Shortly after discontinuing the meds, I would become increasingly anxious, despondent, and even suicidal at times. The anxiety would be so bad that I regularly felt dizzy, nauseous, and had to lay down. Going to the grocery store or navigating Target was totally over-whelming and making decisions about what kind of detergent to buy, impossible. I would sometimes just sit down in the middle of the store, before slowly making my way to an exit, usually not having purchased a thing.

The accompanying depression during these times was like living in an iron lung. An airless, constricted tunnel. Insulated from the world—living in blackness and beyond hopeless, I would retreat to my bed for long stretches at a time, only rising to eat and use the bathroom. What had eventually helped me recover from these episodes was resuming my medication regimen, the gift of time, the support of a fantastic therapist with whom I'd been working for over 6 years when I became pregnant, and my endlessly patient and loving husband. While I still had rocky patches and periods where my depressive and anxious symptoms flared, I had been, for all intents and purposes, in remission for years and had managed a decent recovery. I found meaning in my work, enjoyed my patients, and after years of grueling medical training, I had finally achieved a relatively balanced life.

I had continued to take antidepressants prophylactically, to prevent future episodes, but was advised by my obstetrician to wean off the medication before my third trimester due to concerns about possible negative effects on my unborn child. Working in medicine, I scoured the research in this area before deciding to follow my doctor's advice. I didn't want to risk anything bad happening to my baby and I began tapering off the meds at the beginning of my second trimester. I soldiered through the remaining 6 months keeping myself busy and distracted by work. Looking back through pictures of myself taken during this time, I am startlingly slender for a pregnant woman, wan, and have a forced, unconvincing smile. There is no "pregnancy glow" or light in my eyes.

In some ways, my worst fears came true during my daughter's birth. Determined to have a low-intervention birth, I had sought out an obstetrician who believed in women's abilities to birth naturally. She told me that she would "get down on the floor with me" and said that she had had two completely natural births herself. She practiced at a hospital that had a low rate of c-sections and that was, as I'd heard described from friends, the closest you could come to "home birth in a hospital." I was relatively young at the time, and physically healthy. My mother had birthed three children naturally and I reasoned that I would be able to do so as well. I had even enlisted the support of a doula, a birth aide to provide emotional and practical support through labor. And yet, despite our painstakingly researched and best laid plans, everything went haywire within an hour of being admitted to the hospital when I went into labor. What had started out as a "peaceful" natural birth turned very frightening, very quickly. My attention had been turned inward, focused on riding the hard waves of excruciating pain, and before I knew it the room was full of people. An oxygen mask was being put on me, and a small crowd had gathered at the heart-rate monitor, when I felt a hard thrust as a doctor's hand reached up inside me to attach a lead to the top of my daughter's head. I remember hearing the words "c-section," and at the time the pain was so unbelievable that I wanted to do anything just to make it stop.

The birth itself was like being in a car accident. Certain parts you remember watching in horrifying slow motion, and other parts you have no memory of at all. You wake up and wonder what happened and where you are. I remember being rushed on the gurney down the hall into the blinding bright light of the operating theatre. A theatre of the macabre as it went in my case. I remember being hoisted up and onto a table and then forcefully pushed up and over the side of it as the anesthesiologist inserted something sharp and cold into my low back. I remember saying I was scared—could they slow down and explain what was happening to me. "No. We don't have time," was the his gruff response. I remember asking for my husband—where was he? Why wasn't he here? Why isn't he allowed to be in the room with me now? I demanded. My arms were straight-jacketed down with velcro, a pop up screen erected above my mid-section, and then without much warning beyond the sound of ominous mechanical whirring, I felt myself being slowly opened up. Totally unprepared, I hadn't expected to feel anything and I screamed out, not in pain, it wasn't pain, but shock at the sensation of being slowly unzipped.

I awoke what must have been hours later in a dimly lit recovery room. As my surroundings came into focus, I saw my husband slumped in a corner armchair and my first conscious memory was wondering why he was wearing a funny blue suit.

He hated the color aqua. They were hospital scrubs, I slowly pieced together, through the thick fog of my mind. I was bludgeoned with exhaustion and the effects of whatever medication they gave me. (I later learned that I had continued to cry out and was given further anesthesia to sedate me including one, which causes temporary memory loss.) At some point, my daughter had been brought to me to nurse, but I have no memory of this. I later learned that she had been wheeled back to a nursery where she remained in a plastic bassinet for the night.

By the next day, the medication had worn off and I was holding my daughter. She was a tiny red-faced creature with eyes swollen shut. The nurses had swaddled her into a little burrito and I gazed down at her in my arms with wonderment. My husband was there too, and after everyone had left the room, he delicately crawled through the IVs and wires attached to me onto my bed and, finally together, we turned towards each other and cried.

The moment I had been looking forward to more than anything in my life—the moment when my husband and I were to meet our daughter—had been stolen from me. I had no memory of it whatsoever. Just a recollection of terror, crying, and then waking up heavily drugged. Hot tears rolled down my face as I burrowed into his shirt and sobbed. While our daughter had arrived, and was healthy, her birth had been terrifying. I had felt alone in the midst of a storm far beyond my control and felt that I had, at the time, been brutalized. My body had been sliced and my dream of meeting my baby, seeing her face for the first time, gone. Previously active and fit, I could now barely move without wincing. Nurses brought my baby to me and took her away. I couldn't believe what had happened. I was in a dazed shock. It took over a week before I could finally look down at the thick bandages wrapped across my swollen abdomen.

It must have been the second or third day we brought her home when the images started. They were like graphic stills from a horror movie. She'd cry, I'd pick her up, and then I'd see an image flash before my mind's eye of a dismembered baby and blood all over the floor. I swallowed hard, dizzy, and sat back down. I was just really tired, I reasoned, and tried to push it out of my mind. The image just flashed back at me, and I quickly started talking to my husband—trying desperately to change the channel.

These disturbing photo-like visions continued for some time. They almost invariably occurred when I was inside the house with her, and they always featured small bloody body parts on the floor—like the limbs of a twisted and mangled bird run over by a car. When I was outside with the baby in the stroller (we were living in an urban industrial area at the time) I was preoccupied with worry that the stroller's bassinet was too close to the ground. I was certain that her delicate pink body was going to get damaged somehow by its proximity to the dirty pavement studded with potholes and strewn with broken glass. I wanted to hold her all the time—to protect her. I was terrified of her being hurt.

Around the eighth day of her life, the screaming started. It was a shrill, piercing, pterodactyl-like kind of shriek that tore through me, activating an intense internal alarm system. Panicked, I tried to calm her. I couldn't. I passed her to my husband. He couldn't. Nothing, absolutely nothing we did worked for long to quiet her deafening roars. I bounced on the exercise ball, jiggled her in the sling, ran the faucet, shushed, oooo-ed, and kept trying to nurse her. We might get a temporary lull, but she would start again within minutes, if not seconds. Grimaced, red-faced, her back stiffly arched, she looked and sounded like she was being tortured. I felt like I was being boiled alive. Worried sick, I lost all appetite. Food, even wet fruit, was like tasteless dry cardboard that I struggled to choke down. I lost weight rapidly. At 5'7", I was 118 before I knew it. People told me I looked "great," and asked how I had managed to regain my trim physique within weeks. Publicly, I laughed these comments off. Privately, I felt like I was on the continual verge of a heart attack.

The only thing that bought us momentary peace, we discovered through trial and error over time. She would calm down if we swaddled her tightly, gave her a pacifier, put her in an electric baby swing on high speed in a darkened room, and turned on the vacuum cleaner. This worked temporarily and would buy us an hour or two of reprieve. Sometimes she'd fall asleep in the swing and I'd sit in front of it staring at her, amazed at how peaceful she looked flying back and forth in the air cradled by the mechanical arm of the swing. I wished that there was something I could have done to offer her that comfort. Despite knowing, logically, otherwise, I took it personally and felt deeply rejected by her and totally inadequate. I must be doing something wrong—I was convinced.

Determined to figure out why she was so horrendously miserable and what in God's name I was doing wrong, I called the pediatrician—again. He was a gentle-faced man in his mid-thirties who spoke with in an even measured tone, but his continual patience, imperturbability, and calm in the face of my upset only angered me. This was probably our fourth visit in as many weeks. Yes, he'd checked her again, and, no, there was nothing wrong with her. He'd had three children of his own and apparently some are just difficult. It will pass. "But there IS something wrong with her!" I wanted to yell back at him. I didn't though. Instead, he asked me how I was doing. Glowering at him in response, thinking, "what, this is MY fault??" I walked out of his office, leaving my husband speechless holding our daughter. When my husband emerged from the building minutes later looking withdrawn and exhausted, I shouted at him instead of the pediatrician. Couldn't he see what an incompetent fool this doctor was?? "God-damn it—I know more about infant sleep than he does!!" I yelled at him, my vision blurred with the flood of tears. In retrospect, I may have been right. I had been reading—a lot.

I'd started with the classic Sears' "The Baby Book: Everything you need to know about your child from birth to age two," from which I concluded that I *was* the problem—if I just carried my baby in a sling all day and slept with her at night, she'd become more "securely attached" and stop crying. I tried. Not true. I moved on to Penelope Leach's encyclopedic "Your Baby & Child," then Harvey Karp's popular "Happiest Baby on the Block," research-based Jodi Mindell's "Sleeping through the Night," La Leche League's "The Womanly Art of Breastfeeding," lactation consultant Kathleen Hughes' "The Nursing Mother's Companion," all American mom Elizabeth Pantley's "No cry sleep solution," Marc Weisbluth's "Healthy Sleep Habits, Happy Child–Fussy Baby version," and more. The brown boxes from Amazon promising to hold the answer arrived daily. Before I knew it, our bedside tables were strewn with books and their pages dog-eared and spines cracked open to highlighted passages I wanted my husband to see. I read and read and read. Little helped and nothing reassured me.

The benefits of co-sleeping widely extolled by the attachment parenting experts as the cure for the "difficult to soothe infant," we tried putting our daughter between us in bed. Within inches of our heads, she'd sleep for a few hours at a time, usually two, before she'd wake with a violent start and begin wailing again. Yet even when she slept, I could rarely sleep. At best, it was a fitful light slumber and at the slightest twitch from her, I'd bolt upright in bed and try to feed her hoping that I could satisfy her before she'd become inconsolable. Often, while she was sleeping I would lay awake beside her, fixated. Her skin, delicately flushed, was unbelievably perfect—a healthy pinky peach color with the slightest olive undertone. Her tiny lips pursed into a dewy rosebud, and long dark lashes fanned out below her closed eyes, the thin veins of blue visible beneath the translucent skin of her eyelids. She was a gorgeous, strong baby.

It always happened at night, either while I was up nursing her in the middle of the night or lying awake at night unable to sleep beside her. Staring down at her, demented thoughts flashed through my mind. What if I put a pillow over her head? How long would it take for her to stop breathing? They were dark, twisted, horrifying thoughts that were not "mine" but did nevertheless pass through my mind. I generally cried myself to sleep until I gave out with exhaustion—only to be awoken an hour or so later by her again. These thoughts went on in their acute phase, for almost a month. Horrified, I did not tell anyone.

It was the lactation consultant who picked up on my state in the end. My beloved therapist had relocated to the other side of the country shortly after I gave birth. She met my daughter only once. She had given me a referral for another therapist, but I did not follow up until many months later. I would call the lactation consultant regularly as nursing had also not been going well. My daughter would latch, nurse, and then pull off my breast screaming, milk spewing out everywhere, spraying onto the couch, and finally drenching my shirt as the force lessened. The most basic function my body was equipped to offer, providing milk, she was also unhappy with. We saw the lactation consultant four times. Once in the hospital, and the rest of the times at our home. She was fabulous. One of the last times she returned my call, she said, "I'm really worried about you. You just don't sound like you're doing well at all." I broke down at that point sobbing with relief that someone had finally put words to what I was going through. I was not doing well and I knew it. "I know," I told her through tears. "I'm not okay." She asked when my follow-up appointment was with my OB and I didn't have one. Somehow the 6-week postpartum check was never scheduled and we were now almost 10 weeks out.

She called my doctor's office and booked the follow-up appointment for me—a small task that, at the time, would have been completely overwhelming. After the lactation consultant's call and the floodgates released, I had in a fit of sleep-deprived fury, angrily shouted at my husband telling him that he had NO idea what I had been through or was going through. As if to prove my point, I told him about the thoughts I'd had. Humiliated, ashamed, totally lost, I sat in the back seat of the car next to the baby as he drove me to the doctor's appointment.

After checking vitals, a nurse brought the three of us into the exam room. Overwhelmed with shame, I sat in a corner far away from him, hung my head and waited. A young Asian-American woman, looking all of 18, entered and introduced herself as the doctor. A resident. She was probably 10 years younger than me, and a kid was the last person on earth I wanted to talk to. I took one look at her and I slumped back down disappointment. I began to cry. Again.

Despite her apparent youth, she picked up on my situation right away—postpartum depression? she said. I nodded, though I didn't think I was depressed per se. She wanted to start me on Zoloft, and I grimly took the script from her. Later that evening, my doctor, having just returned from vacation called me at home. We talked through the pros and cons, and I filled the script the next day. I was worried about nursing and the medication getting into my breast milk. Not that my daughter seemed to be enjoying nursing, but I was having some success pumping and getting milk into her through a bottle. My doctor convinced me that the trace amount of Zoloft that might get into the breast milk would do my baby far less harm than having a mother in the state that I was in. I'm not certain how much the Zoloft helped, but what really seemed to help in the end was, awful as it may sound, earplugs and selective use of sedatives to help me sleep. For many nights, I went into a separate bedroom, put in earplugs, and took an anti-anxiety medication. And slept. My husband dealt with the baby during these evenings, giving her pumped milk from a bottle that I'd prepared. Eventually, through re-regulating my system with sleep, and through getting back on an antidepressant, the anxiety lessened. The thoughts stopped. The gory images halted. Eventually, around month five, she stopped crying so much, too.

My daughter, now almost 3, remains in many ways a firecracker. She is a passionate, energetic, determined, funny, and fiercely independent little kid. She wants to do things her way. No, she does not want help. She wants me to "go away, mama," and then in almost the next breath, says "mama, I hold you," and wants to be picked up so she can rest her head on my shoulder and suck her thumb while twirling the ends of my hair with her free hand. She has learned, slowly, how to self-soothe. And I have also learned, perhaps equally slowly, how to do so as well.

My husband has become a true and equal partner in parenting and has been the cornerstone of my recovery. He gets up with our daughter, dresses her, and starts breakfast while I get needed sleep. He drops her off at daycare and they have special games that only the two of them play. I love watching the delight on her face as she hears the door open in the evenings when he comes home. Papa! she shrieks with joy. She adores me too, and while I am equally in love with her, truthfully, I continue to remain exasperated and exhausted by her at times. She is a wondrous, strong, magical little being, whom I mostly just want to inhale. And she is a wild force of nonstop energy. I have learned, over time, that she will be as she is. I cannot always comfort her, though 90 % of the time, I now can. I've also learned that it's a lot easier to comfort her and be there for her, having found solid ground to stand on myself.

The path to this place did not look at all like I thought it would. Looking back on this time, I still feel deeply saddened and aged in many ways. A child was lost, but through this journey a mother woman was born.

References

Brockington, I. F., Macdonald, E. E., & Wainscott, G. G. (2006). Anxiety, obsessions and morbid preoccupations in pregnancy and the puerperium. *Archives Of Women's Mental Health, 9*(5), 253–263.

Russell, E. J., Fawcett, J. M., & Mazmanian, D. (2013). Risk of obsessive-compulsive disorder in pregnant and postpartum women: A meta-analysis. *Journal Of Clinical Psychiatry, 74*(4), 377–385.

Speisman, B. B., Storch, E. A., & Abramowitz, J. S. (2011). Postpartum obsessive-compulsive disorder. *Journal Of Obstetric, Gynecologic, & Neonatal Nursing: Clinical Scholarship For The Care Of Women, Childbearing Families, & Newborns, 40*(6), 680–690.

Little Rays of Sunshine

32

Kathy Sattler

Kathy is a 52-year-old mother of two living in Pennsylvania. She has been diagnosed with bipolar disorder and narcotic dependence and in this chapter discusses how her mental illness and being in and out of treatment impacted her parenting. Today she describes coming "full circle" in her relationship with her children, and she works as a certified peer support specialist.

My name is Kathy, and I am foremost a mother of two successful, grown children who I have a close relationship with today. I had challenges along the way as a parent and as a person with a mental illness, but my love for them always prevailed. My story is a reflection of that time.

I am from Wilton, Connecticut, where I had the privilege of going to school from kindergarten to my senior year in high school without moving. I lived with my parents and a brother who was 2 years younger than I was. I was very different than everyone else in my family in my behavior. I spoke very quickly, had elated behavior noticeably more than other kids, and engaged in very impulsive behaviors. As a teenager I required very little sleep, unlike most kids who could sleep until noon if you let them. I was also very creative and a perfectionist, which was reflected in my grades. I had a very likeable personality and was always a people-pleaser, which unfortunately in some cases led to me putting myself last.

I went to the University of Connecticut, and in 1990 got my Bachelor's Degree in marketing. I met my husband when I was working at a bank and we had our daughter 3 years later. My marriage was idyllic prior to her being born, but rapidly crumbled thereafter. I had a very rough introduction to motherhood as my daughter had colic. The perfectionist in me was determined to stop her crying and soothe her at all costs. I would never let her "cry it out" as my husband wanted me to, and this caused great tension between us. It was the beginning of a great divide.

I was a stay-at-home mom and therefore felt I was an expert on my daughter's care. In my eyes whatever I did was the "right" way, and then there was everybody else's way. I let my husband know that constantly, and he soon felt inferior as a parent so he backed off. He was a great father mind you, but he backed away from me and let me handle the details of child care. I was slowly getting more and more neurotic, focused on making sure things were perfect. I would change my daughter's outfits every time a stain would get on them throughout the day and was constantly picking up toys to make sure the room looked clean after she played in it. I devoted every second of every day to my daughter and her care. I sacrificed friends, my hobbies, the housework (I hired someone), my identity, and my husband. My husband and I rarely, and I mean rarely, had a date night away from her in the first 3 years of her life.

When our daughter was 3, our son came into this world. While having two kids was a rough adjustment at first, this was the best thing that could have happened to me. My son didn't have colic and was the easiest baby in the world. He taught me to relax for the first time in my life. I let the toys pile up, the stains get on the clothes, I nursed him in public, and didn't have anxiety like I did with my daughter. My daughter was like a little mother to him which was adorable, and there was never any jealously between them, thank God. The three of us from that point on developed a bond that would withstand many good times, incredible memories, and lots of difficulties too.

It was when my son was two that I was diagnosed with hypomania. At that point I was staying up into all hours of the night cleaning, jumping from one project to the next and not finishing tasks, my mind was racing, I couldn't sleep, and my husband and I both knew something was wrong with me. I went to my first psychiatrist and I was put on a mood stabilizer. I felt "toned down" for the first time that I could ever remember and it was an odd feeling for me. I was used to being so overly productive, but it was good that the neurosis had stopped, for my children and my husband.

My marriage was stressful as my husband traveled a lot for his job and we moved every 2–3 years, which was an upheaval on all of our lives. He became very emotionally abusive to me and nothing that I could or would ever do was right. I started to get migraine headaches on a daily basis and I went to a doctor who prescribed narcotics to relieve them. Soon I got rebound headaches from taking so many pills and my body created headaches just to get more pain medication. It was a vicious cycle, and I was soon seeing the doctor for more and more pills. I was an addict before I knew it and I was doing anything I could just to get rid of that pain and to feel that high, which made me forget how much my husband hurt me. I changed the amount of the refills on the prescriptions and the amount of pills. I even went to different doctors and told all of them I had migraines just to get them to write prescriptions, which I would then alter. I was lucky I didn't go to jail and lose my kids.

My addiction lasted 8 years which is a v-e-r-y long time in a marriage and in kids' lives. My mood stabilizer didn't work anymore with me taking so many narcotics and actually exacerbated my mania. I was out of control. Impulsivity was the name of the game for me. I lived in the moment and did whatever I wanted, whenever I wanted to. I spent money like it was water, and luckily my husband made a lot and my father gave me annual checks from a trust fund. My impulsivity fueled the shopping addiction so much that I charged $50,000 a year on credit cards over 3 years, until I got caught by my husband. My kids wanted for nothing. Christmas was every day in our household. We got every new video game as soon as it came out, every new Barbie as soon as she was on the shelves, and went to every new movie as soon as it was premiered. That was just the tip of the iceberg; I treated my kid's friends to everything we did as well. So, I was the coolest mom in the neighborhood needless to say and on a first-name basis with everyone.

There were no boundaries anymore it seemed, for the kids or me as they grew up. My husband was busy traveling and that was our peace on earth because he was my "buzz kill." He enforced structure like we couldn't eat out, have lots of friends over or stay up late, and he talked sharply to the kids and me. The house felt like a morgue when he was home and we couldn't wait for him to leave again on a trip. I'm sure we made him feel like he was a stranger in his own home as well. The kids and I had our own routine. I was always ridiculously high and happy all the time, and until their teens they got great grades, were good kids, and we got along great. But, they walked all over me and didn't view me as much of an authoritative figure like they did their father. I didn't get the respect I felt I deserved because I was the nice and reasonable parent. I would soon learn that nice guys finish last.

My mental illness spiraled out of control during the time of my addiction. I went from being manic to being depressed, but mostly manic. My kids didn't know which way the wind was going to blow with me. I would often overreact if anyone spoke meanly to me, violently crying and sobbing on the floor, curled up in the fetal position as if I was stabbed. Words hurt me that way. I tried to kill myself by overdosing on Ativan not once, but two times while my kids were growing up. I blamed my son once in my suicide letter for the reason I was killing myself, because he was so cruel to me. I know later, that must have devastated him. While delusional from being manic and high, I often thought anything was possible and I pushed myself to the limit. I once was so sick with a ruptured ovarian cyst; I kept popping pills for the pain, and even though I was burning up with a fever and could barely walk, by the time I finally got to the hospital I was admitted for a week and almost died. Another time I did something so reckless that I thank God to this day that the three of us are alive. I drove my mini-van while I was high (as I had done many times before), but this time I drove over a friend's lawn, damaged mine, and had no recollection of it until she told me. That story to this day still terrifies me.

On the other hand, being manic most of the time made me constantly happy, and my natural giving and loving personality flourished. I taught my children to read when they were three and a half years old. We took field trips to museums, the zoo, aquarium, library, and concerts. I was very involved with their schools as well and was room mother for both of their classes for many years. I read to children at the school library every week on a regular basis, volunteered at the concession stand at my son's wrestling matches, and ran many fund-raisers for the schools. I threw my manic energy into good causes like helping at the fostering kittens, being a Girl Scout leader, and running multiple school fundraisers. My joy for life was infectious and people were drawn to me. It was a good feeling to be productive and I didn't want that to end, so I kept on getting high. I was everyone's "little ray of sunshine."

There were two times I tried to overcome my addiction and stabilize my mental illness. The first time was when my children were young and we were living in Michigan. I was running out of suppliers for my prescription needs and my symptoms were more bipolar at this point instead of being just manic as in the past. I was going to a neurological institute for treatment in Ann Arbor, and they wanted to admit me to the hospital for detox/rehab. I went there for 2 weeks and came out very shaky. I was off of the pain medication and back on my mood stabilizers, but now I would have to get used to not feeling high, which ended up being short lived. Within 2 months I was finding new doctors, getting pills from friends to get high again, and my mental illness symptoms were in full swing.

The second time I tried to get clean I was faced with an ultimatum. Either I give up prescription pills, or I would lose custody of my kids. In 2003 I was separating from my husband and he was rightfully concerned about my having sole custody of our kids while being addicted to narcotics and not being on a mood stabilizer. So, my psychiatrist weaned me off the narcotics by prescribing less and less each week, until eventually I took none. I was clean and stayed clean. Over the next 6 years I got divorced, raised two kids, stayed clean, kept my mental illness stabilized, and got my Master's Degree. I continued seeing the same psychiatrist for therapy once every 2 weeks. She helped me with parenting issues and mental health challenges that my daughter had along the way as well. My daughter developed bipolar disorder as an adolescent with entirely different symptoms than I had ever had. She was very depressed, and on the flip side, she was angry. We did some family sessions as my kids got older which were helpful for all of us to understand each other better.

In the fall of 2009 my daughter went off to college and there was a huge void in my life since it had just been the three of us for so many years, and now she was gone. A friend of mine suggested that I try Internet dating. I did, and it ended up being the turning point in my life. I met a man who said he was from Brooklyn, New York, and we spoke on the phone and chatted on the Internet for about 2 weeks until I found out he was really from Nigeria. We spent about 6 h a night Isnternet chatting and I had to get up at 5:00 am to get ready for work at the time. So, I was only getting 2 h of sleep a night and went to see my doctor, who gave me Provigil to stay awake during the day. I didn't know that Provigil was very addictive, like speed, and would enhance mania and make my mood stabilizer ineffective if abused.

Over the course of 4 months I started taking more and more Provigil to stay awake until I was addicted to it. I became delusional from lack of sleep and racing thoughts. I let this man extort almost $80,000 (my remaining divorce settlement) from me, and in the end he convinced me to embezzle an additional $8,000 from the bank I worked at. The truly sad thing was that I was so manic and out of my mind that I told no one, not even my psychiatrist, that I was doing any of this. I was arrested in December 2009 and committed to a state psychiatric hospital because the police thought I was insane when they took my statement.

When I was in the hospital I detoxed off of Provigil and was put back on my mood stabilizers; then reality set in as to what I had done. I was in psychotherapy two times a day to help me, but the pain and heartache were unbearable. My daughter had told all of my friends, her friends, their parents, and even my hairdresser what her "crazy" mother had done. She moved out of our townhouse and in with her father. My father stopped speaking to me and the only supports I had left in the world were my mother and my son. I came out of the hospital a month later and my son and I started our lives together with a bleak future for me.

I couldn't get a job anywhere with an arrest record and now my only income was child support from my ex-husband. I didn't realize at the time how much my actions and my mental illness had affected my son, until his grades started dropping and he resorted to a life of drugs and crime. We kept this hidden for a while, but when his father eventually found out he sued me for custody of him and won. Now I had no son, no income, no home, and no hope.

Eventually I got housing with help from my parents, and on January 4, 2012, I was admitted into Behavioral Health Court, an 18-month forensic recovery program, which was divided into three 6-month phases with each phase becoming less restrictive. In each phase you see the judge and get drug tested as well as go to psychiatric visits and have a Recovery Coach. I was blessed to be a part of this program in lieu of going to prison for 7 years for committing a felony by theft of deception.

In Phase One of Behavioral Health Court I learned about WRAP (Wellness Action Recovery Plan) and started attending meetings in my community. I also became a volunteer at a state hospital in the recreation department working with patients on a men's ward. Soon I became a Domestic Violence Counselor and got a job working the hotline at the Women's Center in my community. I felt a renewed sense of meaning and purpose in my life and could respect myself. I became hopeful and educated myself on how to better my life, which felt gratifying.

I had a few minor setbacks in Phase Two which led to sanctions and one major setback which led to my going to jail in October of 2012. When I was inducted into Behavioral Health Court I took an oath to never drink alcohol or take narcotics. In September of 2012 when my molar cracked, I was in so much pain that I made a very poor choice and took Vicodin. Then I got it refilled, lied about it, got caught, and went to jail for 3 weeks. I was off of my high blood pressure, migraine, and anxiety medications while I was in jail, and it was not a pretty picture besides the dire living conditions. But, I took personal responsibility for my actions and vowed to turn my life around as I had hit the lowest point in my life.

When I got out the first thing I did was go to a Narcotics Anonymous meeting and got a sponsor. I continued to go to 90 meetings in 90 days. I attended my weekly WRAP meetings and soon I was progressing through the phases of Behavioral Health Court as I did my work and advocated for myself with the help of my supporters. My supporters were my therapist, my psychiatrist, my family, and my friends at WRAP and, at the hospital, also my Certified Peer Specialist.

On July 29, 2013, I graduated from Behavioral Health Court having successfully completed all three phases. I became a Certified Peer Specialist in August 2013 and a WRAP Facilitator in September 2013. I got a job as a WRAP Facilitator in October a CPS in November, and I continued volunteering at the state hospital 3 days a week. For my ongoing wellness, I attend a weekly WRAP support group in my community, see my therapist on a weekly basis and my psychiatrist bi-monthly, and take my meds daily. I am proud to say that after I graduated from Behavioral Health Court I could have gone out and gotten drunk or high, but I have remained clean and sober and even quitting smoking!

What I have learned in my recovery journey is that you have to: Forgive yourself because it starts with you, Accept yourself because you're worth it, Value yourself because no one else will, Trust yourself because you've earned it, Love yourself like there's no tomorrow, and Empower yourself because you've proved it. Always remember that our past was meant to guide us, not define us. Through it all I believe I was truly an amazing, loving, devoted, educated, kind, fun, and dedicated parent. I still am. I did my best as a wife, but I gave it my ALL as a parent. They are my little rays of sunshine.

Healing Daughter, Healing Mother

33

Nicole A. Barclay

Nicole is a 43-year-old mother of two from Pennsylvania. In this chapter she talks about how she managed her bipolar II disorder and obsessive–compulsive disorder while learning to speak openly and honestly with her children about her symptoms. After her daughter was diagnosed with OCD, she describes how together they began learning about the disorder and successfully became engaged in exposure therapy.

I grew up in Erie, Pennsylvania. My mother is French and dated my dad when he was stationed in France with the U.S. Army. Pretty, French woman meets handsome officer, falls in love, moves to the United States, gets married, and lives happily ever after. I have one younger sister 9 years my junior, and we are best friends. In fact, both of us are married (I have two children and she has one) and live in Erie not far from our parents and grandmother. It is a loving and supportive family.

It seems like I've always known about mental illnesses. Do you remember when you figured out that what was normal for your life was not what others necessarily lived? For example, I thought everyone spent their vacations visiting battlefields, forts, and museums. It wasn't until I was married that I learned that an entire vacation could be based on sitting on a beach.

That's how it is with mental health in my family. I thought everyone knew about depression. There has been a suicide in every generation on my dad's side of the family starting with my great-great grandfather. Growing up, I watched family members deal with their depression, and my parents talked about it a good deal. The number one rule in the house was, "Don't kill yourself even if. . ." then you plug in what might upset you, e.g., you get a bad grade, your boyfriend dumps you, your parents don't understand you, etc.

For the first 2 years of college, I had a pattern with my depression and what later would be diagnosed as hypomanic episodes. The depression would get bad enough that I'd call and make an appointment with a therapist at the campus therapy office. The appointment was always at least 3 weeks out. I'd then feel immense relief that there was hope and that I was doing something to fight the mental anguish, and I'd fly into a hypomanic episode. Then as the therapy date approached, my anxiety would soar at the idea of rehashing the depression and losing my newfound happiness, and I would cancel the appointment. The depression would eventually return, get unbearable, and I would make another appointment and so the pattern would begin again.

My family knew my anxiety was high and had helped me get medication for it, but I tried to hide the depression from my family. Why I downplayed my depression escapes me now. A fear of looking weak? Fear of looking like I was feeling sorry for myself? I was functioning—straight A's, honor student, piano performance major, and French minor. I knew there was help, but denial was my friend and I mistakenly thought it was mind over matter. As if I could just figure out which muscle to flex and it would go away. I may have known about depression, but I didn't understand it.

I met my husband Steve in my junior year of college. He was able to get me to attend the therapy sessions I set up. I told him what the pattern was and asked him to stop me from canceling it as the date approached. He talked me down from my anxiety attacks, and I managed to get to the day of the appointment. He then walked me to my appointment and met me after as well. He escorted me to and from all my appointments that semester.

I was diagnosed with major depressive disorder and put on an antidepressant. My mood lifted and my anxiety lessened, but I found my psychiatrist appointments were difficult for me. For one, I was so adept at hiding my depression from people that it was painfully awkward to begin sharing how I felt. I had tried to push away the feelings for so long that words escaped me to describe it. When I did finally find the words, I found myself downplaying my feelings because I didn't want to seem like I was whining or weak. Irrational as it is, I also didn't want to offend the psychiatrist by telling her that the medication she prescribed to me wasn't good enough—as if she had given me a gift and if I wasn't appreciative enough she'd take it away. I also didn't know what "normal" was for me anymore. I knew I felt better, but I didn't know if I could feel better still. It turns out I could feel better, but that wasn't accomplished until I was 35 and correctly diagnosed with bipolar II and obsessive–compulsive disorder after transferring to a new psychiatrist. But, I am getting ahead of myself.

Right out of college, I married Steve. After 3 years, we decided to try to have a baby. I became pregnant when I was 26 and began to arm myself with as many supports as I could find. First, when I was nearing the end of my pregnancy, I started up again with my therapist Barb. I knew that the enormous change that was coming would be difficult and challenging. Besides the usual first-time mother thing, I was going to have to deal with my disorders being triggered. And, I hate change. Barb prepared me for possible, normal psychological phenomena like postpartum depression, inability to bond with an infant immediately, resentment of the infant and/or father, etc. We talked about my fears of making mistakes and messing my kids up. I have since come to accept that every parent messes up to some degree and the best we can do is avoid the big ones.

My body is rather predictable in certain ways. If something *can* trigger depression or hypomania, it will. I gave birth to my daughter Penelope and postpartum depression hit me like a locomotive. The "hormone soup" my body had become was exacerbated by my decision to breast-feed. I had been off my medication for a year, and my doctor refused to put me back on while I was breast-feeding.

The OCD hit as well, so I was stubbornly refusing to stop breast-feeding and was only eating a small menu of food so I wouldn't give the baby gas. I had mistakenly eaten lentil beans the second day home from the hospital and had one long, unpleasant, odorous night. Steve had to endure me saying that I had poisoned my baby. Every time I nursed her, I cried. (I don't eat lentils to this day.) The next day I researched what MIGHT possibly give SOME babies gas, made a list of those foods, and avoided them like they were poison. I wanted to do everything exactly right as a mom but having never been one before, I was struggling and had no solid answers of what to do. I do not handle being uncertain well.

Two months passed, and I started having debilitating vertigo, went to a doctor who ordered an MRI to rule out a brain tumor and multiple sclerosis. I fixated on the symptoms of brain tumors and MS and became convinced I had one or both and would die and leave my newborn baby girl to grow up never knowing her mother. Since this was the first big OCD attack of my life, I was able to convince Steve as well. For two long, tortuous weeks we waited for the results, which came back negative. (I was diagnosed 16 years later with vertigo migraines which are triggered by hormone changes and lack of sleep.) Through all this the family stood by and Penelope flourished.

I knew that I had two things to keep in mind as a mother—one I could control and one I could not. First, knowing that what I do and how I live will speak louder than what I say, I needed to watch my phobias, obsessions, and fears and try not to pass them on. Second, I acknowledged that there was a strong possibility I would pass along the family genes.

I needed to work diligently on my healing journey to limit negatively influencing my children's worldview. Please note I wrote *limit*. Hiding the episodes was not an option. My kids were going to encounter them no matter how much I worked. Children can sense intuitively when something is not right, even if they can't put it into words. Trying to convince them that nothing is wrong when they feel there is, I believe, teaches them to ignore and disbelieve their intuition—a terribly dangerous thing. In a world where predators flourish and have more opportunities through technology to engage children, having a child ignore their intuition makes them an easy target.

I felt that it was important to talk honestly and openly about my depressive, hypomanic, and OCD episodes. Since it is common that kids take responsibility for the behaviors and decisions of their parents, it made sense to me that the same thing could happen where my children blamed themselves for my episodes. Besides, if my kids ever started having symptoms that escaped my attention, I didn't want them to be frightened. I wanted them to know what it was, that there was help, and feel comfortable telling an adult.

The second time around as a mother of a newborn was easier. I had learned that lack of sleep was a trigger for my disorders so they didn't sneak up on me. I was prepared for the postpartum hormone soup and the vertigo that accompanies it. Knowing what to expect and having had the chance to develop my mothering skills made such a difference. Also, I didn't breast-feed so I could start my medication right away. My son Mark was born and all went much better though I did not completely escape the depression or the anxiety.

Penelope was four when Mark was born. We continued our talks about my sad times and often repeated that it wasn't anyone's fault and most certainly not her fault. We talked about the medication I took and, in age-appropriate language, explained that my body didn't produce the right chemicals so my emotions were affected. It was a matter of waiting for them to subside. She was also aware that I went to a therapist to talk about the things that bothered me and contributed to my depressions. She would ask me questions about it from time to time and even asked if she was going to get depressed as well. I told her that I didn't know, but that if she did, we would take care of it.

Around that age a boy in her school vomited. Between that and a brother who spit up sometimes, she quickly developed a phobia of vomiting that was bad enough to keep her from eating certain foods because they reminded her of vomit. For a short time she wouldn't eat at all. She would become so anxious that if anyone *looked* like they might be sick she had to leave the room. It was the first sign of OCD.

Barb told me to go directly to a counselor in our area that was phenomenal with childhood anxiety and was, in fact, so successful that she was training other therapists because the demand for her time was too great. Barb explained that the process was called exposure therapy—that we would trigger an attack and make her sit through it without allowing her to engage in her anxiety-reducing behavior (her compulsion). This therapist even had a recipe for fake vomit made out of actual food that the child was supposed to mix up and put his/her hand in. The minute she explained it, my anxiety went through the roof! I could not handle even the thought of doing that. We never saw that therapist.

Penelope began fixating on things to the degree that they immobilized her. And once she became anxious about something, it was usually impossible for her to let it go. We talked about it and sometimes were able to help her work through a particular challenge. Unfortunately, for everyone involved, her attacks triggered my anxiety which in turn triggered my depression. We would resonate together and amplify each other's episodes. Often I'd fixate on thoughts of "what am I doing wrong as a mother," "I'm failing," "I've inflicted this disorder on my baby," etc. By the time she was in the fifth grade, the anxiety began impacting her school work, and we realized that she needed some professional help.

I was still unwilling to even consider the expert Barb had recommended, and instead went to a woman who worked specifically with kids. My daughter is very smart, and she maneuvered around the help this woman tried; she'd stonewall, refuse to talk about the reasons she was there, and generally goof off. There was some improvement but not much. I was happy to have a professional involved, but it soon became apparent that this woman, however kind and capable as a therapist, was not the person for my daughter. I was finally convinced I needed the expert. I was stressed enough that anything was worth some relief. The expert herself was not taking any new clients, but she directed us to a woman whom she had trained. Enter Jennifer.

Jennifer was wonderful and quite adept at handling Penelope's attempts to control the appointments by refusing to participate and trying to sidetrack the conversations. Penelope hated going there, and I knew it meant that we were on the right road. She was out of her comfort zone; Jennifer was rocking the boat. Penelope hated going to appointments and was angry at, no, furious with me.

Both Penelope and I learned how OCD worked—how the brain mistakes something as dangerous that isn't or exaggerates the danger of something. The brain then sounds an alarm and the person feels a need to do something about the danger. The activity (the compulsion) that reduced the anxiety only reinforces the brain's initial mistake. It tells the brain, "You were right; there WAS danger" which makes the brain sound the alarm again and makes the person feel they need to continue the anxiety-reducing behavior and on and on it goes (the obsession). It was a revelation into what was going on with my own OCD. Eureka! I was learning how to deal with it!

Then came the work. The idea behind exposure therapy is to get the person to sit through an attack without engaging in the anxiety-reducing activities. They need to learn that they can endure the anxiety and survive. Little by little, the anxiety about those triggers lessens as well as the other triggers that you aren't addressing. Obsessions across the board reduce in intensity.

Jennifer had to counsel me so that I could brace myself for the exposures. They were going to elicit extreme reactions from Penelope, and we already knew that her episodes were intense triggers for me. For just about any mother it hurts to see your child in pain physically or emotionally, but it was vital to just sit with her and watch her be anxious, even panicky, and not soothe her. Soothing also reinforces the brain's mistaken alarm and is the worst thing one can do. Jennifer would spin Penelope in the swivel chair to induce nausea, and Penelope would scream and cry. I cried. It seemed inhumane. My resolve would weaken, but Jennifer (and Barb) reassured me that this was necessary, and I trusted them implicitly.

For homework, we were to engage in two exposures every day. That was quite a fight, and I dreaded them. Mark loved the ones when his sister and I would sit in the kitchen, and he was told to go to her room and touch things. It was a fight nearly every day to do the various exposures, and I became depressed because of how emotionally exhausting the whole process was. Thank goodness for my support system.

Then Penelope, that clever child, had a great idea—well, great and not so great. Since I also had OCD, after she did her two exposures, she could subject me to one. It was awful. But as painful as it was, it was an excellent idea. It took the fight out of doing the homework, it helped me reduce the impact of my OCD episodes, it made her laugh (and me, too) as I struggled like she did, and she got to get me back for making her suffer. The therapy worked—all without medication. To this day she uses the skills she learned and has been able to anticipate attacks and walk herself through them. I'm doing much better as well for the same reasons.

Steve taught the kids how to deal with my problems—how to make me laugh through them and how to love me through them. To this day they come to me, wrap their arms around me, and tell me, "Everything is alright. I love you even when you are depressed." The hypomanic episodes can actually be fun. Mark told me one day that it's like he has more than one mom; there is the fun mom who likes to play and cuddle, the depressed mom who is tired and no fun, and the I'm-too-busy mom who is fussy. It was funny and cute and gave us a chance to laugh at the various sides of my personality. I was told I am most often the fun mom.

In 2006 I had a breakdown. I hadn't found a medication that worked well for me. I fell apart one day as I was unpacking the car from a week-long vacation in Virginia for a wedding. I sat in the car and felt there was no point in anything. I considered cutting myself, but couldn't think how I would hide that from my family and especially Penelope. I also didn't want to teach my children that it was an option. I thought of ending my life but couldn't bear the idea of leaving my children without their mother. So I laid down on the hallway floor in a fetal position and called my sister at her work. She came immediately, took me to my psychiatrist's office, and another medication was started.

I don't remember how I talked to the kids about that. A few weeks later I had stabilized, and I called Barb. I asked if I had been close to being hospitalized. She told me she trusted that I would have admitted myself if I had needed it. I talk openly about that breakdown and about how I feel when I'm in episodes. The kids ask questions and they get straight answers. We discuss ways to handle symptoms and take care of ourselves—identifying triggers and how to avoid them or deal with them when they occur and having plans to "baby" ourselves when we are likely to have, or are in the midst of, an episode.

Penelope is an extremely intelligent and academically minded young lady. She was accepted to a high school for exceptional students and brought home all A's despite her challenging course load. She thrived and was enjoying it all, but it was stressful. Steve and I kept a close eye on her.

Midway through her sophomore year, I noticed her sitting in front of her computer with a 100-yard stare. I put my arm around her and asked what was going on. She shrugged her shoulders and said she was having difficulty focusing on her homework, wanted to do nothing, not even her favorite pastimes, etc. The day had arrived; the day I had been watching for. I put my arms around her and told her I had bad news and good news. The bad news was that she was depressed. The good news was that we could take care of it.

We talked about positive thinking and its place in the treatment of depression. That while negative thinking isn't the cause of the depression per se, it would make it worse. We talked about the cognitive distortions as defined by David D. Burns in his book, *Feeling Good: The New Mood Therapy*—All-or-nothing thinking, Overgeneralization, Mental filter, Disqualifying the positive, Jumping to conclusions,

Magnification or minimization, Emotional reasoning, Should statements, Labeling and mislabeling, and Personalization. She began using methods to "talk back" to this negative side of her brain. We kept talking about depression and answering the many questions she had. There was some improvement, but like before, I knew we needed to get professional help.

She started with Connie who worked specifically with youth. Penelope learned that she showed signs of ADD (attention deficit disorder) which was another big Eureka moment for both of us. We had both felt that there was something wrong with her concentration. She went from blaming herself, which was negative thinking that added to the depression, to understanding ADD and learning skills to deal with it. And as with the OCD therapy, I learned more about myself. I had a similar tendency toward AD, as did many of my family members. What a load off our shoulders once we knew what we were dealing with! Her mood improved some, but she still had "can't brain" which is what she dubbed her depression. She was doing a marvelous job of not blaming herself and attributing her problem to a chemical imbalance in her brain.

All of this was taking a toll on me. Once again, I slipped into a depression. I felt so sad to see my child suffering. I wanted to take it away from her and carry the burden myself. While intellectually I knew it wasn't my fault, I couldn't stop feeling that I had inflicted this on her—that perhaps she would be one of the unfortunate in the family to get so bad she took her life. Barb gave me one of the best gifts. She said that this was Penelope's journey, not mine. She had been placed in my care because I would be the best mom to her. I would be the best support to walk this road. I would help her reach her potential, but I was not responsible for the outcome.

Penelope had some periods of improvement, but as her junior year approached the depression and anxiety really began interfering with her life. It was time to look into medication. I found her a nurse practitioner and she started medication soon after. After a week or so the change was dramatic. Steve said, "We have our Penelope back! I didn't realize how much I missed her."

And that brings me to present day. Unfortunately the medication has not continued to work as well for Penelope so we need to look into increasing or changing it. It is not an easy or pleasant road, but there is support from both sides of the family. The lines of communication are open and working. In helping Penelope navigate her diagnosis, I have learned much about my own and have found healing. After 25 years of therapy (and counting), I am finally figuring out how to ride the depression and hypomanic episodes out instead of expecting the medication to "cure" them.

As part of my healing journey, I have reached out to people I saw were depressed, including friends, friends of friends, and numerous family members. One of the biggest obstacles for people was letting go of the notion that depression was not mind over matter—that it is a disorder. I would tell them that trying to control depression by sheer will was like a diabetic trying to will their body to regulate their insulin. I shared my story so people could see they weren't alone. And whenever I could, I would help them find the resources to get well. Mental health is an integral part of our daily life. There is no stigma or shame or hiding here. I have even heard my kids explaining things to their friends and helping them deal with their own depression and stress. I must have done something right. Every day I thank God for the many blessings I have especially my husband and children.

Learning, Loving, and Giving Back

34

Michelle Reshatoff

Michelle is a 39-year-old single mother from California. In this chapter she discusses her early experiences with symptoms of depression and mania, living in various levels of supportive housing, and fighting against her mental health treatment team. She now works in the same housing agency that once supported her and takes pride in her relationship with her son.

My name is Michelle. I am 39 years old and I live in a small, quaint, and friendly town in Northern California. I was born in the San Francisco bay area but moved to my small rustic town when I was in sixth grade. I went from a being a busy street-smart kid to a kid in the country in a blink of an eye. The small town I grew up in didn't even have a stop light or a population estimate on the street marker. I have an older sister. Growing up, she and I fought similar to what I assume most normal siblings do, but she has proven to be more than any "normal" sibling, more like an ally for what was to come. After our parents moved us from the city to have a "better" life, everything fell apart, from their separation to warring against each other over financial, emotional, and ego issues, and eventually a temporary reconciliation, another separation, and eventual divorce.

During high school, I started to have bouts of severe depression. My freshman year of high school was my sister's junior year and I got the typical razzing from her friends. Something in me couldn't turn it around. I talked to the guidance counselor weekly and I think he was sick of me. I made a sad attempt at hurting myself and it was noticed at school and a note went home. Professional counselor said I needed medication. OK, so we tried medication. My doctor put me on an antidepressant. A few months went by, and I was at school, and I started freaking out, I literally thought I was going to lose my mind. I couldn't think or breathe. It took everything I had to pick up a pay phone and call my mom to collect at my grandmother's house in the bay area. She told me to stop taking the medication and find someone to talk to. I honestly don't recall what happened after that. If I am correct, this was my first bout with mania and anxiety.

Fast-forward to when I was 20 and living in Kentucky. I had followed my heart there and had a rocky relationship with a young man. I went through periods of being in love and then breaking up with him because (from what I now know) my undiagnosed symptoms were out of control. Months later, I had terminated a pregnancy from another boyfriend who I had started seeing, and my life was spiraling out of control. I was completely devastated. I had already had one previous emergency room run-in with my ex-fiancé over emotional issues that didn't end well, so this time, when I needed help, I wanted it on my terms. I saw a commercial for a hospital and I called them and went in for an evaluation. They transferred me to another facility where I was again put on medication. My uncle put me on an airplane back home to California to be with what was left of my family.

When I finally got back to my mom's home, things were really rough. I was there less than 2 weeks and she called the sheriff to have me evaluated. I couldn't stop crying and was freaking out one night. The officer who talked with me was very gentle and brought me to a hospital unit. The nurse was kind and offered me food. I was scared. I had no clue what was going on. I ended up never going back home to live again. This began a life long journey of struggle, grief, pain, and joy for me.

I was sent to a facility to live, kind of like a halfway house for people with mental illness, only I didn't have a problem, EVERYONE ELSE did. Surely there was nothing wrong with me. People acted weird, talked weird, smelled funny, and looked odd. I had NO clue what was going on around me. I had hard lessons to learn in education, non-judgment, and tolerance. Mostly, I didn't know what was happening around me, and I was angry at my mom for leaving me and dumping me off. I swore at that moment, if I ever had children I would be a better parent and stand by my child.

I eventually moved on to other housing options. I was kicked out of other housing models due to my difficult and stubborn ways. I landed in transitional housing through the National Alliance on Mental Illness after leaving the hospital. I lived in a group housing situation with four other roommates and it was overseen by case managers from our county. I was 23 at the time. I was on medication after medication, and not very compliant. I was soon after diagnosed with Ovarian Cancer. I almost died. WOW! Could it get any lower? Twenty-three, bipolar, chemo, next to homeless, oh, and it was Thanksgiving too. I cried a lot. I had several surgeries, including one to remove my right ovary, and another to remove a large cyst on my left ovary. I did major chemo where I was admitted into the hospital for a week at a time each month and then did weekly blasts when I was out. After all that, there would not much chance of having children. And I bottomed out emotionally, it was all that I could take. I partied like I was going to die. I was angry and caused a lot of problems. I was a frequent flyer in and out of the hospital; the night nurse knew me by first name, with law enforcement knowing the drill too. You guessed it, I got kicked out of my housing again. I survived though.

I was fortunate enough to be rehoused and it was a real challenge this time. Amidst all my issues I had gone through, I had applied for housing and disability. I had been turned down many times for disability. A mental health disability is not something you can see immediately or that is apparent right off the bat. Most people don't even see it in themselves. I was so out of control. I didn't even know why I was applying nor did I see the need for medication, but I knew I was way out of control. Within a couple of months, my disability and my housing came through though. I moved into a small studio in town and started working on myself. I had something of value to protect: my independence.

I lost control real bad one more time. I ended up hospitalized for over 2 weeks, the longest ever. It was then that I came to grips with the reality of my illness and decided to come clean and work with my treatment team instead of against them. I decided I liked having nice things like a car, shoes and clothes, and FREEDOM. To this day, I still keep that promise to be honest and not hide anything. It only went up from there.

I had gotten a great job and lived in a cute apartment for a few years. I was absolutely in SHOCK to find out I was pregnant. I had not planned, tried, or even given a single thought to having children after all I had been through physically and emotionally. To be honest, it was a manic kind of idea, and we barely knew each other and it never worked out after. I almost passed out when I saw the results of the home test. REALLY? ME? NOW? WHY? My biggest concern was my medication. I ended up going off all of them immediately with no intervention. Everyone always says no medications, but fails to provide a way to not take them. A few days later came the emergency room visit and a volunteer trip to the hospital to figure out the medication thing. We were off and running. People close to me said "why don't you let this one go, you can always adopt later." I was insistent; I felt this child was my only chance at a family. It was my miracle.

Parenting is not easy. Anyone that tells you anything else is fibbing. It is the most rewarding challenge that I will undergo in my entire life. I hold sacred the responsibility that I have been given to raise my son. He is a gift to me, one that most people do not understand the magnitude of nor appreciate the value that they hold. I am in a very unique position to be able to appreciate being a parent a little more than the average parent does. I do not take for granted one single day of his life or my well-being or ability to parent him. I hold in high esteem the gift that I have been given.

I am a single parent. My son is 10. For a long time, I couldn't connect with my son on a basic level. I thought that if I just kept telling him I loved him, it would all be ok and work out. Eventually, the words came at all the right times and the situations all worked themselves out as they needed to. Together as a team, we struggle with things like his ADHD, school issues, homework, daily chores, friends, and social stuff, and then there are the more personal issues like "mom, why isn't my dad with us?" There is all of this while I struggle daily to keep my balance emotionally in order to provide a stable and constant figure for him to rely on. I want to provide consistency for him, the kind I never got as a child. My parents fought and substances were used by my father in order to maintain an order of semblance in his life. I want my child to have a voice in this world and I want to teach him to use his effectively, to speak up appropriately for what he believes in.

My mental health recovery has given me the ability to see my child as just that, a child. Yes, I have expectations of him: honesty, respect, to be polite (sometimes). But in the same instance, I see him as a person, just like you or me. He is human. Having been through a mental health issue allows you to not only see but to catch an issue sooner than an average person would. My son has ADHD. He is on medication, and I recognized a bad medication issue sooner than another parent might have. On the other hand, having the issues I have, I carry a lot of guilt about my son not having a better or "perfect" parent. I am very hard on myself when I have my off days. I still have those days when I need to relax or I am not on top of my game as a parent. My home is far from perfect, the laundry is piled up, and dishes need to be done. However, what I do know is that my son is loved and taken care of with all that I have and that is me.

The biggest thing that has hurt me has been my fear and insecurity. I let it overwhelm me. I start to doubt myself and I don't feel like I am doing enough as a parent, or that because I take time for myself to tend to my illness, that I am being a bad parent. When I let my weaknesses show, I feel like I am failing my son as his mom. The biggest thing that has helped me over the years is the people on my treatment team telling me and affirming to me that I am a good mom. They give me feedback and say that I have a kind, loving mother's soul. Some people on my team have known me almost since my diagnosis.

I believe that a mental health treatment setting should be positive and comforting. I have never been forced into treatment due to threat of my son's removal; however, this is a fear of mine and keeps me motivated to stay on track. I prefer to seek treatment on my own schedule, as I need. Yes, in some 'cases treatment is definitely needed. Treatment and interventions were often needed earlier in my life. Force is something I fear. It traumatized me when I was younger. The fear of losing my child is enough to set my anxiety spinning out of control. However, I am aware of this fear, and in a way, it keeps me in check. I know that if something were to ever happen to my child, I would absolutely die inside, beyond being able to recover from. I maintain a positive and healthy life, even when I don't want to, specifically for him and his benefit. I feel that there is no reason that he should have to live a negative life just because I have a dysfunctional day or a bad go of it for a few weeks. It has taken me a very long time to build this positive feeling about parenting, to be able to feel secure about myself and my child. I still need reassurance to know that both he and I will be ok. Sometimes, I feel like a child myself, lost in all of this, not sure if I am making the right decisions, and fearful that the wrong decision will affect my boy in a negative way.

I have almost no one to ask about the major parenting decisions in my life. I rely heavily on my older sister. I don't want to burden her too heavily, as she doesn't fully understand what it's like to walk in my shoes and the struggles I face as a parent with a mental illness. It seems I have to work twice as hard to ensure my child is raised properly. I fight with myself the most. The guilt and second guessing are the worst. I try to check in for a reality check with my sister and a friend to make sure I am level and doing a good job, not too over the top or out of control.

People have given me feedback and say I am a good mom. I do my best. I know there is a lot of room to grow. As soon as I hear the slightest hint of negative feedback, I take it very personally and give it a lot of space in my brain to ruminate. What I have to realize is that I have done well so far. For the last ten years, I have lived with a mental illness, coped with my anxiety and fear, become a mother, and raised my son. In between, I have attained my first-level college degree and maintained several jobs.

Being a parent with a mental illness is difficult, but not impossible. I fully believe that this wonderful gift (my beautiful child) was given to me to help save my life. He was designed for a purpose, with me specifically in mind and for a reason. Mental illness is not easy to overcome or manage, but it is not impossible either.

I wouldn't say I have overcome all my issues; I just don't let them overcome me. I reach out and ask for help when I start to feel those bumps in the road, before they become mountains that I can't get over. Having been through all that I have been through, I now know that it is better for me and my son, to ask for the help I need rather than wait until things get so bad that I have no choice.

Now that I have gotten on track with my life, I decided it was time to move forward and do something productive. I have had jobs before and attended college. This time, while looking for employment, I found myself in a unique situation. I attained a job where I am able to give back what was given to me all those turbulent years when I struggled the most. I work in mental health housing. I work for the same agency that gave me supportive housing when I was younger. This time I find myself in a new role. I teach life skills and give assistance to those (like myself) who need a little bit of extra time and space to work things out. I am that ear that everyone needs to bend and the supportive person who resolves the day-to-day conflicts. I also enforce the rules with kindness and support. I fully believe that I have been given the opportunity to give to others what has been given to me. Some will take it, some won't. I can say quite honestly, with my whole heart "I have been there" and know that I am speaking the truth. Others tend to believe me because I have that lived experience.

I try to always teach humility and gratefulness, both to my son and to the people I work with. My son knows what I do for work. I think it teaches us both a lesson to not take each other for granted and to love and appreciate each other and the small things in life even more. My absolute favorite small thing in life is to come home and spend some quality cuddle time with my son and talk about our days. All the "other" things of the day melt away when I see his little face.

I am at peace with my life as it is right now. I know who I am. For the first time in my life, I can look in a mirror and be satisfied in knowing that I am who and what I should be. I am content.

The Best Mother I Can Be

35

Dareia Figueroa

Dareia is a 30-year-old mother from Finland. She is a mother of three who has been diagnosed with depression and anxiety. In this chapter, she describes being physically separated from one child who is being raised in Finland, the impact of multiple relationships, and her struggles with being a single parent in the context of symptoms of mental illness.

I was born and raised in Helsinki, Finland, and I moved to the United States when I was 22 years old. I was raised by my mother. My father was a heroin addict who's now on methadone treatment. Life wasn't always peaches and cream for me, but regardless of the absence of my dad, I believe I had the best childhood I possibly could with my mother. We grew up being best friends and still are to this day. Even though she lives overseas we're best friends and keep in touch several times a day.

I became a parent for the first time when I was 21 years old. I married a guy who I thought was the one for me and soon after the wedding we found out that I was expecting. My first daughter was born healthy; however, after 2 years she started showing signs of developmental delays. After several visits to different doctors she was diagnosed as having a severe learning disability and intellectual disability.

A few days after I had given birth I noticed a big change in my mood. My doctor assured me everything was fine and I was just going through the so-called "baby blues." After a couple of weeks my symptoms just got worse. I had to ask my mother to move in with me to help out with the baby because I was depressed to the point where I didn't feel like taking a shower or even look at my own child. My mother suggested I go see a psychiatrist. After a 45 min session I was diagnosed as suffering from postpartum depression. It was devastating. I felt like my life was over. I didn't see any light at the end of the tunnel. I got prescribed plenty of different medicines trying to make me feel better and "fix the problem" and I was also seeing a psychiatrist on a regular basis. This continued for a long time and after I got the news of my daughter being mentally disabled I just lost it. I started self-

Motherhood, Mental Illness and Recovery, DOI 10.1007/978-3-319-01318-3_35,   269 medicating myself with alcohol because it seemed like the easy way out of everything and made me feel better for the night. I knew this couldn't go on too long. I felt like I needed a break from everything, even from myself. I was working as a bartender at the time and I asked my supervisor to double my shifts at work. I saved every cent I earned and booked a flight to New York, hoping that this escape to a new country would help me with everything and give me the break I so much wanted. It worked. The second the plane landed I felt like I was in a better place.

My vacation lasted 4 weeks and then it was time to go back home. My mother had been spending every day with my daughter and saw how much I'd changed when I returned back home. I told her everything about my trip, how much I loved it in New York, and that I'd decided to have a long-term goal to permanently move to New York. I had already made some connections so I didn't see my journey to relocate being a struggle. We had a long conversation about my daughter and how my mother would be her legal guardian and stay in Finland with her. I was okay with it. It was a hard decision, but I had to be selfish and think of what was best for myself. To stay in Finland and be depressed and struggle with raising my daughter, or to leave her to my mother and move on with my life and make it better for myself. Until this day, I haven't regretted my decision. It is hard at times when I miss her and wish she was here with me, but I quickly snap out of it all when I realize that without that life-changing decision I probably wouldn't be here anymore. My daughter is currently 8 years old and doing great. She receives the best possible care she can in Finland and my mother is happier than ever to spend her time with my little girl.

I've been suffering from panic attacks ever since I was 17 years old. I can't pinpoint the exact event that started everything; I feel like it was a combination of everything that had happened to me. My teenage years were pretty much average. I hung around with my friends, got in trouble in school a few times, and had plenty of boyfriend troubles. I finally dropped out of high school. I didn't see this as an issue since I always wanted to be a bartender anyway, and with that career path, the college degree would have just collected dust. Once I legally moved to New York I married my boyfriend at the time. We had been dating a few years already, and again, right after the wedding I found out that I was expecting another girl. I couldn't have been happier and everything seemed perfect. I enrolled myself to a community college that provided GED classes and after a few months I passed my GED with great grades. I didn't feel depressed at all and this was the first time in a long while that I felt truly happy.

My husband worked a lot and things started to get worse really fast. Being in a different country all by myself wasn't easy. I missed my mother and my daughter and at times I felt like I couldn't get over of how lonely I really was. I quickly realized the symptoms of depression were starting to creep up on me and I sought help. I started seeing a therapist again and I was terrified by the possibility that once again, I would be hit by postpartum depression after I gave birth. My psychiatrist suggested I start Xanax for my anxiety and diagnosed me as suffering from mood and anxiety disorder. I refused the medication because I was pregnant. Couple of months went by and I gave birth to a gorgeous little girl; at the first second I saw her it felt like God had sent one of his most beautiful angels to me to save my life. I felt like my hopelessness and depression flew out of the window the second she laid her eyes on me. I honestly had never been happier. I quickly became the parent who spent every second with their child and couldn't live without them. Everything was perfect once again and I was smiling. Little that I knew things were about to get worse.

My husband started working even more and I felt like he neglected our daughter and me a lot. The loneliness and isolation of being a stay-at-home mother quickly welcomed my anxiety back. I felt like I was suffocating. I couldn't afford to be depressed because I knew no one else would be able to take care of my daughter like I could, but the anxiety attacks got worse by the minute. I felt my heart racing, I was sweating, and sometimes I felt like an unknown power was holding me down and not letting me breathe. Once again, it was time to get treatment. I started seeing a different therapist at a different clinic and I got prescribed Xanax, Zoloft, and Ambien to help me sleep. I was okay with all the medications since I was no longer breast-feeding and my daughter slept throughout the night. I feel like the therapy helped me the most, the fact that I was able to talk to someone about everything without being judged. Sometimes I couldn't talk to my friends because they would look at me and feel sorry for me and nobody wants to receive "pity" looks. Things totally fell apart inside my home and I had to tell my husband to move out. The relationship was abusive and toxic at that point. My husband couldn't understand my pain and my frustration nor did he want to participate in my treatment. Instead of helping me, he was constantly putting me down by telling me I was a failure as a mother and worthless as a human being, a God's disgrace. I was constantly crying and I didn't see any way out, and I actually started to believe what he said about me being worthless. There were days when I was scared my daughter, who was about a year and a half old, would realize that I wasn't okay. I was scared that she would grow up being like me, depressed and emotionally unstable.

After several appointments with my therapist I finally had the courage to rise from my misery. I enrolled my daughter to a day care next to my apartment and started college. I also met a new boyfriend who helped me to pick up the pieces and helped me to put the pieces back in my puzzle again. I felt good once again. I was still on my medication and I had no intentions of discontinuing it since I was in a good place. Whether it was the weekly therapy session or the medicine or both, it was working. Like they say, if it's not broken don't fix it. I was in a stable place once again and life was good, for a minute. My boyfriend and I had talks about starting our own family and I felt comfortable with the idea of once again starting new and moving on. My boyfriend was there for me in every possible way and I felt very safe and secure with him.

Before I knew it I was pregnant again. That's when I can say that I had one of my worst anxiety attacks ever. I realized the fact that I was still using the medications that may not be the best to use while expecting had something to do with it. I also realized that my past two pregnancies were both c-sections and that would auto-matically put me in the "high-risk" pregnancy category. My boyfriend and I were fighting a lot over everything and I got extremely scared about the whole journey ahead of me. I immediately stopped the medications and told my therapist about everything and to the best of her ability she tried to help me out. I felt like my attacks got worse. I felt depressed, nauseous, hopeless, and almost like giving up. I even thought about abortion several times but never actually went through with it. This was all too much to handle for my boyfriend. It seemed like he just stopped caring about my well-being. He saw me in pain several times, he didn't help me out with my 3-year-old daughter, and all of the daily work of keeping the house clean fell on my shoulders. I felt like I was expected to be a superhuman being, doing everything on my own. On top of everything I had an infection that quickly went to my kidneys and I was being hospitalized several times a month. My boyfriend didn't even come to see me at the hospital. This was the final push for me to leave him. I told him to leave my apartment and he didn't hesitate. Maybe at this point, he had had enough of me and my complicated pregnancy. I decided to concentrate on school and my daughter and adapt to the whole situation being a single parent and pregnant.

I'm currently 6 months pregnant with a high-risk pregnancy and I have a risk of going in preterm labor. I have days where I sit down and cry, and just wonder what the real purpose of everything that's happening to me is. I believe that everything happens for a reason, I just can't see the reason yet. I believe that God gives his hardest battles to his strongest soldiers and I believe that he's not giving you more than you can handle. That's like a mantra that I have to tell myself every time I feel like I'm losing hope again.

I remember an incident that describes my struggles with my anxiety disorder. I had had a long day at school and I got home. I went to do some regular grocery shopping, cooked dinner, and cleaned my house. I was extremely tired. I went to pick up my little girl from day care and started doing her homework with her. She told me she was thirsty and I went and got her a glass of apple juice. I was sitting by my dining table typing my homework and she stood next to me watching. Suddenly she dropped the glass and the glass shattered on the floor and there was a puddle of juice on the floor. My daughter is a very smart and kind little girl so she quickly started apologizing for dropping the glass. Everything happened so fast from that moment. I felt like this outspoken rage crawled inside of me and I literally felt like I couldn't breathe, I noticed my hands shaking from anger and I had blurry vision. I started screaming, "Why, why Carissa did you do that? Why would you drop the glass right now? Why is this happening to me?" I burst into tears. They were tears of anger and tiredness and hopelessness. I hit the dining table with my fist because I felt like I was going to explode at that second. I had nobody to help me to clean the mess; I felt so alone. This whole incident took about 60 s and my vision came back and I saw my little girl standing next to me crying, looking me in my eyes, and begging for forgiveness. I felt like the worst mother ever. I was so disappointed in myself. I bent down to her and hugged and kissed her. I told her I'm so sorry that I lost my temper and that mommy isn't mad, it was an accident, and it's ok. I asked her to forgive me and told her mommy is just so tired sometimes and so sorry. She told me, "It's ok mommy, I forgive you. Everything will be fine, I promise." I kissed her again and went to get a mop and started cleaning the mess. That incident explains my daily struggles with my anxiety disorder. It's not always easy, but believing that tomorrow is going to be a better day helps.

I believe that my anxiety disorder has made me a stronger and better person. My therapy has taught me to realize the early symptoms when it comes to my depression and it has helped me to deal with my anxiety attacks without medication. I have never been hospitalized or separated from my kids because of my mental health. There have been times when my therapist suggested I go in to a hospital to "relax" and get a time out and she has been worried about me being burned out. I never accepted her advice because I have always felt that no matter how hard life is for me at times, I can do it and be fine. My daughter brings me the best joy in this world and I wouldn't want to stay a minute away from her. Even though I go through a lot and sometimes I feel hopeless, I never gave up on life. I decided a long time ago I wouldn't let depression or anxiety to hold me down or take me into a casket. I chose to be stronger and better than my conditions and I chose to do everything in my power to overcome the difficult times.

My biggest challenge when it comes to parenting is my temper and my mood swings. My daughter is having her fair share of normal toddler temper tantrums and sometimes dealing with that makes me angry, sad, and hopeless. It is hard to pull myself together at times and remind myself that this will pass and tomorrow is a new and hopefully better day. I'm working on that much more by trying to stay positive and not letting her screaming affect me in a way that it would trigger my anxiety attacks.

My daughter is three now and too young to understand the medical terms of my condition so I haven't had any conversations about it with her yet. Once she gets older I will definitely bring up some issues and explain my behavior to her more. I see that my daughter is very loving and caring and extremely smart and mature for her age. My biggest fear and concern is for her to have to go through the same problems that I've gone through. Some of the things I have gone through I wouldn't wish for my worst enemy. I hope she won't feel neglected, and I hope she will feel my love toward her and understand how precious she is and how I truly believe she saved my life by becoming my daughter.

I would love to share more awareness of parenting with mental disabilities. My diagnoses aren't that severe, but I do feel like I've had my fair share of struggles when it comes to parenting with a mental disability. Especially since I am a single mom and doing everything on my own without anyone's help, I have learned a lot and I feel like I have grown to be a better person because of everything I have gone through. There is always hope for everyone even though sometimes when going through difficult times in life you can't see the big picture. I would like to help others to concentrate on this moment and believe for the better instead of giving up. I believe in myself and that I can be whatever I choose to be. At the same time I can raise my children alone and be the best mother for them that I possibly can. I'm trying not to put myself down by thinking about all the negative things, but instead I'm concentrating on all the positive things in my life. I always remember my dad apologizing to me for him not being there for me when I grew up, for me seeing him shooting heroin in his veins, and for him just ignoring me and going in and out of jail. I always tell him, "It's ok dad, I forgive you. And guess what? You were the best dad to me you possibly could have been and just because of that, you were the perfect dad for me. Because of you, I am the woman I am today and I would never change anything about you." I hope one day my kids can say that same thing about me.

No Perfect Parent

36

Tiffany Williams

Tiffany is a 30-year-old mother from Washington, DC. In this chapter she discusses her depression following the birth of her daughter and offers what she learned through outpatient mental health treatment regarding coming to terms with becoming a mother and understanding emotions related to her own childhood experiences.

My name is Tiffany. I grew up in Washington, DC, with my older brother. We were raised by my mother in the inner city. Drugs, violence, and hardship were a way of life for me and those around me. My mother was a heroin addict until I became a teenager. She's been drug free for 12 years now.

I was 24 years old when my daughter was born. My daughter's father and I met when I was 21. I was enthralled by him. He was everything I was looking for: intelligent, charismatic, and came from a good family, all of the things I desired to be. Because of my need for validation (something I never received) I began lying about who I was. I made up a person who I thought he would approve of and wanted to be with. He didn't find out the truth about who I was until the birth of our daughter. I lied about my age, my occupation, my education, and why he could never meet my mother. The truth is I was ashamed of my mother. He came from a two-parent family that was financially stable, and I assumed he wouldn't approve of my family dynamic which is very dysfunctional most of the time. I also lied to him about my financial obligations; due to my bad money management my car was repossessed, bills became behind, and I lost what little I had. All of this happened a month before giving birth to our daughter. During this time, he began to discover the truth.

After having my daughter, I became severely depressed. Because depression wasn't something ever discussed around me and I wasn't familiar with it, I wasn't sure what I was going through. But I knew my constantly feeling and looking horrible, not wanting to leave the house, and having no desire to communicate with anyone weren't normal. I only had strength to take care of my daughter because I didn't want her to feel what I felt the majority of my life—rejected or neglected. All of my childhood issues came to the forefront. I was petrified. Due to my own fears and not having an example of good parenting, I was fearful I was going to inflict my pain, shame, regret, doubt, and overwhelming sadness on my daughter as she became older. My fears began to overwhelm me.

I started therapy when my daughter was 6 months old. I didn't understand the full concept of therapy, but I did know I had many fears regarding being a first-time mother and a tremendous amount of sadness related to my own childhood. After several sessions with the psychologist, I began to better understand my behaviors, actions, and words. Through constant words of encouragement I was able to grow and evolve in many areas. I began to speak life into myself, I started church and developed a relationship with God, I began to care and take pride in the way I looked, and I accepted the fact that I'm a slow learner and it may take me some time before I finish school. I became more social. I learned to cultivate friendships and do things outside of just being a parent. I started living!

I received services from an outpatient mental health clinic for my depression for 2 years. The weekly therapy sessions I received helped me tremendously. I finally had the courage to step out on my own. I was able to acquire my own apartment, returned to college, and obtained employment in a mental health setting helping others who faced similar challenges as I did. While receiving services at the outpatient clinic, I was taught how to cope with life stressors and what it means to parent effectively in terms of raising my daughter to have her own identity. I also realized my daughter would learn to love who she is by watching me love myself.

Parenting doesn't come with a handbook. I was extremely fearful in the beginning and I was overwhelmed because I wanted to be the "perfect parent." After learning there's no such thing, I begin developing friendships with other moms and dads. I learned through others, reading countless books pertaining to African-American parenting and attending support groups. I learned how to love my daughter in a whole new healthy way. I now know and accept I won't do everything right, but I'm ok with that! Moreover, knowing that my daughter is becoming older and more aware, I'm consciously aware of the way I respond to difficult situations.

Once I began to believe in something higher than me and faced my fears I was able to thrive instead of survive. I had to come to terms with dropping out of school in the seventh grade, molestation, being left due to my mother's incarceration, having to live wherever I could during my teenage years, never feeling good enough or pretty enough, always having to lie about who I really was, not being validated in relationships with men, etc. After going through therapy and doing the hard work of my life, I was able to become self-sufficient. I learned most importantly how to love the good and bad about me which has helped me to better parent my daughter.

Part V

Voices of Mothers: Multigenerational Impact

A Day in the Life of Bipolar Disorder

Pam Kazmaier

Pam is a 60-year-old mother of two from Arizona. In this chapter she describes one day of her life with bipolar disorder and the repercussions that day has had on her children and family. She hopes increased awareness will decriminalize mental illness to reduce stigma and shame.

Today was a good day. From the outside, I look normal. I got up and got the kids off to school, and saw my husband off to work. I cleaned the house and even organized the linen closet. I threw some clothes in the wash. I drove to work and felt, at the end of the day, I had done a good job. I'm writing this after helping the kids with their homework, while they're eating dinner, with a group of friends, at the dining room table. Normal, everyday stuff.

Some days haven't been so good. My dad was diagnosed with manic depression in the 1960s and started on lithium. He didn't believe he was ill. He was always raging. Nights were the worst. He'd storm around the house, in the dark, yelling, moaning, and saying he was going to commit suicide. As a kid, I was helpless to do anything. I'd bury my head under my pillow. This went on for years. Sometimes my little sister would come to my bed, and we'd hide together, in the dark, trying to comfort each other. Dad was never happy or well. We were relieved when he died. My mom had psychosis after surgeries, and one doctor said mom had bipolar disorder also. Mom used tranquilizers and alcohol to self-medicate. We never had much money. Sometimes I wonder how I survived.

When I was a teenager I spent a whole summer hearing voices. I didn't understand that's what it was, then. It was terrible. I was trying to take a typing class. I was bothered with visits from three men who wouldn't leave me alone. They pestered me all summer. They'd tell me how stupid I was. How I was never going to make anything of myself. They made fun of me. They would talk to each other about me. They'd laugh at me and point their fingers. They were bald and had pink skin, sometimes green. They'd watch me constantly. I felt discouraged. During breaks, a friend tried to talk to me. They'd block her and I couldn't hear what she was saying. This happened again in my twenties. I never told anyone. I thought they were real.

Throughout my twenties and thirties I worked at a great career in nursing. I graduated from college. I got married and had two sons. I thought I had PMS. I couldn't sleep at night. I was conscious and awake all night long. I dreaded the nighttime. Instead of getting tired, I had energy surges.

There's a difference in being tired and being sleepy. Normal people don't know that. I'd be tired but not sleepy. During the day, I'd be irritable, exhausted, and jumpy. I asked a doctor for sleeping pills. He refused. I asked other doctors. None of them asked about my family history of mental illness. None of them recognized the mania. I started using alcohol to sleep. It worked pretty well. I drank a lot. I also got very religious. Over the course of 30 years I joined 17 religions. I saw psychologists to help with the anxiety. Talk therapy didn't help.

Sixteen years ago, I went to a psychiatrist. That was difficult. The hardest part of having mental illness is being ashamed. It's the only illness we make fun of. I didn't want to have a diagnosis that had anything to do with mental illness. I felt sorry for my husband and sons. I didn't want them having a family life like I did. I tried different kinds of medicine. Some made me very sick. Nothing helped for a long time. Then I had a breakdown.

Caring for a son with bipolar disorder, while having bipolar disorder, is dangerous. My son Zach was 4 when he was first diagnosed. For years, we went to psychiatrists, tried medicines, and had our blood drawn. Neither of us slept for 11 years. My son hallucinated and tried to commit suicide by jumping off the top floor of the mall. I found him with ropes around his neck. He was on stimulants and antidepressants that made him worse. I kept a navy blue suit in the back of his closet for his funeral. His public school system did a terrible job of educating children with mental illness, though a great job with 1/3 of the kids who are "normal." The hardest part of raising Zack has been the daily war with the school staff who are uneducated in regard to psychiatrically ill students. I have written weekly letters of advocacy for my son and attended meetings. I grew exhausted. Bit by bit, I began losing my mind.

The summer of 2003 I began to feel something big was around the corner, but I didn't know what it was. I began making all kinds of preparations as if I were going somewhere, somewhere for a very long time, somewhere I wasn't coming back from. I felt a real urgency to get my affairs in order. I made all kinds of preparations and appointments so that my kids had their affairs in order. My son was being weaned off one of his medications. He was unstable for all of September. I had just made sure his new school year would be a good one. He had a great IEP. I had had such high hopes. His school year unraveled within a few weeks. Teachers were threatening not to keep him.

I was panic-stricken; I called his psychiatrist. I e-mailed her. I was at her office four times that month getting different medicines for him. His mania scared me. His doctor laughed at it though and said, "You're going to have to learn to live with it." I knew we couldn't live with it. I called four hospitals to get him help. One hospital said we were on the wrong side of the county line. One hospital wouldn't take him because he was under the age of 13. One hospital wouldn't take him because he wasn't also a substance abuser. The last hospital said they didn't take children. I slid the white insurance book across the kitchen counter to my husband and begged him to get our son a new doctor. He refused. I sank into despair. There was no way out. Our situation was hopeless. I remember the exact moment I snapped. Just like a rubber band that gets stretched, especially when it's old and stiff, maybe one that's been weathered a little.

I felt like I was treading water in the deep end of a pool with my son on my back. I had treaded water as long as I physically could, and we both began to drown. He was getting bigger and stronger and heavier, but I was weakening and couldn't support us. I just couldn't continue. It was too much for too long. I was way past the breaking point. There had been so little time over the years, for myself, I had forgotten that I was even there at all. I had died somewhere along the way.

Looking back to that day, I got up early as usual, nothing out of the ordinary, except that I wore no makeup, and just let my hair fall in gray threads. I wore black. No color at all. My husband and older son were at church. My younger son came up to me and said, "Mom, let's kill ourselves!" He was smiling. We were like two weak ice skaters holding on to each other for support. When one falls, he pulls the other with him. It never occurred to me to call anyone for help. Some days with bipolar disorder don't make any sense. There is no logical explanation for what happened next. I felt like I was falling backward down a hole. The room got dark, even though it was morning. I couldn't focus. I was very slowed down, uncoordinated. "Ok," was all I said.

I felt it was my duty as a mother, to go with him to the other side, so he wouldn't be alone. If he was finally going to kill himself, I must get over there too. I wanted him to feel relief. I didn't have the ability to get us to the other side. Maybe we could just sleep. I told him we could take our meds. We could take a little extra.

In the past, I had followed the advice of a therapist who told me when I was having a bad day, take my meds early, take extra, and go to sleep. Her theory was a person didn't really want to die, just black out. It had worked for me. I had never tried to help anyone else do this. I didn't want to kill Zack, just give him relief from his mania.

My son was used to taking his medications four times a day. I didn't have to help him. I was concentrating on swallowing as much medicine as I could. If he was going to the spirit world, I needed to be there for him. It was like I'd hold his hand as he crossed a busy street. I had stopped him, so many times over the years, from taking his life. This time, I was going with him, so he wouldn't be alone. A few months earlier, my brother's son had committed suicide, at the age of 14. I had felt sad that he had died alone.

I was getting sleepy as we wrote our notes to say goodbye, in case we didn't make it back. They'd be better off without us. Their whole lives revolved around our mental illness. Without us, they could live normal lives. We pushed a heavy dresser in front of the bedroom door and locked it. We didn't know if we were going to have enough time to get to the other side. We took a picture of Jesus off the wall and laid it between us and lay down on the bed and held hands. It was a picture of Jesus holding a little boy as he is helping an older girl up out of the river. We slept. I lost consciousness.

When I first tried to open my eyes, all I could see was white. Then I recognized the metal curtain track. I never got passed the ceiling. I couldn't use my left hand. It was tied to the bed. I was so sick. The next 3 days I was in and out of consciousness. I remember my husband saying our son would be ok. Occasionally people would come to the bedrail and ask questions: doctors, social workers, a chaplain, and policemen reading me my rights. I remember a visit from a friend who said, "Why didn't you call me?"

Actually, I had called her. I told her many times: Zack killed animals, set fires, kicked in doors, and threatened to kill us and blow us up with the propane tank. He wasn't sleeping. He was suicidal. He cut himself with knives just to see the blood. He collected knives. I protected my older son by installing a lock on the inside of his bedroom door, as he was frightened for his safety. Zack didn't fit in at church. He didn't fit in at school. We never had a fun family time in all our life. I had told my husband and my friends. I told church leaders and scout leaders. I told the doctors. I told the ladies who drew our blood. I told the secretaries and receptionists. I told the specialists. I had called family over the years. No one could help us. Every day was a fight. Looking back now, I should have changed his psychiatrist. We later found out her license was suspended due to drug abuse.

After 3 days in ICU I was shipped off to a psychiatric hospital, alone. My husband had had enough of me. He didn't accompany me or help me. All I had on was a hospital gown. I was barefoot, cold, and terrified. I had no socks, no underwear, no shoes, no hairbrush, no makeup, no clothes, no money, no family, and no friends. I sat in the lobby for hours before being admitted. It was the middle of the night. I overheard the staff laughing about other psychiatric patients and the funny ways they had tried to kill themselves, through hanging. That scared me. I had been on psychiatric medicines for 12 years. Now it was several days without them, having been totally purged in the ICU. My teeth were chattering. I was cold. My skin was crawling. I was paranoid. I tried several times to phone my husband, but he never answered. Later he said he had had enough and I was on my own. He had seen an attorney who recommended Kevin to divorce me, take full custody of the children, and put me away. I couldn't blame him.

Early in the morning I was admitted to a locked ward. There were crickets, and the bathroom fixtures dripped, dripped, dripped all night long. There was a red light over my bed that never shut off. The mattress was only an inch of plastic, as was the pillow. I dreaded the nights. I wasn't given any medicine and I never slept. It was torture, never being able to rest or sleep, being manic, without meds, the red light, the dripping, the crickets, the miserable plastic, the cold, and my skin cold and crawling, being jumpy. Being locked in with other symptomatic patients.

I was absolutely frantic about my son. He was in the same horrible place somewhere on a children's unit. Was he sleeping? Was he eating? Was he drinking? Was he as scared and lonely as I was? I was hysterical to get to him until one of the staff told me he was doing well. He was eating and drinking and sleeping and had made friends. He was *sleeping? He had friends? That was new!* He had night terrors for 11 years. Our entire family had not slept for 11 long years.

The first thing Zack's new psychiatrist did was change the medications ordered by the old psychiatrist [which had caused Zack to be manic/suicidal]. This hospital psychiatrist stabilized Zack quickly by discontinuing the antidepressants and stimulants that had induced instability in Zack. Zack was immediately placed back on the Tegretol, the mood stabilizer the old psychiatrist had discontinued in September (which had destabilized him to the point of mania/suicide) and was placed on a new medicine, called Geodon, an antipsychotic. He went home and back to school in a few days. Each day, my son improved. It has now been 9 years. He has not been suicidal once! The antipsychotic medication "Geodon" has been a miracle! Zack is now doing well. He graduated from high school with his class in 2010. He is over six feet tall, lives on his own, and is fun to be around. He is moving forward. Zack has goals for the future. He still goes to the psychiatrist who stabilized him so quickly.

I had to stay in the psychiatric ward for a few weeks, and then I was arrested and handcuffed, booked, and chained to a bench in jail. I was indicted on a class five felony of Dangerous Crimes Against Children, carrying a mandatory 34-year prison sentence. I pled guilty and spent 5 years on supervised probation, rather than having a trial. Many people with mental illness end up in the criminal justice system. It's devastating. The reality of mental illness is discrimination and blame. It's the only illness we *blame* people for having. It doesn't happen with a heart attack, just a brain attack. The police and courts don't understand how much worse they make life for those with mental illness. For 2 years I went back and forth to court as a defendant. I'm shamed, embarrassed, and defeated. I am a social reject. I'm an outcast. I feel lower than low for my bad judgment of that day. I wouldn't mind serving the rest of my life in prison for what I have done to my children.

If my case had gone to trial, it would have cost thousands of dollars we didn't have. Our medical and attorney bills took our life savings. My sons and husband would have had to take the stand and repeat their original statements against me. My husband told the attorney I wasn't worth the $50,000 it would have taken to go to trial. This whole incident was a huge embarrassment to my husband who was a lieutenant and bomb commander with the local police department. I pled guilty and became a felon. I've had to surrender my nursing license and could no longer pass a criminal background check. My voting rights were stripped away, along with my self-esteem.

I feel badly my husband has had to be married to a person with mental illness, raising a son with mental illness. I read somewhere that 80 % of the marriages raising a special needs child end in divorce. My husband warned me he can never go through this again. Our marriage had been a strain. If I knew then, what I know now, I'd never have proposed to him so very long ago. He is a good man and deserves more. I felt like a ball and chain to him.

I took classes with the National Alliance on Mental Illness. I found better psychiatric care. NAMI gives Arizona a "D" for mental illness services compared to other states. In our state, the public psychiatric system is better than the private.

For a couple of years I really struggled to get back to normal. Then I realized, "*back, wasn't normal.*"

Our family was out of balance. I've tried to take better care of myself. I got angry for a while. I quit our church. Church is harder on women than men. I actually think it's set up for men. They like having the women do all that hard work for them. I found a job. I got my own bank account. I started exercising. I got my hair done. I freed myself from the slavery of housework. It was killing me. My husband is stepping in and being a parent. Imagine that. My boys began doing their own laundry and cleaning their own rooms. They're learning to cook. All that work and sacrifice were unhealthy for me. My enmeshment in their lives was impeding their development and independence. Hopefully I am no longer an over involved, problematic mother.

For the first time in many years, I want to live. I'm happy waking up in the morning and having a job to go to. I have pursued my goal of working in mental health rehabilitation. I have gained more education and became a Certified Psychiatric Rehabilitation Practitioner. I encourage our members that there is life after a nervous breakdown, psychiatric hospitalization, and criminalization. I have a paycheck again. I'm on a medicine that doesn't make me sick. I moved to my own place. The memories of living there were too much for me. My house is a quiet retreat, decorated in soft, soothing colors. I rest there, feed my birds on the patio, and water my plants. I read a lot of books by women who have also overcome many challenges. I listen to women's music. I do yoga now. I take care of myself, a new concept after 55 years of taking care of others. I am making progress, moving forward. Life is good now. I have learned we women have to take care of ourselves because no one else will. I believed a lie for a long time: love a man, nurture him, and he'll take care of you. That is such a lie and women believe it all the time. I'm taking care of myself now. The breathing space between my husband and I has given us a renewed friendship with each other. We've been married now for 32 years.

I enjoy seeing Kevin, Mike, and Zack. We talk or visit every week. On holidays I spend more time with them. We're all doing well and making progress in our lives. We're more honest and open with each other and support one another. Our living arrangements sound odd to others. When a family struggles with mental illness, extraordinary choices need to be made. We have gone through hell with bipolar disorder. We've learned the wrong medicine can be dangerous, but the right medicine can be life changing.

Like Rosa Parks who drew a line in the sand and refused to go to the back of the bus, I've taken a stand in my life too. It's time to stop blaming people with mental illness. Mental illness is a medical condition, not a legal/criminal matter. A criminal history denies a person work, an apartment, and recovery. The hardest part of having mental illness is being ashamed. This shame prevents patients from taking the medications that are 80 % effective. I made a bumper sticker that says: *Mental illness isn't a sin or a crime—it's an* **illness**.

Family Secrets

38

Valarie Anthony

Valarie is a 49-year-old mother from New York City. In this chapter, she describes her time in the New York City foster care system and her experiences being abused and neglected by family and foster care providers. She also discusses her family history of mental illness and the challenges of motherhood in the context of posttraumatic stress disorder.

My name is Valarie. I was born in Brooklyn, New York, and was raised in Brooklyn and Queens. I am told that I lived with my parents and siblings in the Crown Heights section of Brooklyn for the first 3 years of my life. My parents separated when I was 3 years old and they would eventually divorce. I do not recall living with my parents and I never felt emotionally connected to either of them, but this is what I was told and what is documented in my foster care case file.

The earliest memory that I have from my childhood does not involve either of my parents. It was when I was 5 years old and living in a Brooklyn foster home. In this memory, my foster mother is forcibly guiding my small hand over an open flame at the kitchen stove. This was punishment for my refusing to eat a bowl of cereal after I saw a roach crawl out of the box and into the bowl. I'm reminded of that incident every time I look at my left hand. Although the burn mark is very noticeable and other kids have noticed it during my childhood, no adult professional ever seemed to notice it.

I was 3 years old when my three siblings and I entered the New York City foster care system after my mother suffered a major mental breakdown, following the mysterious death of my newborn baby sister. At the time that we went into foster care, I recall being told that there was a house fire and that my sister did not survive. As a result, my mother suffered a nervous breakdown. I have never been able to recall anything related to the fire, and as an adult I began to question if the fire ever occurred at all. Since I was a 3 year old, I was never given specifics about the fire or the whereabouts of my sister's remains. I was always left with the assumption that

Motherhood, Mental Illness and Recovery, DOI 10.1007/978-3-319-01318-3_38,
© Springer International Publishing Switzerland 2014

my sister was left at the apartment. Years later, I would learn a different reason for going into foster care. The story about the house fire turned out not to be true.

It is documented in my case record that on this particular day, my mother asked a neighbor to call an ambulance for her as she was not feeling well. My mother reportedly became impatient waiting for the ambulance and the neighbor observed my mother climbing down the fire escape with 4 of her 5 children, which included 5-year old Dan, 4-year old Andrew, 1-year old Chad, and me. I always thought it was odd that we went down the fire escape instead of going through the apartment door. The fire escape incident explains my fear of heights, especially fire escapes.

My mother took us with her to the local welfare office, where she had recently began to receive benefits after separating from my father. At the welfare office, her case worker noticed her bizarre behavior and arranged to have my mother transferred to the psychiatric ward of Kings County Hospital. From the hospital, she contacted her friend Mary, a woman she had met when she was pregnant with Chad. The two women had kept in touch and my mother reached out to Mary, asking her to take care of her children for a few days while she was in the hospital. Mary agreed to take us in, and when it appeared that my mother's hospitalization was going to be on a longer-term basis, Mary enlisted the help of her two tenants, Gina and Betty.

Aunt Mary owned a three-family house in the Crown Heights section of Brooklyn, not too far from the apartment we lived at with our parents. Aunt Mary resided in a one-bedroom apartment located on the first floor, while Aunt Gina resided in a two-bedroom second floor apartment and Betty resided in a two-bedroom apartment located on the third floor. Of all three women, Gina seemed to be the most capable parental figure, followed by Mary. Betty appeared to be the worst. Her life seemed to revolve around chaos and drama. Chad and Dan moved in with Mary, taking the bedroom located in the rear of the apartment, while Mary slept on the couch. She purchased a bunk bed set for the boys to sleep in. Andrew resided in Aunt Gina's apartment and I resided in Betty's apartment.

I noticed how nurturing and caring Aunt Gina seemed to be, not just with Andrew who resided in her home, but with all of us. She was a little older than the other two women and reminded me of someone's favorite grandmother or aunt. She seemed very knowledgeable on many different topics and always encouraged Andrew to focus on school; he would eventually go away to a prestigious New England boarding school during his adolescence. I remember that Aunt Mary was always playing music and singing, teaching me how to dance, and encouraging me to learn the newest dance steps. Although she had a drinking problem and we would sometimes find her passed out drunk on the couch, she did the best job she could in taking care of my youngest and oldest brothers, ensuring that they were always fed and taken care of.

Betty appeared to be the opposite. She had a 16-year old daughter, a 3-year old son, and a 4-year old daughter also living with her. She would give birth to another daughter several years later and she always seemed to be short on funds. She also had other children who were in the care and custody of their fathers. I would later learn that Betty was also an ex-offender, having spent time in prison for embezzlement.

Betty's daughter Pat had the front bedroom, while Betty and her boyfriend Jim had the larger bedroom that was located in the back of the apartment. Three-year old Ken and 4-year old Dana slept on the living room sofa. There was nowhere for me to sleep, so I slept outside the apartment in the hallway. Sometimes, my brother Chad would spend time with me in the hallway, playing with me and keeping me company. When it was close to his bedtime, Aunt Mary would always call him and tell him it was time to bathe and get ready for bed. I noticed that Betty always seemed stressed and didn't seem nurturing at all.

Despite the extra help she received after adding me to her welfare budget as an Unrelated Child, Betty seemed to have difficulty managing her household and providing quality care to all the children in her household. In Betty's home, I rarely ate food, and when I did eat, it was neither healthy nor filling. I don't recall ever having a hot meal in the home or eating at the table. There were no toys for me to play with, I never celebrated birthdays or holidays in the home, and I always lived in constant fear of Betty and Jim. In addition, I experienced Selective Mutism which didn't seem to go away until I was 8 years old, the year Betty decided to enroll me at the elementary school near our home.

At school, I developed a very close relationship with Ms. Rogers, the school guidance counselor. Ms. Rogers took a special interest in me, talking with me, braiding my hair, and encouraging me to have healthy meals during lunch hour. She noticed that I was walking on the balls of my feet, so she referred me to the PTA Fund so that I could receive a new pair of shoes, but Betty refused to allow it and I continued to come to school every day in shoes that did not fit. Eventually, Ms. Rogers contacted Betty to advocate on my behalf. After several attempts to get Betty to cooperate, Ms. Rogers placed a child abuse hotline call as she already suspected abuse and neglect.

After several visits with the Child Protective Services investigator, the allegations were substantiated and the foster care agency contacted Betty, informing her that her home was an inappropriate foster care placement and that she failed the most recent Home Finding Study. They also informed Betty that in 30 days, they would be transferring me back to Protective Custody until another foster home could be found. Betty, angry that she failed yet another Home Finding Study and feeling rejected, contacted the agency and told them to transfer me out of her home as soon as possible. I was immediately removed from her home and transferred to the Queens home of my aunt and uncle, where I resided for the next 10 years, enduring physical and sexual abuse by my uncle and emotional neglect by my aunt.

When I was not at home, I appeared to be happy and well-adjusted. Like most foster children, I had no choice where I would live, with whom I would live, or how long I would stay in a particular placement. I somehow slipped between the cracks of the system as I grew and developed, enduring all kinds of abuse and neglect within the foster care system. Instead of feeling like a family member, I seemed more like an unwelcome guest in other people's homes, even when they were the homes of relatives.

I "met" my mother when I was about 8 or 9 years old. All the siblings would gather at the foster care agency to celebrate birthdays and holidays. I observed that my mother's behavior was kind of strange and I felt uncomfortable being around her. By the time I entered adolescence, I would learn that my mother was mentally ill and that there were frequent hospitalizations to treat her schizophrenia. Throughout her adult life, my mother reportedly was noncompliant with her medication due to side effects, so she never recovered from her mental illness. My siblings and I continued to reside in foster care, and my mother would eventually have seven children in the foster care system. Agency social workers would step in and find foster parents for each new baby. The last three were eventually adopted out.

I was a preteen when I began seeing my first therapist. My great uncle began sexually molesting me the first night I arrived at the home. There were "grooming sessions" several times a week, followed by sexual abuse. I was 8 years old when this began, so by the time I developed into preadolescence, I was scared, uncomfortable, confused, and very angry.

My aunt reported my "behavior" to the caseworker and he eventually referred me to a child therapist. As a young person, I felt that the adults in my life were clueless. Some seemed to feel that I was developing schizophrenia like my mother, while others didn't know what the issue was. I felt like there was no one who seemed to notice that I had the classic signs of child physical and sexual abuse. I think this frustrated me even more because I felt misunderstood, misjudged, and misdiagnosed. During my senior year in high school, I began seeing a different therapist, who seemed to be right on point. She seemed to know what I was going through. In one session, I observed her crying a sea of tears, and then she asked me why I wasn't crying. Because of my dissociation, I was able to talk in therapy about incidents that occurred in the home as if I were talking about someone else.

Just as the new therapist began planning to involve my aunt and uncle in the therapy sessions, my aunt abruptly terminated the services, telling me that I no longer had to go to therapy. To the foster care caseworker, she would blame me for the termination of services. It was documented in the case file that my aunt told my caseworker that I refused to attend any more sessions, which could not have been further from the truth. I remember discussing with the therapist the plan to involve my aunt and uncle in the sessions and I was finally ready to confront my uncle about his abuse toward me. I always felt that my aunt was nervous about the skeletons coming out of the closet. She knew of the sexual abuse, but she never did anything about it. During my adolescence, I told my aunt of the sexual abuse but she responded by calling me a little slut. Not long after, I was transferred out of the home and into several foster homes and foster group homes.

I resided in over 12 foster homes and two foster group homes over the course of my childhood. Because of the physical, emotional, and sexual abuse that I endured while living in foster care, I had an unhappy childhood and experienced early signs of Post-Traumatic Stress Disorder. I recall experiencing symptoms of this disorder as early as 8 years old, but I was never diagnosed as a child, nor was I treated for the abuse and neglect that I endured. For a long time, I worked hard to bury my secret past and didn't actually address these issues until much later. It has taken me several decades to no longer feel ashamed because of my foster care experiences. This process has finally allowed me to make peace with my past, the woman who abandoned her children, and the imperfect child welfare system charged to look after us.

After high school graduation, I went away to college in Massachusetts. During vacations, I resided in foster homes in Queens and a group home in the Bronx. One of the "house parents" at the group home documented in my case record that I "had the classic signs of child abuse syndrome," but no one from the group home or from the foster care agency did anything to help me address it. Her statement seemed more like an insult or gossip, rather than the words of a caring and concerned child welfare professional.

I "aged out" of foster care just prior to college graduation and decided to remain in Massachusetts, where I began my career in the field of Human Services. When I was in my mid-1920s, I enrolled at graduate school and completed the program at age 28, the youngest in my class. I made the decision at that time not to reveal to colleagues and friends my history of foster care because at the time it wasn't acceptable, especially in the corporate world to admit to having a less than ideal childhood. So I created a persona that I revealed to the world. At the same time, I was able to bury the secrets of my past.

I was in my early 30s when I became pregnant with my son. Prior to becoming pregnant, I doubted my abilities as a parent and was content with working and socializing. After I became pregnant, I did a lot of reading on parenthood and decided to try to be the best parent I could be. I bought him the best clothes, the most expensive diapers, and even tried my hand at making homemade baby food. My son's father chose not to remain a part of his life, so I had no choice but to raise him alone. I feel that my experiences in foster care, as well as my family's history of mental illness, helped me deal with the challenges of motherhood. As a human services professional, I had many resources available and learned all I could about parenthood prior to giving birth. Unfortunately, I no longer had contact with my family members, so I did not have the benefit of older relatives' expertise.

When my son was 2 years old, he began to display signs of trouble, and at age 7 he was diagnosed with Pediatric Bipolar Disorder. He has been hospitalized on multiple occasions because as a child, treatment doesn't always work. Whenever he would grow and develop, the medication would stop working and it was necessary to bring him back to the hospital for assessment and treatment. It was at this time that I started to confront the secrets I had been keeping. I often wondered if my family's history of mental illness was related to my son's issues. I began seeking the services of a therapist for myself and at that time was officially diagnosed with Post-Traumatic Stress Disorder. I was never separated from my son and I often felt successful that I have always been able to keep him at home. I feel that my mental health issues never interfered with parenthood, but my ethnic background and marital status did. As an educated African-American single parent, I feel that I've had to work twice as hard as two-parent families to provide a quality home for my son and I have been successful at it, but I've had to deal with outsiders who do not necessarily understand different cultures and different types of families, placing my family at risk for involvement with Child Protective Services.

I remember when my son was very small, a nurse at a Connecticut-area hospital reported me to her supervisor for physical child abuse after noticing several large "bruises" on my son's back. My son and I were subjected to questions and body checks during an "interview" by a nurse manager and a physician at the hospital. The "bruises" the nurse observed were actually Mongolian Spots, which are common in Latino, East Asian, and Native American infants, as well as Polynesian and Micronesian families. They look more like very large birth marks rather than bruises. My son's Mongolian Spots were present since he was about 2 months old. I too, was horrified when I first saw them, but I met with his doctor and asked questions in a calm and intelligent manner, learning that they are harmless spots that will eventually fade.

As a preschooler, my son was classified as a special needs student and he has had an Individualized Education Plan throughout the years. During the elementary grades, I have observed and listened to comments made by school staff, as well as agency staff alluding to the fact that my single parenthood may not be sufficient in raising a child. I was constantly asked by these "professionals" why I wasn't married. The questions were more like a statement of my inadequacy as an adult, rather than a question.

Today, my son is a 16-year-old high school Junior. He attends morning classes at an alternative high school and attends afternoon classes at their career development program, where he is enrolled in the A + computer technology program. My son is a computer and electronics wiz and hopes to eventually attend college and major in computer technology. The challenge that I often experience with him is that he is easily distracted by friends who may not necessarily have future plans and goals. I remain actively involved with his treatment and maintain ongoing contact with his treatment team. I continue to encourage him to do his best at school, with the main goal of graduating from high school.

The advice that I can offer mothers facing these challenges is to stay involved with school and treatment teams, attend all meetings if possible, and document everything. I would suggest that mothers keep a portfolio or notebook for school meetings. I usually keep an updated photo of him in his book and offer to let others at meetings view the book, as well as his photo so that they could really get to know him as a person. It would also be a good idea to develop a list of resources.

When I first moved to our county from New York City, I created my own resource manual using a loose leaf notebook. I researched all the agencies and schools in the area that I thought would be useful, keeping a list of contact people, addresses, phone numbers, and services provided. I would also advise parents to stay on top of their own mental health issues, surround themselves with positive people, maintain an ongoing social support network, and get plenty of rest, nutrition, and exercise. This will help you function better. I would also advise parents not to drink alcoholic beverages or take illegal drugs of any kind.

The more alert and clear-minded you are the better you will be in confronting any issues with your son or daughter. It is very important to take care of your emotional, physical, and social needs. Also, keep in mind that the best way to advocate for your child is to learn all you can about your child's condition, as well as resources available.

Find Your Light

39

Shannon McCleerey-Hooper

Shannon's recovery journey includes being a daughter of violence and substance abuse, a mother, a family advocate and caregiver to a brother who was a quadriplegic for 22 years, a personal struggle with hyperactivity and deep depressive episodes, and, most recently, a mother with a child who carries a diagnosis. She works as a Senior Peer Communications Specialist in California and has also dedicated herself to educating others about behavioral health and recovery through her many presentations, workshops, and conference talks on the topic.

"Find your light!!!" were three words I heard at the age of nine, echoing from the back of my elementary school theater house. Little did I know that the director was telling me something very profound and life-altering. As I stood there in my rag-a-muffin costume as Oliver, the title role of my very first musical theater production, I sensed the darkness she was talking about and "cheated" my way downstage a foot to feel the heat of the hanging Fresnel, a warmth I will never forget or take for granted.

A few weeks before, I was sitting in my beanbag chair in my new suburban bedroom, thinking about ways I could just disappear, die, and not cause any more distress or frustration to my family. How can I do it so it wouldn't hurt, so I wouldn't make a mess, and what to write to my siblings to tell them that I did it to make their lives better. Not until I was in my thirties did I truly understand that this was not a normal way of thinking for a child, for anyone. Those thoughts and designs would come and go many times throughout my life.

When I was 3 years old, my mother, married to a career Army Captain, lost her hope for a life of love and peace and fell into despair. She suffered a severe mental breakdown that left her wandering the streets near the beautiful Santa Barbara coastline. Authorities and family found her crawling on her hands and knees in bushes near a cliff side. Over the next few years she spent time in and out of the

Motherhood, Mental Illness and Recovery, DOI 10.1007/978-3-319-01318-3_39,
© Springer International Publishing Switzerland 2014

hospital and eventually attempted to take her own life. The story that was told to me and my three siblings was that she had abandoned us, that she was a bad mother, and that she was crazy—this all coming from a person who would impact my life, in ways much more traumatic than the disappearance of my mother. I didn't see her again until I was 6 years old.

Dad was an angry man by the time I came on the picture. My eldest brother was nine, my other brother, eight, and my sister was seven. When mom left, dad didn't even know how to make toast. He was lost, frightened, betrayed, and ill-equipped to care for four small children. Dad is an alcoholic who knew combat, control, training, and discipline. We became his little Army unit, he the Drill Sergeant. This made for a formula of fear, intimidation, and violence that would shape our lives as torn-down "probies" to be molded into soldiers of survival. I was a "hyperactive" child of the 1970s and the only way to keep me in one place was to force me to submit through physical pain and humiliation. No wonder that, by nine, I was cycling through episodes of undiagnosed depression and insomnia plagued me. I never told a soul for years that I slept very little and the tiniest of noises would bring me instantly to life, out of my bed, standing and ready for what might be coming.

My father remarried a woman who had two children of her own and did not care for me, because I had "too much frenetic energy" that I was "an annoyance." She was verbally and psychologically abusive to all of us, driving my eldest brother to college campus living, 3 weeks after high school graduation. Her contempt for my dad's kids and her abrasiveness, compiled with my father's heavy hand, pushed my second brother into alcohol and drug addiction. He ran away from home at 15 and never returned. My sister followed my brother 6 months later after being caught with drugs and alcohol in the home and I witnessed my father break a chair on the wall over her head. I stayed. I was 11.

While living in complete dysfunction over the next several years, I threw myself into school extracurricular activities (to stay away from the house as much as possible). I had become a leading lady in all the school musical theater productions, a principal actor in all things Drama, an accomplished violinist, a member of an elite chamber choir, and an English language junkie. I was the fun, impulsive, outgoing, and all-around ball of positive energy to my huge circle of friends—the family I built for myself. When I would isolate, I would hide in the warmth of musical comedy. I would put on headphones and listen intently to soundtrack albums, obsess about every word and every note, and fantasize about a life on the Broadway stage. The upbeat persona worked for me and kept me from sitting in depressive states and having thoughts of dying early. I thought it could keep me safe from anything else that could potentially traumatize me further. Well, the Universe had other plans. And to this day, I will never understand why so much pain is required to find a higher place of consciousness.

While at the high school, having our final dress rehearsal for *Carousel*, my stepmother came to the dressing room area where I was applying makeup. This was shocking and way out of character, as she had never participated in any way with my extracurricular activities. She approached me directly and my first thought was,

"Ah shit. . .what did I do now?" She asked me to come outside with her. All the rest was in slow motion. She proceeded to tell me that my brother and sister were involved in a serious car accident and that she would come back to get me after rehearsal to take me to the hospital to see what was going on. And being a 16-year-old, you just don't have enough reality to understand the gravity of what was happening. I ran the show and she was there waiting in the parking lot.

When I arrived at the hospital, my father's facial expression was something I had never seen before. He was as lost as I had ever seen him. He was in "business mode," taking notes and listening intently to what doctors and nurses were saying. I was directed to take a seat in the hallway. Now, I had not seen my sister in about a year and my brother since he had run away from home three and a half years earlier. I caught a glimpse of my sister whose big brown doe eyes were just as lost as dad's, but she was frozen—traumatized. She had bandages all over one of her legs, on her forehead and hands. There was blood on her shirt. I didn't even know what to say, so I stayed silent for a while. Dad stood with arms folded and turned to me. I finally asked, "Where's Patrick?" My father was talking to me, as if I was under water. Trying to explain what had happened, he ushered me into a hospital room where my brother was suspended in a hospital bed facing the floor. He had broken his neck and was paralyzed from the chest down. They called this "traction" and I, too, was frozen. They had drilled holes into the sides of his head and had installed a "halo" so his head would not move. This was the beginning of a completely separate "time space continuum" in my recovery journey. It would last for 22 years and play a huge part in my journey of hope and recovery.

In spite of all the "life" I had already experienced at 17, I went on to college and got a degree in Musical Theater. I was part of a new life that had nothing to do with my suburban neighborhood, my old friends, my fucked up family, or my deepening depression. I ran away, leaving all of that and them behind—without a word. Later, I learned that I hurt a lot of people who loved me when I left. My self-preservation was self-centered and something, for which I have since made amends.

In 1988, I experienced what I lovingly call "The Triple Whammy." I had my first real crisis. After being in three acting classes, being three different people, rehearsing for a show for 3 h on a musical theater leading role, and triggered by an altercation at a Sunday family get together—I forgot who I was. I forget who-I-was, in the most literal sense. I was in a dissociative state, crying uncontrollably for what my roommate says was about 6 h. She was so frightened by what was happening to me, she took me to the university health clinic. When I woke in my own bed twelve hours later, I felt like I weighed a thousand pounds and could not move. I had only fuzzy memories of the day before. I only had a paper from the health clinic referring me to a campus counselor and therapy group for Adult Children of Alcoholics.

After about a hundred therapy sessions, a marriage, and a divorce it was 1991 and I was starting my life again, and again, I ran away from the college circle of friends and dove into the experience of living alone for the first time. I was deeply depressed, binge drinking, being sexually promiscuous, and putting myself into very dangerous situations. Amidst all this ugliness, the one thing that never left me was "the warmth" of that light on stage. I used my time in theater to work out my emotions and be somebody else for a little while. It was really working and I was in a very good place by 1994.

I met my husband, my darling Eric, while performing in *A Funny Thing Happened on the Way to the Forum* for a college summer program. He was the Stage Manager and I did not like him. Hilarious as it is, we will celebrate our 20th wedding anniversary in 2014. I became a mother so quickly after I married him, I did not have time to really think about it. I had never wanted children. I always feared I would fail to control my impulses and hit my children.

I was never nurtured by any member of my family. The only nurturing I experienced was from the mothers of my friends. These mothers knew I was being emotionally tortured by the people who were supposed to protect me. They knew, and in visits with them over the years, they divulged that they would have family discussions about how they could help me without putting me in further danger. That image makes me tearful as I write this. Bonnie was the mother of my next-door neighbor and best friend of 36 years, Tracy. She made me feel so welcomed and loved that, over time, I would be that kid who would come over, open the refrigerator, and say "What's for dinner, Mom?" and she would shoo me away from the kitchen and tell me to set the table. She loved me like family. Their home became a sanctuary. When she left this world to be an angel for us, I felt the loss of a daughter whose mother had passed. I also had a friend, Dawn, my acting rival in high school, who is still one of my dearest friends. Her parents would hug me and hold me just a little longer than other people, because they knew. I guess, at times, they were as hopeless as I. They were the mothers whose actions I branded onto my heart. Their love and wisdom have stayed with me as I have nurtured friendships and raised my children.

In college, we nurture our gifts. We meet people who impact the rest of our lives. Relationships, lovers won and lost, counselors, impactful faculty, and friendships, all who change us. One of these friendships was a randomly placed dorm roommate, Shelly. We became friends immediately. She was reserved, quirky, and sweet—didn't cuss until she met me. After our dorm life we lived together on and off from 1984 to 1992. We were very close. When I found out I was pregnant, she was ecstatic. She could not wait to become an "Auntie." She planned a baby shower and rubbed my belly every chance she had to see if Andrew-Devon would kick. (We pre-named the babies long before they were the size of Bartlett pears.)

On the day of the baby shower, her husband of just a few days stopped by the house to drop off decorations and balloons for the party. He rushed away from the door stating that Shelly had collapsed from an ongoing lung problem she had been experiencing over the few months prior. Though I had reservations and anxiety about having the party, I sent my love and asked him to call me for a status as soon as he knew more. Friends and family chipped in to keep the party going, because Shelly wanted it to go on. Twenty-five people came and went from my home, but I heard nothing from her husband. She was at a hospital a whole county away, so it was not as simple as going a few miles to the hospital to check on her. I finally called her father. He told me that she was suffering from cardiopulmonary hypertension and throwing blood clot into her lungs. The situation was grave. I made the trip out to the hospital to see her. She had been forced into paralysis and barely conscious when I got there. My emotions took over my entire body and I went into premature labor. I was stabilized and sent home.

After a few days of acute care to control the clotting, Shelly was told that she would need open-heart surgery. On July 4, 1994, she successfully made it through the surgery, so we all carried on with 4th of July plans with family. At 5:00 pm I got a call from her husband's best friend, telling me that in recovery she was crashing and they had asked for last rights. My husband and my brother drove me 60 miles to the hospital to say good-bye. We didn't make it in time. I was stopped at the door of the hospital by a friend as he struggled to tell me that my friend Shelly passed away. The devastation was unbearable. I didn't get to say good-bye. How will I live through this? I looked down at my belly and I heard her say to me, "Carry on. You can do this." In my cloud of grief, I moved through my life like I was under water, again. On July 21st—in the cavern of my deepest depression, my first child was born.

My first child, a daughter, my Devon Dear really changed my life. When I brought her home from the hospital and it was time to change her for the first time, I dangled her naked body over the changing table, with my hands behind her precious "noodley" head and my thumbs under her sweet little armpits, and I cried. Eric came up beside me and asked, "Oh, honey, what's wrong?" I said, "What do I do? I don't know how to do this? I don't want to ruin her life." He put his arm around me and said, "I'll show you how." I loved her with all of my being and I knew, on a spiritual level, she was here to change me, to heal me, to bring me into the real world. The first few months with her were hard, as they are with any new mother. The lack of sleep and the anxiety attached to falling asleep exacerbated my adult hyperactive tendencies to start projects, lose focus, and forget what the original plan was. The talking to myself (out loud) and the depression would come in waves. "Lousy mother, lousy housekeeper, washed-up actress, poor time manager. . ." the self-talk would silence the positive, outgoing me. I became isolated and stopped talking to and seeing friends or relatives for months at a time.

In the seventh month of breast-feeding Devon, I found out I was pregnant with my son, Andy. Irish Twins. . .kill me now. I was stunned and terrified. Thought, "Well, I have until December to prepare." Not so much. I had a difficult pregnancy with gestational diabetes and placenta previa. My placenta ruptured 31 weeks in. They had trouble finding a heartbeat, because he was breach and I was bleeding out—and coming unglued inside. As I lay there with hospital staff scrambling to cut him out of me, I thought "if he dies, I will be right behind him. I just won't make it." He was in the neonatal intensive care unit for the longest 12 days of my life. He had fetal respiratory distress, lungs not fully "cooked." He was touch-and-go for the first week. In those days, they did not allow you to stay in the hospital with your premature baby. I would pump breast milk and bring it for the nurses to tube feed him, but I would have to leave. The grief was crippling. But even in this terrible state, I had an epiphany. After about 20 years of cycling depression, I realized—my mental health symptoms were triggered by grief. It was grief. Grief pulled me out of the light. The rest of my life would come to be a series of feeling the grief, experiencing the symptoms, and working very hard to find my light again.

I had the struggles any mother has with two children so close in age. I don't think I slept through the night for 5 years. Ok. . .maybe I'm being a little dramatic. That being said, insomnia continues to be the bane of my existence. My darling husband has always been very involved and helpful with the children. I had always held a job (or two) since I was fifteen. Having "high energy" has always been helpful in my work life. I had been working full-time for a construction company for about 7 years when I had Devon. Eric was doing well with his own business, so we decided it was ok for me to leave my job to be with Devon. For the next 10 years was given the unique and wonderful gift and career of Stay-At-Home Mom. I had a home-based direct marketing business, so I made my own hours and was able to contribute financially.

After being at home with the children for 7 years, living life in a real state of wellness, I was feeling like I was in a good place. My children had a very fun and loving environment free of substance abuse or violence. I had broken the patterns of my childhood and was in a place of security and confidence.

Remember my brother, Patrick? In 2005 after being wheelchair bound for nearly 20 years, his health began to decline. Over the years, my brother had gone from dealing drugs from his wheelchair to being touched by God and living his life for his Savior. He became a positive and loving person, who he, himself, struggled with depression. He talked about ending his own life countless times in the 22 years in his paralyzed state. He managed to exist well with a caregiver and I would visit him frequently. I would care for him for short spells while his caregiver was transitioning a new person to care for him. I was with him each time he was hospitalized for pneumonia, in grave danger for months at a time. Many times I was asked by the doctors to prepare myself and the family for his imminent death. This occurred three times in the last 4 years of his life. I was his go-to gal. We were thick as thieves. Our relationship was light and fun, full of twisted jokes about quadriplegics and deep discussions about faith, spirituality, and music. I loved him so. I was with him at the end, because I wanted to be. While he was making his final ascent into the great unknown of the afterlife, I sang to him, his favorite song "Wondrous Stories" by YES. It was my privilege, my honor to be there to say goodbye and wish him a safe journey. The grief overwhelming, darkness enfolding me, I called my family doctor and asked him to refer me to psychiatrist. I feared that this experience would put me in a tailspin that would render me useless to my children. The help I received was something that pulled me back into the light so much faster and so much more affectively, it astounded me.

Why didn't I do this before? Doctor "Sharly" helped me realize, for the first time, I could shorten my episodes and that I was more than a Depressive Drama Queen. She held a mirror up to my face and asked me to tell me about *Her*. I didn't call myself names, which is what I had done in my head my entire life. This time was different. This is not to say I wasn't extremely self-deprecating as I described my appearance, resembling a drowned gerbil. That really wasn't far from the truth. What I said after would sit with me the rest of my life. I am a mother first. I am a really great friend. I have a huge singing voice. I'm great in bed. My husband adores me. I have a beautiful family. My kids are amazing, and I went on and on. It turns out that, intellectually, I knew all along that I was a survivor, a winner, and a blessing to others. I just never met anyone who asked me to be honest with myself and take responsibility for how I respond to anguish and disappointment. I never had anyone tell me that my brain's chemistry was, as she put it, "just a little whacky" and that there were medicines that could assist me in my recovery process. "People who know about this stuff can help you." What??? Really? I just thought I was crazy and weak. I had always thought that I was somehow incomplete or defective. Apparently, this happens to a lot of people. And I said, with my typical, silly, sarcastic smirk, "So...it's NOT all about me." I went from drowned gerbil to a laughing hyena. Doctor Sharly nearly peed her pants.

I went home with a prescription for Celexa and the hope that had left me when Patrick went to heaven. Hope that had been pushed to the background, in place of the complacency of "just another episode in a series of many more," had found the light. All I had to do was "cheat," with the help of others, to get back there. Eric noticed a change in me just a few weeks later. It was amazing.

This part of my recovery journey went unnoticed by my young children, but as they have grown, I just "put it out there." They would notice that every morning I was taking medicine; they would ask if I was sick and I simply said, "Sometimes, but this helps me stay better." Little ones are satisfied with responses that have simple resolutions, but by the time they were 9 and 10 years old, the questions of "why?" that we all dread became gateways—permissions to explain more. I normalized it. I assured them that is wasn't contagious and that it was like having itchy skin behind your knees (using the example of a relative who shared their eczema story at Thanksgiving). It goes away for a long time and then just shows up and causes irritations. When I do what I need to do to make it go away, it goes away. When I don't—like when your Uncle wore jeans for too many days in a row—it just gets worse and takes longer to go away.

My kids are now 17 and 18. Over the last 4 years, they have witnessed my symptoms at their worst and watched me work to sustain my wellness. They have grown to understand and give me the space I need to work through difficult days. They would tell you that my mental health wellness is something that I manage very well. They joke with me when I am particularly energetic "Has mother taken her meds today?" much like I would kid around with my brother back in our days of wine and jazz enthusiasm. They also understand that their mother cares about people, especially people who are different. They try hard to use respectful language when speaking of "crazy people." They often correct themselves or reply, when gently admonished with "Sorry mom." They, along with my darling Eric, are my biggest supporters. They hug me longer, they check in on me, they embrace my propensity to use dramatic license to describe things or situations, and they have cheered me on when I say I'm too old to perform in theater.

Writing this piece was odd, because I have never put all of this "stuff" down on paper. I have told little pieces of my story to people who ask me questions about my life. I have shared an even shorter *Readers Digest* version of my story to the people I work with and to people I assist in learning about mental health recovery concepts and practices. This experience has been cathartic. It is another moment to find my light. What a warm place it is.

Mental Illness and the Pursuit of Stability Across Three Generations

40

S.J. Hart

SJ is married and a mother of three children. In this chapter, she talks about growing up with a father diagnosed with bipolar disorder who died by suicide when she was a child, and the onset of serious mental illness in her children and herself when she turned 43. SJ talks about the struggle of taking care of her children when she felt unstable herself, and gives suggestions to other parents coping with mental illness in their children.

I am one of four children: three girls and one boy. My brother is the youngest, and in our family the youngest was allowed certain liberties: fewer consequences, more latitude, and a later curfew due to aging parents too tired to be as strict as with the first kids. Often my brother had a sense of entitlement. I have thought about my parents and how their parenting changed between my sisters and brother, as I have struggled with my own ability to set limits and enforce rules as a parent with my own fatigue and periods of instability. Just as I witnessed how entitled my brother seemed to become as a result of my parents being so liberal with him, I have wondered, and felt guilty at times about how my parenting affects my children.

I grew up outside the city of Philadelphia. We were a young family living in a row home, nicely set in a neighborhood of many other row homes. Our family and our neighbors often gathered on our front stoops to discuss a variety of topics, such as school, current events, the weather, and any community rumors. Up until I was the age of 10, this was how life existed. It was predictable. In those 10 years, however, there were also tumultuous times. Back then I would have defined it as an abusive home, with an abusive father perpetrating chaos, fear, and catastrophic violence with the use of a leather strap, metal irons, hands and fists used as weapons, and large breakable items. But looking back now, with decades of education, training, and therapy, I see it more as a result of my father's unstable, severe, and chronic mental illness. There were many inpatient hospitalizations, and I could never make sense of our routine visits. His illness was invisible though he

Motherhood, Mental Illness and Recovery, DOI 10.1007/978-3-319-01318-3_40,
© Springer International Publishing Switzerland 2014

received treatment in a hospital. Why was he there? The answers never came. I did not understand until I was much older. My father was prescribed medication, but it was unclear whether he took it, didn't take it, or didn't take it regularly. Though our extended family provided a net of support, the lessons came early at a young age, about the unforgiving, chronic, and seriously misunderstood mentally ill.

My father was eventually diagnosed with bipolar I disorder (manic-depressive illness), and after years of failed treatments he stole his best friend's gun and shot himself in the head. I was 12 years old. I didn't understand. Who was this man? Where was the kind father I knew who used to tell funny jokes and read bedtime stories? Both that kind man and the unpredictable, abusive one were now dead. This is the legacy I would run from for the rest of my life.

In my early adulthood, I tried to push my family history into the background. I attended outpatient therapy, but it was a bottomless pit of fear, grief, and apprehension, and I could tell this would be a never-ending job. Underneath the bundle of emotions I had was a big heaping dose of post-traumatic stress disorder that brought nightmares, anxiety, on occasion alcohol abuse, and took a very long time to manage with the help of an effective therapist. Despite these challenges I was working hard in school and was hopeful about my future.

During graduate school I met a kind and thoughtful man. He worked many hours while I studied for my Master's degree, and after each exhausting week, we settled in on a Friday night, ordered a pizza, and discussed our goals and future plans. Never in those plans could we have foreseen the tsunami of severe mental illnesses that were coming.

We were married after I earned my degree, and had our first daughter 1 year later. She was the first of our three children born in 1987, 1992, and 2001 after I suffered two miscarriages. Up until 2002 we lived a "typical" life untouched by the serious mental illness I had witnessed in my family growing up. We spent time going to soccer, dance recitals, trips to the beach, birthday parties, holiday gatherings, and much more. Parenting was hectic but joyful. We had a busy and full schedule, surrounded by family, community, and friends. Being a mother and caring for my family defined who I was as a person, as a woman, in ways that separated me from my role in my career. We did not see what was coming down the road like a freight train at full speed, causing devastation and profound grief. Nor could we ever prepare for the acute onset of my illness at the age of 43.

My oldest daughter (14) had an acute onset of bipolar II in 2002, and in March 2005 my middle daughter (11), youngest son (3), and I all suffered an acute onset of several mental illnesses. They consisted of symptoms of bipolar disorder, anxiety, post-traumatic stress disorder, obsessive–compulsive disorder, and attention deficit disorder. We all had a different mixture with anxiety being the only one we had in common, often driving the symptoms of all the others.

I became nonfunctional as I slowly watched my children decompensate right before my very eyes. I had thoughts of suicide all the time, could not sleep, and yet at the same time my children were frightened and looked to me to relieve them from their catastrophic suffering. These were moments of mothering no woman should ever experience. I was helpless to comfort them and unable to help myself.

My husband, sister, and mother-in-law took over the care of our newly formed psychiatric unit. I offered what I could in terms of information I learned from treating my oldest daughter and shared our requests for certain medications with the psychiatrist. We had been very careful to find a good psychiatrist for our oldest daughter, and with myself and two other children needing help, the issue was multiplied. With our current insurance, we were able to choose clinicians who would collaborate with us and listen to our needs.

I did not sleep for 21 days at first, and I knew instinctively my mind would break if I did not shut down my brain and rest it. Along with the insomnia came terrifying pictures that were manufactured by my new brain: pictures or short movie clips of shooting myself in the head, driving into a truck on the highway, hanging myself from a noose in my home, taking full bottles of lethal prescriptions, driving into a tree, and so many others. They remained whether my eyes were open or closed. It was the first time I fully understood a biochemical suicide created from within the brain not from external hopelessness and depression.

My primary care physician at the time did not get it, so I went back to my psychiatrist and he prescribed sleep medication. We worked very closely together until I was sleeping for short periods of time with the help of pharmaceuticals, in order to strengthen my mental health and take care of my very sick children.

Though chronic brain illnesses are no different than other severe chronic illnesses, the one glaring difference is the void of compassion and empathy for the mentally ill. I have been taught that stability is defined as more stable days than unstable days. For us stability also seemed to depend on other factors as well: whether thyroid and other hormone levels were stable, stress, the additives we consumed in food and beverages, sleep, and many other things that were not always discussed.

My instability had several presentations. I had crushing depressive episodes where I didn't shower for weeks, couldn't sleep, had lack of motivation, lack of initiative, feelings of discouragement, and often hopelessness and fears about the future. Sometimes I became pressured when speaking where I just couldn't stop talking, was making impulsive decisions, and I had to be careful sending e-mails and making phone calls.

The mental health treatment settings most helpful to me have always been outpatient. In community settings I can speak with other parents in the same situation as mine, with children suffering from mental illnesses and long family histories of mental illnesses. Some of my closest friends who have a family history of completed suicide and serious mental illnesses are understanding and I don't have to explain a thing. They get it. They live it. They have ideas, and when they don't they know where to refer, they listen to me cry and hold my hand. I was most frustrated with my one inpatient stay, as I found the professionals talked more than they listened; this has been the experience with both myself and my children.

It wasn't easy living in a household where so many of us were ill. I found out quickly, perhaps too quickly, that with such large quantities of pharmaceuticals in our home the risk for an accidental overdose increased quite a bit. Our son had two overdoses and I had one. After one such incident, a social worker interviewed us in the emergency room, bringing tears to my eyes, heaviness in my heart, and a sick feeling in my stomach. Though there was no threat to remove our son from the home, it was another glaring reminder of the stigma of mental illness. And with that diagnosis come the looks, the judgment, the assumptions, and the discrimination.

It is very difficult to adequately describe the suffering of having severe symptoms of mental illnesses and mothering children with severe mental illnesses. Early on in our new normal, I was encouraged by a group of moms to focus on stabilizing myself, so that I could then help stabilize my children. It was hard since my illness came on abruptly when I was 43. It actually took almost 3 years to come close to stability, though my depressive symptoms remained for years. During that time I came close to burning down our kitchen once trying to cook dinner. Before getting sick I was an excellent cook. The losses just kept mounting.

During those times I helped my children prepare for school and do everything they always had even though they continued to be horribly unstable. My daughter was severely paranoid and seeing a "vision," while my son was raging and spent most of his time in a small padded room at school. We requested many school meetings to build a team of professionals around our children and our family. My husband and I were well aware of our enormous need for help and needed to work with professionals that would also respect our guidance.

The successes we had often reflected the involvement of others. Special education, psychiatry, therapy, social skills, modified school schedules, and any and all services available. We lived in a community with a public school setting where we could request all types of evaluations in order to receive broad services. We requested evaluations for every child by the psychologist at the schools they each attended.

The challenges were still enormous. Our oldest daughter refused medication and was involved with the police, ultimately getting pregnant by an abusive mentally ill boyfriend. Our second daughter had an acute onset of mental illness at age 11, but with a broad team went into remission for 6 years, developed her musical talent, connected solidly with the director of the music department, and played in all of the concerts and band events throughout high school. On occasion when she was angry about having a mental illness, she would stop taking her medication. Though she could go for short periods of time, eventually the paranoia, depression, and visual disturbances would remind her of the importance of taking her meds in spite of her grief and anger about having such a profoundly stigmatizing illness. Although she had a boyfriend all through high school, she never fully disclosed to him her illness. So there was always a secret. And for many of us with mental illness our culture supports silence and secrecy.

While she struggled our oldest daughter was often running loose in the streets of our community. She eventually graduated high school, though the 2 weeks prior she did not come home, and became more and more symptomatic. My husband and I could not break through to her, and when we were finally able to commit her to treatment we got looks and stares from friends and neighbors who were mocking and judgmental.

We have believed for many years there is a genetic component to mental illness and presumed there was a lack of concrete evidence proving that. Our children ask us on occasion about genetics, and whether we would have still had children had we known there was a genetic component. We don't know what to tell them when they ask if they should have children—the questions are never ending and always heartbreaking. Yet despite the difficulties, we have moments. Those moments are deceiving but we recognize that is all we may get. And that's our legacy.

The many things I would tell mothers

1. Mothers must be close to stable in order to work on stabilizing and advocating for their children.
2. Mothers and their partners need to create a team that includes educators, clinicians, psychiatrists, primary care physicians, family members, occupational therapists, physical therapists, guidance counselors, administrators, school coaches, etc.
3. Call an Individualized Educational Program (IEP) meeting as often as necessary and be clear with requests.
4. Have your child sit in on the last half of the meeting to visually see all of the people on his/her team, and explain that each and every single one are there to help.
5. When there is a meeting dictating protocol following a crisis, especially if the crisis is regarding safety or a full-blown rage perpetrated by your child, ask someone to bring a snack for the group so that your child understands he has an illness and is not a bad person. They many not tell you how mortified they feel from an incident of uncontrollable rage. But they are deeply affected.
6. Always have 3–4 identified people in the building that are the "go to" team members, in case 1 or 2 are out.
7. Give your cell phone and email address to all of the people on the team. Make sure you or someone close to your family can be accessible.
8. Join a group for yourself with other mothers with mental illness, parenting children with or without mental illness. Groups can be in person, online in a group or a chat room, and through professional organizations. It is essential that your support also comes from people who live it and get it.
9. Find time for yourself. Managing your severe chronic illness is exhausting, and you have to recharge your battery.
10. Educate others as often as you can. You have done nothing wrong. It is empowering to use your voice, and it teaches your children not to hide. Use nonclinical words. Your children will learn how to express and describe their symptoms to teach others and understand what they cannot understand. They are different and live in a culture that is intolerant and uneducated. It is best to understand from you.
11. Research and question until you find a psychiatrist that fits your needs. Remember they work for you.

12. Remember to be careful with medication and trials and adjustments. Everyone responds differently, and modifying slowly with the guidance of a medical professional is safest. Research medications thoroughly.

Though I have had many hopeless days where I fear what the day will bring, who will call with devastating news, whether I will have the police in my home again, whether I will continue to experience unconscionable insults in every media form of our culture, the one thing that often helps in those moments is this. In a moment of quiet, in a moment of calm, in a moment of educating others, in a moment of mothering….it is a moment. And the ones that mean the most are the mothering moments. Regardless of instability, irritability, compulsive decisions, I experience mothering moments. And those are the moments that mean most to my children...and to me. When my son asks me to scratch his back at bedtime, and when my daughter calls from college asking for advice, those are the moments that I am not a mother with mental illness. I am their mother. I am a mother.

Coming into the Light

41

Samantha Pierce

Samantha is a 37-year-old mother from upstate New York. In this chapter she discusses her struggles with depression in the context of raising five children, two of whom have been diagnosed with autism. She also talks about the impact of the Nurtured Heart Approach® on her parenting and relationships with her children.

This story is as much about my children as it is about me. I was born in the island nation of Barbados. I was 7 years old when my family—my mother, father, two younger sisters, and I- moved to the United States to pursue the American dream as so many immigrants before and since us have done. Growing up in New York City in the 1980s and 1990s was certainly an experience. We are a people of faith so church activities were the center of social life for my family. My father also eventually served as an assistant pastor in our church. My parents took the kinds of jobs that new immigrants typically take until they were able to find something better. My mother eventually became a certified nurse's aide while my father spent more than 20 years in New York City classrooms as an aide and special education teacher.

I did well enough in school to take the placement exam for the three specialized high schools in New York City at the time. After 4 years at the Bronx High School of Science I went off to college in Syracuse, New York. Now that was some culture shock moving from the big city to a declining rust belt city in upstate New York. I completed my degree in environmental and forest biology in 5 years, as opposed to the usual 4. I married my husband, a graduate student at the time, right after graduation. I didn't realize it at the time but I had been struggling with depression for years and I was about to jump out of the proverbial frying pan and into the fire.

My oldest child was diagnosed as autistic when he was two and a half years old. My husband and I had spent quite a bit of time studying the *Diagnostic and Statistical Manual of Mental Disorders* and having academic discussions about

Motherhood, Mental Illness and Recovery, DOI 10.1007/978-3-319-01318-3_41,
© Springer International Publishing Switzerland 2014

autism before this point so the diagnosis came as no surprise. We were cast adrift in a strange new world as parents of a special needs child with no idea what to do next.

Becoming a wife, a mother, and then the parent of a special needs child within the space of 4 years was a significant stressor on my already chronically depressed state. But I wasn't thinking about taking care of myself. My needs took a backseat to those of my child. Like many parents in our position my husband and I turned to the Internet to see what information we could find about helping our child. This wasn't an especially good move in terms of my emotional state.

Online I found parents talking about how damaged their autistic children were. They talked about how their children were poisoned by vaccines, how they were stolen away from them, and how their children were trapped in a world of their own by autism. They talked about how angry they were that all of these awful things had been done to them and to their children. I was horrified. My child wasn't poisoned or diseased, he was quite healthy. He hadn't been stolen away from me, he was as he always had been. He wasn't trapped in a world of his own, he was giving us a fascinating new prospective on the world. I wasn't angry that my child was autistic, I was satisfied that my suspicions had been correct.

I withdrew from the online autism community because there was clearly nothing there for me. I avoided the real-world autism community as well. I didn't want to join in on railing against vaccine manufactures and doctors who supposedly knowingly poisoned my child. I wasn't interested in talking about all of the "biomedical" treatments I was trying to detoxify my supposedly poisoned child either. The anger and pessimism I found in the autism community made me run the other way. This self-imposed isolation and the alienation I felt from what was presented as *the* autistic community added to the mental health struggles I was still unaware that I was having.

A little over a year later my second child was diagnosed as autistic shortly before his third birthday. I didn't cry when my first child was diagnosed, but this time I did. Not because he was autistic but because I realized that he would have to live in a world that saw him as broken, diseased, poisoned, and lost. I cried because by now I had realized that some of the biggest challenges in getting him help would come from the very people tasked with providing him with that help. Things were not looking good for my baby and I felt as if I had no one to turn to for help or hope. My anxiety for my children and my doubts about my ability to properly care for them grew in leaps and bounds. I was beginning to feel that I was failing them because I wasn't doing the multitude of things that therapists and parents claimed I needed to do to save my children from autism.

I didn't feel that my friends and family were much help to me when I was suffering what I now recognize as a depressive episode. None of them had the knowledge or the tools that would have helped them recognize what I was going through or to get me the help I needed to deal with the challenges I was facing. Finding the *autistic* online community, the one that included the voices of autistic people, helped give me some hope. Here were parents and autistic individuals themselves talking about autism. They weren't talking about kids being poisoned by vaccines or curing them with special diets and untested treatments. They spoke about strategies for acquiring services like speech and occupational therapy. They were talking about the good things about being autistic. They spoke about the value of autistic individuals to society. They spoke honestly, but with respect for the autistic individual, about the challenges of raising autistic children and being autistic. I felt I had finally found a home for myself and for my children that respected them and appreciated them for who they were.

In the off-line world I was increasingly isolated, alone, anxious, and depressed. My husband and I added three more children to our family understanding that siblings could be the greatest allies our autistic children would know in their lives. I experienced a bittersweet relief when it became apparent that each new addition to the family appeared to develop typically. I often found myself feeling like a first-time parent all over again. My younger children did, and still do, all sorts of things with ease that their older brothers had a difficult time learning. Realizing that many of the difficulties I had parenting were due in some part to having children with disabilities did not serve to alleviate my anxiety about being an inadequate mother.

At one point in my parenting journey I remember saying to a friend, "If I'm not depressed I certainly deserve to be." Years of struggling to care for my children in an environment that I felt was devoid of the emotional and practical support of family or friends had taken a toll on me. I had put my needs, particularly my need for affirmation as a mother, on the back burner. In my path to treatment I didn't even focus on taking care of myself. What finally got me into treatment was convincing my husband to be evaluated to see if he was on the autism spectrum. In my attempts to look for a reason for my misery I was convinced that this was the case. This was perhaps one of the best things I have ever done for myself.

The psychologist who evaluated my husband took one look at me and recognized that I was depressed and in need of treatment. I had known, but not acknowledged this for a long time. But I had finally come to the point where I was ready to be done with being in the emotional void that had been my home for so many years.

Armed with information from the psychologist who was supposed to solve my problems by helping my husband, I went on to solve my problems by helping myself. I got my own therapist and spoke with my primary care physician about appropriate medication. The discussion I eventually had with my family doctor about starting medication was perhaps one of the most awkward I have ever had with a healthcare professional. I say this as a woman who has birthed five children. There are few instances that leave you feeling as exposed and vulnerable as when you are in labor surrounded by half a dozen unfamiliar faces poking and prodding you. But talking to my doctor, who I had known for nearly a decade at that point, about my mental health challenges was more difficult for me than going through a pelvic exam during labor.

It has been a few years now since that first session with the psychologist. I have finally learned the value of self-care and I protect my mental health with extreme prejudice. Once I finally got into treatment I was on the road to recovery. I was so glad to be doing something to help myself that I was committed to doing whatever it would take to stay healthy.

I think what really helped me was my grounding in the principles of Christian faith. No matter how dark or difficult my life or my parenting challenges were there was always a part of me that believed that God had something better for me, that joy was supposed to be a part of my life, and that the sorrows I experienced could not last forever. I flailed for many years looking for a way to do right by my children. I struggle still against forces in my life that equate motherhood with martyrhood. I don't want to be a martyr or a warrior mother. I just want to enjoy life with my children again.

Regardless of how depressed I was I always focused on teaching my children that they are a precious gift from God and that they are capable of doing great things regardless of what the world may have to say about their abilities or disabilities. I sought out therapies and interventions for my autistic children that would recognize their inner greatness. I eventually found what I was looking for in the Nurtured Heart Approach®. The Nurtured Heart Approach® is an individualized, person-centered, relational approach to fostering healthy interactions with others. Anyone can use NHA® in professional and personal settings. NHA® digs down to the intrinsic value of the individual to build on a positive foundation to create success.

I got my first taste of NHA® one wintery Thursday afternoon when the program director of a local agency visited my honors abnormal psychology classroom. Part of my recovery from depression and anxiety was returning to college to study psychology. The program director provided a very effective demonstration of how NHA® can have a powerful impact on a person's life. Her answer grabbed and held my attention. I was hooked in less than 5 minutes. She mentioned that there would be a workshop on NHA® that very weekend. I wanted to know more.

I wasted no time signing myself and my husband up for that workshop. They were providing childcare so I didn't have to worry about what we would do with the kids. Sitting on the edge of my seat more often than not I listened as NHA® was explained. Designed to bring out the greatness of the individual it was what I had been struggling to teach my children about themselves for years. I discovered I was already on the NHA® path. It was a gratifying experience as a parent to find such like-minded people in the world.

I went home and tried out NHA® on my children. They were as stunned by it as I was. One child declared to himself, in that child's whisper that has the ability to reach every corner of a room, "Something is wrong with mommy. She's excited that I'm doing something right!" He was as stunned by the application of NHA® as I was. It makes sad sense if you think about it. How often do we pull out all the stops to celebrate people when they are doing what is right? Unless you are steeped in NHA® you have to admit that that hardly ever happens. NHA® brings to light the power of doing just that. It can transform lives.

In the months following that first workshop I purchased some of the NHA® books and set about dazzling my family with their own greatness. I watched as my children bloomed under the realization that they were indeed formidable human beings. As for myself I was more and more drawn to NHA®. Just to be sure that it was something I really wanted to commit to (I confess to having a reputation for impulsiveness in some quarters) I took another full day workshop. By the end of that workshop NHA® was looking more and more like the way I should go for myself and my family.

There were so many tantalizingly wonderful possibilities with NHA®. Life is a completely different experience when you realize the greatness that you are capable of. Now I get to spend more time enjoying my children. Together we explore the great things we are all capable of. The joy and pride on their faces and the way they stand a little taller when I point out to them the things they do right more than makes up for the challenges we face everyday.

All my children really know about my mental health is that I go to the doctor on a regular basis and I take medications to keep myself healthy. It's a truthful and age-appropriate assessment of my current situation. As they mature I will share some details with them as I deem them appropriate. My primary goal is to show my children that taking care of your mental health is no different from taking care of your physical health. My oldest occasionally complains about all of the classes I've been taking recently. He recognizes that what I learn I bring home and practice on him and his siblings. I always use his complaints to point out how important being his mother is to me.

While I was never physically separated from my children as I struggled with my depression and anxiety I was definitely emotionally separated from them. There were many days where I had no energy to do anything more than the most basic of parenting functions, feed the children, clothe the children, and make sure they were in a safe place. We didn't laugh or play. I very much felt that I was an inadequate parent. The threat of having my children taken from me was always present, but it didn't come from social services. Rather, the threat of losing my children was a common warning I received from family members. I was repeatedly warned that I could have my children taken from me if I did not work harder to handle the housework that I was supposed to be doing. This was held up to me as the mark of a good mother, a clean house. Their warnings did not help improve my mental state at all. They only served to add to my conviction that I was a worthless failure as a wife and mother.

We live in a culture that counts it as a grave moral failing to have a mental illness. I don't want to add to that stigma by hiding my own mental health struggles from my children. Taking care of yourself is as important as taking care of your children. Even though I said for years that a good mom needed to take care of her own needs so that she is well enough to take care of her family's needs I didn't actually do it. I talked the talk but I didn't walk the walk. I caution moms everywhere not to fall into the habit of neglecting yourself. It will be difficult to find the right balance, but we owe it to ourselves and our families to develop healthy self-care habits.

Hard Work and Love

42

Christine Shiffler

Christine is a 47-year-old child developmental therapist living in the Philadelphia area, and she talks in this chapter about her struggles with bipolar disorder and endocrine conditions and her son's diagnosis of autism. Through support from her husband and others through the years, and through therapy, medications, and medical interventions, the author describes how she has coped with these challenges and come to a place where "life is good."

My name is Christine. I decided to write about my experiences to finally release the years of bottled up emotions that I hold and have weighed me down and in hopes that someone else may benefit from something I've written. I am the type of person who puts on a brave face, forges through, and is eaten up with emotions held inside. I am working these things out with my therapist. Loving yourself is hard to do sometimes.

I was born and raised in Philadelphia, PA. I have two sisters, a mother, and a deceased father. I lived with my mother and two half sisters growing up. I always considered my sisters to be my responsibility. I was the oldest of three. We had a tumultuous childhood. Our mother had many struggles with depression and alcohol. At age 11, I first started medicine for depression. I was hospitalized and given my last rites by age fourteen, after a suicide attempt. I entered a hospital program for adolescents. A few years later I went to live with my maternal grandparents. Those were my happiest memories of childhood. I had not yet been identified as having bipolar disorder, but I was diagnosed with depression. I struggled for years to find the correct medicine and to get help. I had many highs and lows throughout those years.

I married at 25, and found out at age 28 that I had infertility problems. My pituitary hormone levels were abnormal. This was the first sign of problems in my endocrine system. I came to realize I married someone who was immature and dishonest. He robbed me of all the money I had in my bank. This was indicative of

Motherhood, Mental Illness and Recovery, DOI 10.1007/978-3-319-01318-3_42,
© Springer International Publishing Switzerland 2014

our marriage, taking without giving. I finished my Master's Degree in Education and our marriage came to an end when I was 33 years old. I was hospitalized shortly after another suicide attempt.

Finally, I was diagnosed with bipolar disorder, posttraumatic stress disorder, and premenstrual dysphoric disorder. I was placed on several mood stabilizers until I found lithium. I had a friend during this time who stayed by my side and guided me to continue therapy and make all my doctors appointments. Sometimes she even went with me to make sure I was staying on track. The sad part for me was that she died in her sleep. We were living together after my divorce, and she got ill with pneumonia, had complications, and died. It was a painful time for me and I felt even more adamant that I was not deserving of love and relationships.

Life had been full of failed relationships with few positive ones. I felt very lost and unsure of when someone would truly love me. It took about five more years until I realized that *I* need to love me and that is all that matters. This was a hard task for me to fulfill. I had lots of negative self-talk in my head: no one loves me, no one cares, it must be me, I have something wrong with me, etc. I did not give up. I worked hard in therapy and I dedicated myself to my career working with young children with special needs.

Later, I met my second husband. To me he was everything I ever prayed a husband would be. We eloped 9 months after meeting one another. We were initially so happy, but then, his family was not supportive of our union and 1 month after we married I found out I needed a surgery for a rare large tumor in my head. The feelings of inadequacy and fear of rejection rose from within again, but this time I liked me. I felt anxious, but secure enough to state feelings I would have internalized in the past. This made for a difficult start to the marriage. At times, I even felt like I made another bad choice, especially when we argued. I started to believe that my husband didn't really love me. I was not lovable. It was not until we learned to communicate better that I was able to feel better about our union again. By our third year of marriage, I became pregnant.

When I first discovered that I was going to have a child, I was already 3 months pregnant. It came as a complete surprise since I was told that I would not be able to get pregnant. I had been told by numerous doctors that I had hormone problems and infertility. I was 41 years old when I broke the news to my husband. Although we were happy, we were terrified too. I remember time almost stood still for us the weekend we found out I was pregnant. I went to the doctor on my 41st birthday, heard my son's heartbeat, and then believed I really was going to have a baby.

I was worried about the medications I had been taking, since I had not known I was pregnant. What did this mean for my baby and me? I stayed on the lithium since I was already 3 months pregnant. I felt from the beginning I was dealing with a unique set of stressors that mothers without mental illness don't worry about. I started to worry; will my child have this illness too? Will my child be healthy? What will the medications do to my child?

While I felt it was natural to be nervous and concerned, I decided the best thing for me was just to continue to manage my disorder, treat it as much as possible as a nonissue and deal with my day-to-day life as an expecting mother. Sounds easy to do, but it was hard at times to not feel inadequate, unsure, and very nervous about having a baby. Some days my mind would take over and I would start feeling incapable, overwhelmed, and full of all kinds of anxiety (some reality based, others distorted). As time passed in the pregnancy, I started to feel confident that I was stable, I had a supportive spouse, and I knew I worked well with children (I worked as a developmental therapist). I had the tools I just needed to see what I could do with them. I loved children and I knew I already loved my child too. I thought to myself, all I need is love and the desire to be the very best mother for this child I was carrying.

Family members during this time were not supportive and caused as much chaos as they could. No one from my husband's family came to the baby shower. It was hurtful to both of us. All the stress started to affect us. I was trying so hard to be positive. When I gave birth, I had an emergency c-section. I was fearful. I gave birth to my son who was immediately taken to the neonatal intensive care unit. My son was born at 12:42 pm, 5 weeks early. I did not get to see or hold him until 8 pm, and then only for 5 min.

I was feeling weird and disconnected from my own child. I felt this way for a few weeks. That was scary for me. Could I do this motherhood thing? Would I connect with my child? Once my husband went back to work and it was just our son and me together, I started to feel the connection. I felt overwhelmed too. This is when support is needed, I did not have any support. It was just my husband, me, and the baby. I believe support is crucial and can make times of adjustment easier on all involved.

During the first year of our son's life, my husband was laid off from work. Our strength came from knowing we had a child to support. Our child's life was blissful, full of pictures, laughter, and complete joy. However, upon taking our son to his pediatrician on his first birthday, it was discovered he had a motor delay. I knew from working in the field that this could mean more was going on. I was angry at myself for not seeing anything and I was consumed with the thought that my disorder had something to do with it. My son was tested for developmental delays and received services in our home. By 18 months, he was seen by a developmental pediatrician and diagnosed with autism and cerebral palsy.

I was devastated. I cried hard for a few days and fell into a depression. I went through all the illogical thinking and blamed myself for this diagnosis. I was sure it was my disorder, the medications, or something about me that caused this to happen. Through the support of the therapists, my husband, and doctors, I was able to turn around my distorted thinking.

It didn't help matters that some family members acted as if we were making up our son's diagnosis. They implied I diagnosed him since I worked with children with developmental delays. This was a real kick in the gut. Around this time, my husband, who has had two heart operations, was hospitalized for internal bleeding. It was very scary since I only learned of my son's condition 10 days prior to my husband's hospitalization. I thought I could be left alone to raise our son. What was I going to do?

I chose to immerse myself in the therapies that my son needed. He had 25 h a week of therapy in our home. It was very challenging and exhausting. I lived and breathed those therapies in order to make my son the best he could be. It was more difficult for me because everyone had expectations that I knew everything since I also worked in the field. How untrue when it comes to your own child, and the emotional involvement. As time went on and I learned specific ways to reach my child, things began to flourish in therapy. I worked with my son morning, noon, and night so we could reach his goals.

Although I made this choice, I still struggled with depression and anxiety. I felt so much frustration, anger, rage, and feelings of being overwhelmed. I worked all day with the therapist coming to the house from morning till late afternoon. I could no longer go out of the house now that we had therapy. I felt like I lived under a microscope, with everybody checking everything out. I was extremely uptight. Mrs. Clean was my middle name. I had no assistance, my husband worked and was not home until dinner time, and I was all alone with all the responsibility. I felt isolated and overwhelmed. I just bottled it all up and just kept moving forward for my son. I did not want my son to feel left out, unaccepted, different than everyone else the way that I did growing up. I really struggled during this time, on a daily basis. I even got drunk a few times, until I realized being sick and dealing with a special needs child were not going to help. I just went through the motions some days. At times, I was living my own personal hell.

Then, my son started preschool. I was able to get a new job as a developmental therapist and I used all the knowledge I had gained from working with my son and helped other families with children with autism. Things went well for about 6 months. After that, I went through series of four operations in 14 months. Family members said I was not sick, just trying to get attention. I was infuriated. They had never been supportive and were still saying disparaging things about me. I was really hurt and angry.

I came to find out that I have an autoimmune disease and that my endocrine system attacked itself. I had breast, uterine, thyroid, and a tumor in my brain interfering with pituitary functions. The depression returned with a vengeance. During this time I was sometimes unable to get out of bed. I had a very hard time dealing with the day-to-day routines. My son would say "get up!" I would listen and feel badly. I could not move some days. Would this affect him later? Was I a bad parent? I found out that thyroid dysfunctions can enhance your depression and moods. I had my left thyroid removed. Things got so bad my nurse practitioner added latuda to my lithium. It helped and so did therapy.

I told myself this was just a condition that had to be managed. I was holding on to this idea and trying to believe. I just needed a fine-tuning of things during this time in my life. Nothing in life stays the same, things change. I was admitting I needed help and I sought it out, but kept wondering, why am I not feeling better? Why couldn't I have the drive I had when he was younger? What was wrong with me?

My husband took over a lot of the things I would normally do. He was great at helping with homework, getting my son ready, sending him to school, etc. I was able to concentrate on feeling better because I had the support I needed. Support is very important when you feel so badly. We could have used more support, but we just did not have any, no family, or friends. We believe our families were overwhelmed and fearful of things they did not understand. All we could do was to deal with things the best way we knew, with doctors, therapists, and groups. It all helps, if you work it and try to learn new ways to deal with new situations that arise in life.

As a parent it is crucial to communicate, listen, try things, adjust things, and most importantly love. My treatments for bipolar disorder have taught me how to do all these things and to do them well. As a parent with a mental illness, I am fortunate, I have learned these skills, and have practiced them over and over again. I have the confidence to know that life happens and you need to adjust to those things. The same is true for parenting. My son may have a condition that needs to be managed like I do, but our love for one another and my willingness to give him all the tools he'll need to succeed makes for a great parent–child relationship.

Today, I see that sticking it out though the rough and hard times and seeing things through to completion make for successful parenting. I see my son go off to school with confidence in him. He knows his likes and dislikes. He has a clear vision of himself and yet he is kind and compassionate. I know and see that all the hard work and time does pay off. I am clear and know I did the best that I could and continue to strive every day. It has not been easy, life can be a struggle, and I still battle depression, but dedication does work for me and my son. By being a parent, I think I developed a better appreciation for what is important in my life. Health and well-being come first; you need to take care of yourself first. The best way to be a good parent is by learning to love yourself before you can truly love anyone else. Loving yourself means taking care of your health physically and mentally.

Currently, I am still seeing doctors for my physical health problems. I go to therapy once a week and see a psychiatrist every 3 months for medications. I belong to a group for people with bipolar disorder on the Internet. I have one good friend I confide in and lean on. We have a few relatives that are supportive and in my son's life. Support is very important, and I am grateful to have these supports intact. My husband is laid off from work again, but we are making it through. He now has a great deal of stress worrying about us. It is even harder to cope because I feel like I need to keep it together especially now. At times it can be tiring and exhausting to keep things going. But the truth is, there is no alternative. I have a child now, who needs me to keep it together as best as I can so he can have the opportunities he deserves to have in life.

My son is a happy, easygoing, 5 year old now. He has accomplished many goals in his young life. He has graduated from physical therapy and no longer needs leg braces. He runs and plays nicely with other children. He has just started to talk this past year, and his vocabulary is building. It was wonderful for me to hear "I love you mommy "for the first time! I get the chills even writing about it. He is receiving occupational therapy and speech therapy at school. He is in kindergarten and rides the "big boy" bus.

Life is good now. It takes hard work but you can do anything you put your mind to. I feel proud of myself and my son. I would not change a thing in my life, because it has led me to the beautiful place I am in today. Although I feel being a parent is one of the hardest jobs in the world, I know that it has made me more aware of my own disorder and more insistent on staying on track with my medications and therapy. If my son can be so young and work so hard to be successful in his life, how can I not do the same? On days that I feel I can't, I take a good look at my son, think to myself, you have to keep motivated, and you have more capabilities and therefore are more responsible to do your best. Yes, I am hard on myself, but it is all worth it when I look at my child happy, smiling, living a full life.

An Unquiet Mom: Much More Than a Memoir of a Mother with Bipolar Disorder and Substance Abuse

43

Jamie Carr and J. Rebecca Weis

Jamie is a 30-year-old mother of two living with bipolar disorder as well as alcohol and drug abuse. Through commitment to her own wellness, she has been sober now for over 3 years and has found treatment that works to keep her mood stable. Through her work as a peer advocate, she has dedicated herself to helping families stay together and supporting others on the road to mental health recovery.

Introduction

Jamie's road to wellness has not been an easy one, and she herself had to face scrutiny as a mother by the child welfare and family court system on more than one occasion. Although it is difficult to find estimates of the impact of parental mental illness and substance abuse on child abuse and neglect, we do know that large percentages of children within the child welfare system have parents who have substance abuse and/or mental health problems. For instance, in 1999 the U.S. Department of Health and Human Services estimated in a report to Congress (USDHHS 1999) that between one-third and two-thirds of children in the child welfare system have been affected by substance use disorders. Because substance intoxication and periods of psychiatric instability may have negative effects on children not only through abuse and neglect but also in terms of development (in particular for very young children who are absolutely dependent on their caregivers for basic care as well as for healthy emotional and cognitive development), there is certainly cause for concern; however, The Urban Institute, a non-profit organization, produced a study in 2002 that highlighted that placing children in foster care does not consistently and reliably ensure improved resources for the child (Kortenkamp and Ehrle 2002).

Motherhood, Mental Illness and Recovery, DOI 10.1007/978-3-319-01318-3_43,   319
© Springer International Publishing Switzerland 2014

Programs that support mothers with substance abuse and mental health issues have demonstrated some promising results (Krumm et al. 2013). Although much more information is needed about whether treatment of maternal mental illness allows for "good-enough" parenting to support healthy child development, the STAR*D-Child Report was reassuring in that remission of maternal depression led to improvements in child psychopathology including not only child depression but also behavioral problems (Weissman et al. 2006).

As Jamie will point out in the interview to follow, child welfare workers and family court judges would benefit from a more nuanced understanding of the barriers substance abuse or mental illness pose to mothers AND the types of support mothers need in order to overcome these barriers. There is clearly a need for more research to define effective interventions and helpful strategies—but perhaps even more importantly there is a need for brave advocates such as Jamie who will lead the charge and help more mothers speak up for what they really need.

Mental health and recovery is something I'm passionate about—my mission someday is to do some kind of training for judges. I see stigma a lot in the work that I do and in my own life. I think a lot of judges just see mental illness and say "ok, we're gonna take the kids" and there's no real questioning about what would be best. I am lucky enough to already provide a snapshot version of my story for law enforcement—I've been participating in the Sacramento City police mental health training. I first talk to them as a mental health trainer, but then I tell them my story. I would prefer for my diagnosis and story just to be out in the open. My kids will definitely be aware that mental illness runs in their family. I manage a serious mental health condition and my past is my past. Some people encourage me to shut up but I don't—they are just affirming how pervasive the stigma is in society!

I was raised in the Bay Area, but my parents were from the other side of the tunnel. My parents married young, and they divorced when I was 3. My mom got into another relationship with my stepfather who lived in Walnut Creek, so we moved to this very rich suburb. I wouldn't say we were poor by any means but we weren't rich. My stepdad sang at the bars for a living—he was pretty decent. My mom always had problems. I now define her as an alcoholic although she doesn't because she just drinks beer, but she would drink 18 a day. She was always prescribed things so her nightstand looked kind of like a pharmaceutical company. I don't like painting my mom in a bad way—she's heard me say stuff like this and she doesn't see herself that way so it can be painful for her. My dad was kind of a workaholic. He got this job at a baking company and would work 18 h a day in a bread truck managing his route. He would drive into Walnut Creek to say goodnight to me. I have a brother two and a half years younger than me, and I was always very stern with him. He says he can still hear me saying "Jason, don't go near that!" I wanted to parent him from a very young age. I feel I was born an adult—I was always taking things very seriously and there was no play.

I was a perfectionist people-pleaser from the beginning. I don't know if I was trying to make up for what my family seemed to lack, but I had to get straight A's. My first major meltdown was when I was in preschool. I was tapping the pencil, and some teacher said "Who's tapping their pencil?" I immediately stopped, but I didn't say anything. It was the first time I had been in trouble. I went home and cried all night long. I went to school the next day and said "I was the one tapping the pencil." The teacher didn't even remember what I was talking about. Once in elementary school, I got a "satisfactory" instead of an "excellent" and that was just the end of the world. I was fairly decent at sports, but I quit most of them if I wasn't the star of the team right off the bat. I eventually was a swimmer and into water polo in high school because I excelled at that naturally. I always had to have the teachers like me and I wanted to be liked amongst my peers. I had a pattern of having a "best friend" but then we would have some blow-up. That's what my relationships would look like throughout my life.

In seventh or eighth grade I started seeking approval by being the one who would "do anything or say anything." I had a boyfriend, and I was sexually involved very young. My mom hadn't known about sexuality growing up, so while everything was hidden from her I got the opposite. I knew everything about sex—stuff just not appropriate for my young age. I lived a double life starting in seventh and eighth grade. I was still a perfectionist, but I hung out with people who were up to no good. Because I still got good grades, there were no red flags for anyone. I think I drank for the first time my freshman year. I drank like an alcoholic from the beginning—I suddenly didn't care what anyone thought of me. I relaxed and could be myself. I still managed to do very well in school and sports. I would black out every weekend and kind of thought it was funny. It seemed to me that's what everyone was doing—mostly because that's the crowd of people I was hanging out with.

When I look back on it I think I was always mildly depressed through high school, but I also remember having suicidal thoughts at a young age. I never really acted on it and was always able to be successful, but I hung out with a group of people who were pretty pessimistic about life because that was my mentality. I put all my eggs in the education basket. In my mind I was going to go to college, and I was going to get this degree, and then I would be ok. I'm happy to have grown up in Walnut Creek because people didn't even question whether going to college was a choice. I don't think I even knew that college was optional. I'm not a very good test taker. I get very good grades, but when it comes to multiple choice questions and stuff like that I'm not very good. My GPA and determination got me into UC Davis. I was drinking, but I was also on the dean's list pretty much every quarter. I studied abroad in France and worked as an assistant at a law office. I still always thought I wasn't good enough in anything I did. I still went out with the same boyfriend from seventh grade. He was from a very good family—six brothers and sisters. They did party a lot, and alcohol was always present, but it was just a good family. His mom and dad had been together since they were in the seventh grade and had a loving relationship. I was part of that family, and I think that's why I never broke up with him because I was part of that family.

In college, I was taking an upper division class called abnormal psychology because it fit in my schedule and it satisfied some sociology requirement. I remember thinking "I don't know anybody who's crazy." The professor had listed dozens of books you could have chosen to read, and I chose "An Unquiet Mind" (Jamison 1996) because I liked the title. It was one of the only books I really read in college (not just skimming it), and strangely it ended up becoming my story. I hadn't known what bipolar disorder was. My mom called me on the day of that final and said "Jamie, your brother is talking to the TV. He says he's Joan of Arc, and Regis Philbin on the TV is making fun of him." I said "What! That's classic paranoid schizophrenia. I'm taking a final on it right now." He ended up being hospitalized. He was the black sheep of the family because he never finished high school and could never live up to his sister's standards. Ultimately, he found this super spiritual path and now he's a shaman. He's not always financially stable, but spiritually he is pretty fit. In 2005, about 6 months before I was supposed to graduate from college, I was getting up at four in the morning to work out. I was still getting great grades although I was partying every weekend and I was drinking. I had broken up with my boyfriend of 7 years on a whim and I didn't care. All of a sudden, guys thought I was cute and I was having one-night stands. This was totally not usual behavior for me. I had this boyfriend within a very short amount of time. He broke up with me a month later (probably because I was planning our marriage and children). From that day I just checked out of life. Everything became dark. I couldn't understand my professors, and I didn't want to get out of bed. I kept thinking this has to be a nightmare. I failed my first midterm meaning I couldn't graduate, so at that point I just stopped getting out of bed. I just slept 18 h a day all summer long and couldn't believe I didn't graduate.

My dad came and picked me up. Now I look back on it and realize I was psychotic. As we were driving, I was paranoid that we were going to get pulled over by the police because they would think that my stuff was stolen. I ended up sleeping at my mom's. She would throw a candy bar at me every morning because she thought that chocolate improves your mood. I remember thinking everything was one big prank—like my mom had done some kind of candid camera thing and it had just gotten really out of control. She showed me my driver's license picture that happened to be a good one and said this is my daughter hoping to snap me out of it—I believed this huge story that she had faked my identity somehow. When I went to a psychiatrist, he asked "What's your name?" and I answered "I don't know." He handed me seven pills of Abilify in a sample pack and said "Go home and take this. You'll feel better." I thought he was giving me Abilify to make fun of me. A few months later my dad came to me and said we have to go to the hospital. At the time, he had his hands on his abdomen and I thought he was saying I need your liver because I had seen an ad about liver disease. When they brought me to the psychiatric unit they said "Do you know why you're here sweetheart?" and I said "Yeah, I'm here to give my liver to my dad." I ended up being hospitalized for a couple of days and finally realized where I was. I had a moment I'll never forget when I realized "oh my god I'm in a psych ward." They said I was getting better so I could go home. I was diagnosed with major depression with psychotic features. At that point I'd given up on life and was drinking to die. That's when I started using cocaine because that was rampant at the bars in Walnut Creek. I was seeking treatment at the time, but I was very forthright with the fact that "I'm still using and you're not going to stop me—I'll take whatever pills you want but I'm also going to use because it makes me feel better."

A counselor finally got through to me. I realized my abusive boyfriend and the drugs were going to kill me. I went to rehab in Southern California for 90 days, and when I got out I was starting to see a glimmer of hope that I could get my life back to what it was. That's when I met my husband.

I guess he had kind of had his eye on me from day one. He wasn't in rehab but he was friends with someone who ran the rehab. He had been sober a little longer than me. I was on some medication—I don't know which one—that made birth control inactive. That is how I got pregnant. He already had a daughter who was ten at the time. I was so overwhelmed thinking "I'm pregnant, and I just got out of rehab." It seemed pretty bleak and I was depressed. Actually he was good then, so I said "Ok, this man wants to marry me and he's promising me all these things. He seems like a nice guy who just has a bad past." We got married, and our marriage was good for the first year because we were both sober and we were both working a program with AA. Then that kind of stopped—we both relapsed. I got back into the program 3 days later, and I thought he did, too, but looking back on it he didn't.

This is where the details kind of escape me. I think I've blocked a lot of it out. I just don't want to look back at it. I was bringing my son with me to meetings all the time. Our living situation was kind of unstable. We ended up in Long Beach somehow, and I told him I wanted to move out because his behavior had changed. Looking back on it now I can see that I'm very co-dependent. I would believe his words when he said "I'm sober, I'm sober" even though all his actions were pointing toward not sober. His behavior had changed enough though that I said I was taking our son and leaving. That's when he went and filed in court that I'm a danger to my son. He and his mother took my son for 3 days and wouldn't tell me where they were. I had been trying to piece my life together, so I had gone back and made a timeline with a counselor that went from first drug use through bipolar disorder, hospitalizations, suicide attempts—my husband gave it to the judge. I suppose any judge in his right mind looking at a timeline like mine would question whether a mom with this history could be a responsible mom, but at that point I'd been sober for quite some time. I was being treated for bipolar disorder. I had a counselor and a psychiatrist. I was doing well, and I don't believe I was putting my son in danger in any way. The judge saw my history instead and handed my son to a drug addict. That day I moved back in with my husband. There was never a judgment that was actually filed because he didn't follow through on any of it with the court after I moved back in.

When I found out what he was really doing with the drugs, I did take my son and lived in a woman's house where we rented a room. I was trying to go back to school, so I took a class at Long Beach State called The Sociology of Mental Illness. I went into the class with all these 18-year-olds who were kind of making fun of people who were "crazy," but it was like studying my life. I went up to the professor and said "I just can't do this. I could teach this class, and I can't just sit here." She introduced me to the idea of peer counseling, programs employing people with lived experiences to be peer counselors to help others see that recovery's really possible. I eventually got accepted to a certified peer advocate program; out of about 450 applicants, I was one of 20 chosen. I was trained for a month, and I got my son in daycare. After I finished the training, I found a peer advocate position in Rocklin. My husband called and said he wanted to get sober—I said "of course" like a good co-dependent and didn't see that he was just running from his problems. I almost immediately got pregnant, and my husband was gone almost the entire pregnancy. I was working full-time while pregnant and had a son in daycare. I kind of threw myself in Al Anon, and I got an Al Anon sponsor just because I saw how big co-dependency was a problem for me. I had my second son—they're almost 2 years apart exactly. I went back to work and my sons are four and two now. After my second son was born, I was hospitalized briefly. I'm fairly certain with the doctor I have now that doesn't have to happen again because I'm on Seroquel. I have had some awful side effects to medication, but this is working really well for me now.

I have truly a co-occurring illness in that I have drug and alcohol addictions completely separate of and independent of being bipolar. I have to address both problems. I'm an active member of Alcoholics Anonymous today. I work closely with my sponsor. I'm further than I've ever been in the steps and the promises that are associated with those steps. I've made amends for the things I did in my life in that really dark time. I'm just hoping to be able to clear up the past so that I can be free of it for my children. They can know about it, but it doesn't have to be part of their life.

Today I live in a two bedroom with them. My dad lives with me, which is strange. I've never lived with him since I was tiny, and here I am 30 years old and living with my dad. He's always helped me, and I knew I just couldn't do it by myself right now. My dad is the male role model to my sons. I'm finishing my degree this fall quarter—I'm going part-time to work and will hopefully get enough financial aid to make up the difference. I have two classes to finish.

I've gone through my story but never in such detail. Motherhood being the topic of it makes me feel guilty. Honestly these innocent kids did not ask for this. The thing is I always beat myself up, and I know that. I can hear a million people in my life saying "you're such a good mom" . . . and I am a good mom. I probably overthink it, but I don't feel I have any other choice. Even if I didn't already have bipolar being a mom would maybe induce a manic illness in me—if there were ever anything I wanted to be perfect at it's being a mom.

My goal for my sons is to have some sort of spirituality in their life. I don't know how to do that because I wasn't raised with it. I didn't even know that Christmas had anything to do with Jesus or that it was in any way biblically tied. I was always angry at my parents for not teaching me anything about the bible but they just didn't know. I want my kids to know that they don't have to rule the universe. For so long I thought that if I didn't do this right the world was going to end. There are so many spiritual tools out there I've learned about through AA. I hope my kids don't have to go to AA as a participant, but I hope my kids can learn to rely on something other than just me or themselves—to know that there's a god and God loves them. It's become an important piece of my recovery, and it's the last thing I would have ever guessed because I was so intellectual and thought I was going to figure it out myself. What I've come to know is that I don't know. The second I say I don't know and "can you help me." I've been able to endure some pretty difficult things. Recently it's been the most profound change in my life. By being sober and not even having the thought of wanting to drink, I can really just look at bipolar disorder as something I have to manage. My doctor has an emergency number that's to his cell phone and I'm programmed in it. The problem with the county system, which is what I work in and what I had access to for a number of years, was that I needed medication and I needed an intake almost immediately. I kept cycling in and out of locked facilities because I didn't have access to treatment. Having a psychiatrist who meets with me for longer than 10 min is really important! I guess it's because he has the ability to have a private practice and I have the means to seek out his services today. Managing bipolar disorder and alcoholism is very time intensive! I know now that taking care of myself 100 % carries into how I parent. That took me some time to figure out. I was taking care of their needs, but I was just neglecting myself.

The situation with my husband at this point is still complicated. He eventually did get sober and he came for the kids' birthday this year. I disengaged with him completely for a while—I had to. He's recently tried to pick up the pieces—when he makes a mess, he makes a big mess. Even though I almost had a panic attack about it, I let my kids fly with him and his daughter to Connecticut for 8 days recently. He has a great family, and that's why I let them go, to experience a really close-knit, big family since they won't get that experience from my side of the family.

Self-esteem is still an issue for me. It's tied to the stigma of having bipolar. There are so many reasons to hide your diagnosis. I get that it's protocol, but you get treated differently, like a 100 % differently. For instance, I had my children go to daycare for the week that I was hospitalized to keep their routine normal. Since I wasn't at work, I had to have this form signed called a statement of incapacity—it states that you can't care for your kids everyday because you have bipolar disorder. I walked in with this form and said "I'm sure you've seen this before" and the principal, who's been there for like 25 years, said "No, I can definitely say I've never seen this before." She wasn't being rude, but this is such a hidden thing and we don't talk about it. You go to your primary care doctor, and they ask you if there's any heart disease, but they'll skip over the questions about mental illness. I feel like so much could be prevented. It doesn't have to get to the full-blown problem if you could have picked up on little signs and gotten treated earlier. That's what I hope for my children if they ever have any signs of mental illness.

There are some great services offered for parents in mental health treatment. After I was hospitalized I got some counseling subsidized. I took off work to go for sessions with a specialist for postpartum depression. That was very helpful. Generally when it's county funded the caseloads are just too high and the compassion leaves. The only real help I've gotten is from the people who probably put way too much of their emotion with you. I've been helped in a lot of ways, and I've been mistreated in a lot of ways, too. I just try to take what's good, and today I know what's good so that's what I try to find.

I know my mother-in-law called Child Protection Services after I had my second son. They came to my house and said "We have a report that there are children around a mom who has a mental illness." I said "I'm sorry is having a mental illness and having children illegal"? Of course they said not at all. They didn't do a formal investigation, but they came in and sat down. We talked about my work. They asked about my mom as a source of support, and I said I don't talk to my mom (which was what was going on at that point). As they were leaving they asked about my husband's mom. They looked at a paper and said her name. I said it's a typical in-law relationship—she hates me, I hate her—and the guy rolled his eyes and said "see you later, call me if you need anything." The threat of my children being taken is very scary and very real for me. I'm far enough in my recovery that the fear is dissipating because there'd be no argument for it any more. I have enough proof of my stability.

I haven't actually sat down and had a conversation with my children about my illness, but they know that mommy takes medication at night. That's when they take their vitamins so I've never said mommy's sick—we all just take what keeps us healthy together. I assume I will have a conversation about why their dad's not here with us at some point. I have this book about bipolar for "dummies." My 4-year-old son for some reason loves that one. I don't know if it's because it's bright yellow, but he wanted to bring it to school the other day. He wanted to bring it to share day. At first I said "No, take another book." I got so adamant about it, then he said "But I love it" so I decided it was ok. We walked in, and I laughed about it with the teachers because they know about my illness.

Luckily today the really difficult parts of my illness are in my past. I work with people all the time whose kids are taken by Child Protective Services. I feel like more attention could be paid to helping moms instead of taking children away. They're put in a foster system that is so broken that the children suffer and will be homeless or drug addicted and just continue this cycle. It sickens me. I can't save the world, though. I can just sort of save my little family that I have here.

References

Jamison KR (1996) An unquiet mind: a memoir of moods and madness. Vintage Books, New York, NY

Kortenkamp K, Ehrle J (2002) The well-being of children involved with the child welfare system: a national overview. New Federalism: National Survey of America's Families, Series B, No. B-43

Krumm S, Becker T, Wiegand-Grefe S (2013) Mental health services for parents affected by mental illness. Curr Opin Psychiatr 26(4):362–368

U.S. Department of Health and Human Services (USDHHS) (1999) Blending perspectives and building common ground: A report to Congress on substance abuse and child protection. U.S. Government Printing Office, Washington, DC. Retrieved February 4, 2014, from http://aspe.hhs.gov/hsp/subabuse99/subabuse.htm

Weissman MM, Pilowsky DJ, Wickramaratne PJ, Talati A, Wisniewski SR, Fava M, Hughes CW, Garber J, Malloy E, King CA, Cerda G, Sood AB, Alpert JE, Trivedi MH, Rush AJ, STAR*D-Child Team (2006) Remissions in maternal depression and child psychopathology: A STAR*D-Child report. JAMA 295(12):1389–1398

Part VI

Voices of Mothers: Adult Childrens' Perspective

Shadow Mothers

44

Judith Hannan

Judith is a 60-year-old mother of three from New York City. In this chapter she describes her experiences with her mother's mental illness, her own personal struggles, and how motherhood has helped define her sense of self.

For much of my childhood, my mother was a whisper of her full self. When I became a mother, I developed rules in response to those years. I would not reside in her shadow.

My twenty-one-year-old daughter, home from college for the summer, was leaving to visit a friend for the weekend. "Are you going to come to the door to say goodbye?" she called.

"Of course," I answered from the living room and went to give her a hug and kiss.

I was at the door, too, when her twin brother left for his summer job each morning, delaying my daily meditation practice until the elevator doors closed behind him.

I have been walking my children to the door since they were little.

My first rule for good mothering: *Be there. Be there when the children wake up, while they eat breakfast, at the door when they leave for school. Do not disappear behind blank eyes or into rumpled sheets behind a closed bedroom door.*

As a child, I didn't know my mother had a story and that that story was being written on my character. I only knew what I experienced: her slowly waning animation. By the time I was 4 I had a dropping in my stomach, as if my belly were growing eyes, the kind that can see what the brain can't. When my mother said goodbye to me at preschool, I held my breath until she returned. She never seemed quite the same as the mother who dropped me off, as if my planet had rotated without her.

By first grade, I ate breakfast alone, the sight of my rubbery eggs as unappealing to me as to my mother who couldn't deal with my school-phobia induced tantrums. At the dinner table, where we gathered every night at 6:15—my mother, my father, my sister, and I—a glaze would shroud my mother's eyes that couldn't be penetrated from either side of those walled off pupils.

Motherhood, Mental Illness and Recovery, DOI 10.1007/978-3-319-01318-3_44,
© Springer International Publishing Switzerland 2014

In the third grade, I returned home from school, finally able to cope with a few hours of separation from my mother because my new teacher was showing me how to play the guitar. "I learned a new round at school today," I said to my mother. "Will you sing it with me?" Her back remained a few moments too long hunched over the kitchen sink. An unnamed pain circled within her eyes. I performed like a circus monkey waiting for the clink of my mother's happiness to fill my heart. My mother didn't sing well. I thought I was the source of her tears.

In the sixth grade, when I got my period, my mother never got out of bed to talk to me. She called from her room to tell me the Kotex was under the bathroom sink. I found it next to an unopened box of hair coloring. I had seen my mother remove this box from its hiding place, turn it over in her hands, study the smiling brunette on the cover, and then summon some cryptic determination to put it away, still unopened.

I never searched for the meaning behind my mother's projects. The sight-singing lessons that ended after a few sessions, guitar lessons that continued until the anxiety of performing in recitals brought dissonance to the experience, the canvasses that remained unpainted, her one year as a Brownie leader, one sewing, one involved in the League of Women Voters, one spent redecorating a house.

I was 11 when I came home from my friend Ruthie's, searching for my mother to tell her that Ruthie said she didn't like me anymore. I wanted my mother to act like the lionesses I saw on *Wild Kingdom*. I wanted her to roar and make Ruthie apologize. But my mother was too intent on her reflection in the bathroom mirror. When her eyes finally turned to me, they weren't even curious enough to ask, "Who are you?"

She "went away" a few days later. There were no men in white coats or jackets that wrapped around her like a puzzle. My father drove her to the hospital—the kind with no maternity ward, surgical suites, or emergency room—where she was gone from my view.

> When my older daughter, Frannie, was twelve, I was late picking her up at an event after school. It was the second time that month. "I'm just not myself these days," I explained to Frannie.
> "You keep saying that," Frannie said. "I don't want to hear it."
> **The second rule**: Show no weakness or anxiety. Do not wobble or fall when a child leans against you. Be their mountain.

My memory of what happened after my mother left is as blank as her mind appeared to be. My father told me that he took me and my sister to the hospital to visit. My mother was waiting outside in the garden and when I saw her, I ran to her crying, "Mummy, mummy." I don't remember her hug, but I assume there was one; I always understood that my mother loved me.

I remember only a dream. In it, when my father took us to see our mother, I thought, finally she will tell me what happened. I saw her looking out through an open window. The window was high. My father and sister could reach it, but I could not; no one would lift me up and my mother wouldn't look down.

My mother avoided the electric shock therapy the doctor prescribed. She checked herself out of the hospital and entered the outpatient program at McLean

Hospital. Without knowing why, I understood that these acts were heroic. Without understanding how, I saw my mother emerge, joint by joint, over the lip of her despair. It was like the sudden emergence of Popeye's muscles after eating his spinach, only I didn't know what my mother's "spinach" was.

Was this still my mother—this woman who seemed invincible, who went off to college and graduate school and work, and whose eyes no longer glazed over but penetrated so deeply it felt as if she could read my every thought, detect my every deception? I entered high school, went away to college. I tried to separate, but how could I resist regressing, repeating those younger years, this time with a mother who would not disappear.

When I left home my separation anxiety roused itself. It wouldn't let me sleep, eat, take a shower, and leave my dorm room. It distorted my senses, my balance, and, like an infant, the relationship of my body to the world. It sent me running home as often as I could, where my mother's strong fingers would knead the tension from my scalp. Back at school, I stayed tethered to my mother through the telephone lines; even as I heard the weariness and frustration in her voice, or maybe because of it, I kept calling. I knew she wouldn't hang up on me.

Finding my own strength came slowly. It came from a marriage in which my husband could relieve my mother of some of the burden of my anxieties. It came from practicing bite-sized pieces of life—living on the sixth floor so I'd have to learn to ride an elevator, going on subway rides while my husband held my hand, and taking a Freedom From Fear of Flying class. I regained my footing when we moved closer to my family for 2 years while my husband was in graduate school, when I started therapy, when I entered the workforce, found a career in fund raising, and got promotions eventually becoming Director of Development at the 92nd Street Y.

When I was 30, my mother died of breast cancer. During that time, she never asked for my help, to care for her, to bend my head over her feet to tie the shoes she could no longer reach. As much as I had grown since graduating college, I was still her baby when she died, the one to whom she never said "I am afraid," "I hate my body," "I am going to be cremated."

I was flying with my family when our plane was hit by lightning. As I heard my children screaming, I braced myself against the turbulence and planted myself in front of them where they couldn't avoid my eyes. I gripped them in my presence until the crisis subsided.
    ***The third rule:** Do not be a shadow mother.*

When my children were born, I finally began to tell myself my mother's story. It began with a cliché—a suburban housewife, married with babies at too young an age, no schooling beyond high school, and no internal passion that propelled her into the external world. She could be any of the women Betty Friedan talks about in *The Feminine Mystique*. But that era of the 1950s and 1960s was merely the petri dish in which the specific toxins of my mother's childhood were allowed to grow.

My mother was 6 when her own mother had a stroke, paralyzing her body and scrambling her mind. I learned from an aunt that my mother was locked outside the bedroom door without even a too tall window to give her hope; my mother couldn't see, couldn't touch, and couldn't ask whether she still had a mother. She had two older sisters who had had friends and boyfriends, Hebrew and music lessons, who went to conservatory, and had their pictures in the paper. My mother went to school and came home where she saw her mother wrapped around the hot water heater as if it were providing the warmth of a human, speaking to absent or deceased relatives in Yiddish. A controlling sister—who siphoned off the love my grandfather could have shown my mother—oversaw my mother's childhood but did not enrich it.

My mother married the only man she ever dated, a young genius who went to work every day in a research lab, whose muscled body implied a sense of security, and who could understand and fix anything with physical properties. He could not find or patch the leak in my mother's spirit.

My grandmother's definition was taken away from her. My mother lost hers. Motherhood defined me in a way nothing else had. It was the first job for which I had a blueprint—be the opposite of the mother I had as a young child and channel the one she became later. This binary system perhaps made me a good mother. But I wonder if the shadow I ended up casting over my children was too big. As I saw them off in the morning, made sure we had meaningful dinner conversation, was there for every hurt, and hid every one of my own insecurities and doubts, I didn't always leave enough room for my children's identities. I couldn't grow beyond the mother I needed as a child, having never experienced the full arc of the mother–child relationship.

> When my aunt was dying, I went to see her in the hospital before she was disconnected from the machines keeping her alive. Frannie, now a young adult, said, "I want to come with you."
>
> "I'll be okay by myself," I said. I saw Frannie's disappointment, her potential exclusion from this adult event and from my own sadness. Then I realized I really did need Frannie and it was okay to tell her.
>
> **Final Rule**: There are no rules except for what the moment asks of you.

Motherhood kept me out of the shadows. I had allowed it to be an antidote to my own stunted maturity. The year before my nest emptied, the anxiety and depression of my college years returned. I wasn't leaving home, my home was leaving me. I felt like one of those cartoon characters who run off a cliff and keep pedaling in mid-air before they plummet to the ground. I didn't fall; the floor has stayed beneath me, but it is an uneven surface at times as I grow with and outside of my children.

River of Resilience: A Daughter's Memories of Becoming Whole

45

Maggie Jarry

Maggie had three parents who struggled with mental health. Her mother was diagnosed with bipolar and schizoaffective illnesses, her stepfather experienced schizophrenia, and her father experienced homelessness and severe depression. Inspired by her life experience, since 2003, Maggie has coordinated a national working group dedicated to improving awareness and addressing the needs of "Daughters and Sons" of all ages who have a parent with psychiatric illness. Her central message has focused on breaking stigma against parents with mental illness and the underlying assumptions people have about being raised by a parent with mental illness.

Prologue

Several years ago I participated in a panel discussion in which a noted psychologist said: people tend to think that resilience is an inherent trait within a person, when in fact, it is a series of factors (internal and external) that ebb and flow throughout a person's life, like a river (Gearity 2008). As I was growing up, being resilient (or strong) is what I was told to be. This may have helped me survive situations that were harmful to both my mother and me. However, learning not to be strong was an important breakthrough as I developed into adulthood. When people called me "resilient" in my youth, it felt a bit like a burden. What if I fall apart? What if I am not strong? My resilience has been as much connected to my apparent internal strengths as to the ability of people around me to see and support me through my weakest moments.

As I share vignettes from my life with my mother there are qualities I think may be difficult for readers. First, my childhood memories rarely flow in a linear fashion. This is in part due to the episodic, repetitive upheaval I experienced with each of my mother's hospitalizations. Therefore, I am not attempting to retell or give full

Motherhood, Mental Illness and Recovery, DOI 10.1007/978-3-319-01318-3_45,
© Springer International Publishing Switzerland 2014

context for the memories I am sharing. Second, as I focus on strengths I think it is possible for readers to interpret my mother's illness as not being severe. In sum, she had at least 18 hospitalizations and spent almost 30 years either hearing voices or worrying that "the voices might come back," which is how she phrased it. In her later years she experienced sexual abuse and in her young adulthood she had been raped. My mom's unprocessed pain from these events impacted my relationship with her. Neither her memories of rape nor her experiences of sexual abuse were therapeutically addressed through her years in psychiatric treatment, which started in the early 1970s and ended in 2007. It was at that time that my mother died at age 60, while hearing voices, alone. It is almost impossible for me to look back toward my love for her without feeling sadness. When I reflect I see many missed opportunities. Opportunities I had to be with her in my young adult years, when I was struggling for my own stability, and missed opportunities of mental health systems to be more supportive of us. Therefore, when I mention grief within the context of my story, it is grief for my parents as much as for myself.

Lastly, I will be referring to "Daughters and Sons" with specific meaning to indicate people who have a parent with a mental illness of any age. I cofounded and am part of a movement called the Daughters and Sons Initiative. The web of people involved with the Daughters and Sons Initiative stretches across the United States, into Italy, Quebec, and Australia. We are inspired by and loosely connected to two groups in Australia—COMIC (Children of Mentally Ill Consumers) and COPMI (Children of People with Mental Illness). In 2003 we began referring to ourselves as "Daughters and Sons" because terms that are often applied to us, such as "adult children" or "offspring," were connected to models of thought that did not reflect our experience, nor the universally human component of our relationship to our parents. We use the phrase "Daughters and Sons" to encompass people of diverse backgrounds and of any age who have had or currently have a parent with a psychiatric illness. Daughters and Sons share qualities in common, including a struggle with identity formation, foreboding sense of stigma, and hypervigilance that mental illness will emerge in our lives as though it were our destiny. Yet we have differences in our stories, depending on the ability of our parents and other adults around us to recognize and discuss our experiences.

Leaving Home

The year was 1994. Mom and I met at a restaurant in a mall for lunch. We were talking about an upcoming move that I was to make from Tucson, Arizona, to Alaska. I had just graduated from college. At age 24, I'd been living on my own for 7 years and I was struggling. College had been stabilizing, but without it a question loomed: where should I go? I could not return to my mother's apartment and I was uncertain about job opportunities in Tucson. In theory the trip to Alaska would take me away from Arizona for a year, but ultimately, I never moved back. Although I loved my mother deeply there was no "going back." Mom and I both knew that for me to stay at that moment would likely lead me into a downward spiral. Mom was living in Section 8 housing. Neither she nor I had financial resources beyond ability to pay for basic needs. Mom and I had survived a lot. Yet despite her abundant love, she could not offer me respite. Poverty was not the only issue we were facing. Unfortunately, my mother's illness had led to a series of relationships with men who were abusive. It is painful for me to write about the abuse we suffered and this is the first time I have disclosed this part of our history publicly. I am doing so because, frankly, I know that it is common. Years later I did cursory research for a grant proposal that helped me understand the demographic situation of my mother and into which I was born. Women who experience mental illness experience abuse from perpetrators at alarmingly high annual rates, yet this is rarely discussed by sexual abuse advocacy groups. I hope even mentioning this briefly draws attention to this important subject, but I will not focus on it here. It is simply enough to say that neglecting this part of my mother's health had ramifications that caused constant suffering for her and for me. She was vulnerable and so was I. Although I loved her deeply, I needed to protect myself from various people who preyed on the vulnerability of us both. Although we struggled with these issues, we also spoke openly with each other about them. I remember vividly that mom said, "I will miss you so much." I knew I would miss her too, but I doubt that I understood how much. After leaving Tucson it took me almost 10 years to feel stable and financially able to visit home regularly. When I did visit I could not stay at my mom's apartment. There really was no going "home." Mom and I talked daily via phone until she died. "No trumpets sound when the important decisions of life are made. Destiny is made known silently." This quote from Agnes de Mille hangs on my cubical wall at my job in New York City. Almost 20 years from the day of that lunch, this memory of my mother saying "I will miss you so much" still makes me sad. I missed her immensely and I miss her even more now that she is gone.

However, I have learned to counsel my memories with words of forgiveness. When I left Tucson I was struggling with typical 20-something confusion and discontent, but also something more. My feelings of disconnectedness had become so acute that I was feeling deep inner turmoil. Looking back I realize that, were it not for resiliency factors of friends and a general optimism to persevere, I might have become suicidal. In fact, during my year in Alaska a friend in Arizona committed suicide. My friend's death awakened me to my own depression, which I was fighting. The way I had moved from Tucson to Alaska was dramatic and I had treated it as a form of social suicide. Realizing that what I was suffering from might be serious, I sought out counseling. In the few sessions I had with a therapist that year she interpreted my struggle as an existential journey. Much as I had found in my college years, when I reached out for help I was often told that I was remarkably strong and showed no symptoms of psychiatric illness. Like most people, my therapist in Alaska was not familiar with the types of issues a young adult struggles with when she has a parent with mental illness. I had developed coping mechanisms that allowed me to appear stable, when inside I was struggling with anguish. After those few sessions in Alaska, I did not seek out and could not afford therapy for another 10 years. During those years I struggled with experiences of derealization and dissociation that would emerge, like swelling inside, taking me on a wave of pain. My surroundings would become unfamiliar and I would yearn to go "home," with no sense of where home was. This pattern consumed my 20s. Often I would feel compelled to make a drastic move in hopes that somehow the next place would feel more real, more like home.

No one offered or suggested that I should seek mental health support in my young adult years. Similarly, mental health support was not available to me in my childhood. As a child I experienced sudden moves from one state to another each time my mother's voices returned. By fifth and sixth grades I was experiencing depression so severe that I would not bathe or go to school. I had just emerged from one foster care placement, was living with my mother and new stepfather, and was experiencing bullying at school. Children in my neighborhood knew that my mother had a mental illness. Many told me that they were forbidden to play with me because of her illness. Others teased me as an outsider, a disheveled kid. Of the various adults in my life, no one aside from my mother asked me about my experiences. I also never had access to my mother's doctors, and in retrospect, I wonder if they ever asked my mother how I was doing. Adult family members seemed to be either unaware that I was impacted by my mother's illness or were just too afraid and exhausted to consider thinking about my situation. Our focus was on mom, her illness, and hope that someday she would not be cycling through hospitals. That focus consumed my childhood. I, too, worried about mom. It was only years later that I was able to look back on these moments and appreciate that I had survived, and some would say, ultimately thrived.

As a public speaker on experiences of parents with mental illness and their daughters and sons, I almost uniformly receive questions from concerned "consumer" parents at the end of my presentations. They are usually worried about their children who are aging into adulthood. Typically they are dealing with feelings of guilt or shame, feelings of not having been a good enough parent, while they are also facing ordinary parenting challenges of having a teenagers or youth who may be lashing out in anger or feeling frustrated in the shadow of their parent's illness. I reassure them that their love and concern for their children will increase their children's resilience, as my mother's did for me. However, I hope this is the case. Many daughters and sons enter their young adult lives without information about their parent's illness, nor accurate information regarding their own (small) likelihood that they will experience illness. The ramifications of neglecting this part of mental health consumer/survivor parent's lives are great for the parents and their children.

The Tools in My "Baggage"

Looking back from the safe perch of my full adulthood, fortunate not to suffer from the same illnesses that tortured my mother, I see her losses and mine more clearly. Each year of my life has been a marker. Certain years I realized I was getting to higher ground, to a stable life on my own. Other years I realized that I was not going to become ill like my mother. I no longer feared the ticking bomb of illness that seemed inevitably wanting to explode inside my body. Eventually I came to realize that I had classic symptoms of complex traumatic stress disorder and I still struggle with moments of flashbacks, hypervigilance, foreshortened sense of time, and feelings of panic in specific situations. Yet, I have come to understand my strengths through my relationships with peers and that has helped me reach recovery. My favorite definition of recovery is from an organization in Phoenix, Arizona, called Recovery Innovations: *Recovery is remembering who you are and using all of your strengths and abilities to become who you were meant to be.* By coming to know other Daughters and Sons as peers I have gained a fuller picture into how my story reflects experiences of other Daughters and Sons and what aspects might be unique. In gaining that context I no longer felt damaged. Rather, I began to feel whole. For me, wholeness is a type of recovery of self-definition. It allows me to remember painful events as part of a larger tapestry of life events, beliefs, and experiences that are woven into my identity. A key to my becoming whole was my search for peers. Through them I realized that my experiences have a context and that there are millions of other people in the world having similar experiences. I am not alone.

In 2003, during the early stages of organizing the Daughters and Sons Initiative I met a fellow daughter, Heather Burack, who was doing research into what she calls the "redemptive" qualities of people who have a parent with mental illness (Burack 2004). Heather was a student at Hunter College School of Social Work and found that research articles looking at experiences of children who have a parent with mental illness were bleak, discussing children as wounded and hidden victims. These frameworks did not tell the whole story of children and certainly did not reflect her experiences. For this reason Heather decided to do a series of qualitative studies of adults who have a parent with mental illness. Through these studies Heather identified the following five "redemptive" characteristics of people who have a parent with mental illness: creative orientation, tolerance of difference, willingness to challenge the status quo, emotional expressiveness, and a sense of humor. Building off of what I learned from Heather, I have come to realize some of the qualities I gained from my experiences growing up.

A host of resiliency factors saved my life, including my mother's love. Qualities I gained from my life with my mom:

1. *Self-Esteem*: I cannot emphasize enough that my mom was a compassionate, great listener. Her central calling in life was to be a parent. She took pride in my brother and my successes and forgave us of any failure, including expressions of anger or frustration that hurt her. She managed to parent my brother and myself against incredible odds. Only one thing was forbidden in our house—we were forbidden to say "shut up." We always had to honor each other's experiences and leave room for expressions of grief. We ended every conversation on the phone or in person with the words "I love you" rather than "good-bye." The reason for this was stated directly by our mom—she wanted those to be the last words we heard from her in case anyone of us should die. We danced on the edge of traumatic, foreshortened time while retaining an abundant love for each other. To our mom, we were the most beautiful children in the world. At one point, after organizing the Daughters and Sons Initiative for about 3 years, I said to my

mother: "Hey mom, I have been realizing that I am really lucky. In all your years of illness you never said a cross word to me or Andrew (my brother)." Mom was silent for a long pause, and then she replied: "Thank you. It was very difficult." Meeting my peers allowed me to get perspective that my mother, counselors, and friends could not give me. I realized that many of my peers could not have conversations like this with their parent who had a mental illness. It allowed me to have conversations with my mother, such as the one I am mentioning here, that were affirming for her and for me.

2. *Belief that small actions can have a big impact:* It is possible to impact the world without knowing what you have done. I learned this through people who helped me as a child, without realizing their impact. Three examples come to mind. First, I spent a summer in foster care with a large Mexican family in Wisconsin. I do not remember the family's name, but they were superb at including me and my brother as part of their clan. My recollection is that my brother and I were their 26th and 27th foster care children, and they had ten children of their own. When I think of that summer I think of going to their nana's house on Wednesdays as "ladies time," eating her homemade fresh tortillas, and watching General Hospital. That family gave me a glimpse into the tight network of large families and Mexican culture.

   Second, 2 years later, I was stuck in a bad situation. My mother was hearing voices and my brother and I were traveling with her through various parts of Texas, trying to reach our grandparents in Arizona. While staying in a hotel in San Antonio, I walked through a small shop. I was 11 years old and in the midst of one of the most traumatic episodes of my life. Chatting with the woman in the gift shop, I mentioned that we were in the hotel and that my mom was hearing voices. The lady in the shop was helpful to me, simply empathetic. As I looked at various items in the shop, I saw a gold leaf pendant that I liked. She gave it to me. I still have it. That leaf reminds me that people can make a difference, even in a small conversation, and never know that they did. I can never go back to thank her, just as I cannot reconnect with my foster care family because I was never given information that would help me track their name.

   Lastly, by the time I was 14 years old my mother was stable and we were living with her. We were all receiving public assistance, but I wanted to go to a private Catholic high school. Part of my reason was that I had experienced severe bullying in public schools because of my mother's illness. More importantly, my experience of God's presence helped me through some extremely lonely times. Most of all, my grandparents had paid for my brother and I to go to a Catholic elementary and junior high school once we arrived in Arizona. I wanted to stay with the same kids. I was desperate for lasting relationships with kids my own age. The turning point for me was an offer of a scholarship from a person in our parish. Ultimately, that scholarship paid a portion of my school tuition and I worked with my mother to pay the balance. I loved my high school years and have lifelong friendships from those times that continue to feed my resilience. Some of my classmates helped me through later years when my mother's episodes of illness returned. Yet, I do not know the name of the person who gave me the scholarship. I cannot thank him. All of this reminds me that I too can change the world, even without realizing it.

Compassion: I had three parents who suffered through mental illnesses. Although I am focused in this essay on my mom, my father also suffered from severe depression that led him to periods of homelessness and my mother married a man who experienced schizophrenia. Though my stepfather and mother's marriage lasted only a few years, they were pivotal years for me. As years progressed my mother's friends were usually people she met during her time in hospitals, "half-way houses" (in the late 1970s) and Clubhouses (in the 1990s). People who had mental health experiences, survivors of psychiatric hospital environments, consumers of mental health services, and diverse people living in poverty wherever we lived were the people I first came to know in life. I would not trade those experiences or the insights they gave me for the world.

Growing up in the 1970s and 1980s with people who experienced mental illnesses allowed me to understand suffering and humor. I was never afraid of the people I came to know, and I gained a dynamic worldview from these relationships. Most of all, my mother was compassionate. She cared about her friends and people in our neighborhood. Most significant for my resilience, after the first ten years of my mother's struggle with her illness she came to recognize that she began to manage her illness' symptoms with medications and preventative activities. This became a situation of trade off because the medications changed her. She gained weight, was often thirsty, and was slow in her responses sometimes. However, she was available and her ability to recognize that she had an illness allowed her to discuss it. She also realized that her illness had impacted me and my brother. She took time to talk with and listen to us about our experiences.

In my adult life I realized the enormous pain my mother carried in her, feeling that somehow she had hurt us through her inability to protect my brother and I from circumstances surrounding our family because of her illness. Surprising to many people, even when she was experiencing her worst symptoms (a cacophony of voices, twenty to thirty at a time), our mom was able to remain loving and affirming to us as children. My saddest days were when she would be taken away to a hospital. I worried about her and often felt I had no one to talk to when she was not present. I often had to wait for her to get better, which could take 9 months to a year, before I could receive accurate information regarding what had happened to her because all of the adults in my life, aside from my mother, were unwilling to talk with me about her illness.

3. *Questioning Reality*: Facing the symptoms of my mother's illness when I was very young (starting at 6 years old) helped me to begin asking metaphysical questions. My experiences may not have been typical for a child, but the synaptic connections I made as I faced symptoms of my mother's illness may have laid groundwork for my intellectual pursuits in theology and other subjects as an

adult. I wondered about what humans are made of and thought we must be more than our physical bodies because my mother looked so different when she was hearing voices. By this I do not mean to make a statement regarding the root cause of mental health problems. Causality related to types of mental illnesses is a complex subject. The causes and experiences of people, even with the same diagnosis, can be radically different. Rather, I want to highlight that, although I didn't learn to play as a child, my intellect and capacity for conceptualization developed rapidly during these childhood circumstances. These abilities helped me become a leader in college and later in my career.

Listening to my mother talk about her experiences in hospitals I also learned about power dynamics within mental health systems. Mental health consumer culture, to me, includes a certain level of us-them dynamics along with dry humor regarding tragic subjects. The humor I witnessed as a child is most similar to humor I have experienced hanging out with American Indian friends. You can only survive if you laugh—at yourself and at people who seem unaware that they are denying your story, your life, as having any worth. This may seem extreme, but it is something I learned amongst people who were surviving before "recovery" began to be a focus in mental health systems in the 1990s. My mother struggled for her recovery during an era when people like Judi Chamberlin, author of "On Our Own," were beginning to develop their voice. Yet she never knew about this type of literature. I learned about groups like the National Empowerment Center after my mother's death. She would have joined such groups had she known about them. Reading "On Our Own" recently I was surprised that so many issues that Chamberlin was writing about in the 1970s remain issues today. Reading her words I felt like I was talking to my mom again. I felt comforted, yet sad.

As context, in 1979 my mother had been told she was the worst case of her particular illness that one hospital had seen and that she would "never get out." She worked hard to prove the doctors wrong, but recovery was never a part of her vocabulary. She told me about being locked in solitary confinement for long periods of time with food being given to her under a door. She spoke of being held down by several men so that she could be forcibly medicated. I heard about these stories as I was growing up and I was traumatized as I visualized the experiences she was sharing with me. Collectively, her experiences in mental health systems of the 1970s and 1980s, along with her life experiences before her illness (including rape in her last year of college), led to an overall effect of traumatic stress and distress that she tried to manage. She was not given a recovery framework to consider her potential. She was told she must conform to a system that she eventually feared and referred to as a type of prison. Through these experiences with my mother and her friends I became sensitive to power in various forms. Perhaps also because I lived in the shadow of her illness, I have always had interest in groups of people who are perceived to be invisible and who are not given a voice within dominant power structures. In this sense, I developed something similar to what W.E.B. Dubois called a "double consciousness." Although I do not face issues that people of color face everyday, and I honor that Dubois was speaking specifically of black people's experiences in America, I have a hidden sense of being "other" because of my experiences and my mother's. That I can hide this part of my life is a type of privilege, but it comes at a spiritual and emotional cost. I have chosen not to hide, which means I confront stigma while also (hopefully) opening possibilities for others who have internalized feelings of being inferior, damaged, or somehow less than OK. Becoming publicly open by sharing my personal narrative has been a continual process of "coming out" that allows me to reclaim my identity as whole, while also challenging systems of injustice against people with mental illness and their families. I see this as a continual strength that I gain through my close contact with people navigating psychiatric systems while experiencing mental illness.

4. *Value of Friends, Extended Family and Peers*: A few years ago a friend's mother said: "family" are the people who are there for you. That particular friend's mom had also lost a mother to mental illness, although in her case her mother was hospitalized in the 1950s and never returned home. My friend's mom, along with her larger extended family, had included me in a loving embrace within their family system. Because of divorce and anger between people in my own family, I need to search out relationships with cousins to fill in gaps where my more immediate family was absent. I have been fortunate to have deep friendships with people who have taken me into their family systems, welcoming me at holidays. My brother successfully developed into a wonderful father and husband. I embraced the newness of having nephews and a niece during the same periods of time that my father, mother, and grandparents were passing away. Teachers played a surrogate role for me, encouraging me academically, but also seeing my potential as a person. Growing up I desperately wanted friends my own age, but we moved so often from one state to another that building lasting childhood friendships was impossible. Eventually, with diligence, I was able to develop lasting friendships with people who understood, sometimes even better than me, what had been lacking in my environments and who were willing to give me accepting love.

However, a new layer of experiencing wholeness came into my life when I began to meet other people who had a parent with mental illness through grassroots organizing to create the Daughters and Sons Initiative. In cofounding a support group for adults in New York City and doing workshops and presentations across the United States I began to realize how ordinary my experiences were and are. Of course I was afraid I would become mentally ill! So were each and every individual I met who was a Daughter or Son. I began to realize that some of the things my mother was able to do were not the case for others. I was lucky that my mom had been able to talk about her illness so openly. I began to understand what was typical and what was less typical of people in our group.

Rearranging the House, Unpacking, and Settling Down

One of the popular phrases in the Daughters and Sons Initiative was coined by one of our group members: "Resilience is inherited." Through this member's initiative buttons were developed that use that phrase as a tag line. As the group developed this phrase as a motto, at first I thought, "but wait, resilience is a set of factors, not an inherent quality inside a person!" Then I considered the deeper meaning. Many of us are facing stigma that somehow our parent's illness is inherently within us, waiting to come out. Or we face stigma that we are damaged. Yet, resilience can be part of our inheritance, much like some people inherit family silver.

Although I am still coming to peace with why my mother and I ended up where we did, what I have learned is that there are millions of people who have a parent with a mental illness. Although our stories have differences, we have some experiences in common. Foremost among our shared characteristics is a struggle with identity formation. We live under broad shadows of illnesses that all too often dehumanize us as well as our parents. Some/many mental health professionals continue to be surprised at how many people experiencing mental illness are also parents. This is a key indicator of how deeply hidden are the lives of children who have a parent with mental illness. Optimistically, this also means there is huge, untapped potential for parents struggling with mental illnesses and their children. Potential that mental health and child welfare systems are only beginning to explore.

Sometimes mental health professionals ask me whether issues of Daughters and Sons who have a parent with mental illness are new phenomenon due to deinstitutionalization. My general answer is that having a parent with mental illness is not new. What may be new, however, is the emergence and maturing of a generation of people who have grown up with parents who were deinstitutionalized or became ill in the 1970–1980s. Our generation is reaching a level of maturity in our various professions where we can begin to lend our voices to the larger world of mental health advocacy. Our shared voices, expressed through diverse media, are coming together in a mosaic of stories and shared agendas that cumulatively will provide hope for the next generations of Daughters and Sons.

Ultimately, parenting is as common for people who have a mental illness as it is for the general population of the United States (Nicholson et al. 2004; Sherman 2007). There are practical things that each one of us can do, while we work collectively toward system-wide change. First, we can bring this topic up in meetings, public forums, and conferences. We can ask why data are not being collected. We can talk to people who are receiving services about their parenting and offer them support through information and literature. We can incorporate toys into hospital environments where children are coming to visit their parents. We can develop age-appropriate children's literature to open up conversations with children. We can listen to children, and be amazed by what they know (sometimes more than the adults in their lives want to believe). We can develop pamphlets of instructions for adults regarding how to talk to a child about their family member's mental illness. We can let children know that they are valued for their caring role within their families. We can help parents and children know that mental illness is not an inevitable destiny but rather a confluence of factors. We can find hope by listening to people currently receiving services, asking them what matters most to them in life (Nicholson 2009). In my mother's case, she often told my brother and me that her sole motivation for wellness was her desire to be with us as a parent. How many health professionals are overlooking the possibility that parenting can be tied to wellness?

Despite the qualities I have shared and my various personal and professional successes, sometimes the trickle of a memory still leads me through a familiar landscape. If I am not careful and if the memory gains momentum, it can twist and turn, leading me to a canyon of grief. That I grieve deeply is part of my strength. I think the grief that drilled itself inside me as a child also broadened my capacity to understand people in the world. To paraphrase a class I took on foster care parenting: I became a loss expert. I transitioned the skills I had learned in my youth to help my own community—the Daughters and Sons—and discovered my wholeness through the mirroring of peers.

Once my journey as national organizer for Daughters and Sons began in earnest in 2003, I began traveling across the United States to national forums. Along the way I began unraveling the belief systems of a complex mental health system that had failed to recognize the mental health impact of my mother's illness on me and had failed to see my mother as a full person.

My hope is that supported parenting will become valued in mental health systems as much as supported employment (Nicholson and Deveney 2009). Eventually, I hope the systemic problems that keep Daughters and Sons hidden will be overcome as people who have a parent with mental illness continue to tell our stories. By purposely sharing our stories we break stigma, realize we are not alone, and shed light on a large gap in our current health systems. Each story is a drop toward collective change. Together we are becoming a river of resilience that carves out a new destiny for ourselves and our families.

References

Burack HD (2004) Listen carefully and you can hear our voices too: redemptive aspects of growing up with a parent with mental illness (Professional Seminar Paper). Hunter College School of Social Work, City University of New York, New York, NY

Gearity A (2008) Panel discussion on "Growing Up in A Home with Mental Illness," sponsored by the National Alliance on Mental Illness – Minneapolis, Minnesota. March 26, 2008

Nicholson J, Biebel K, Williams VF, Katz-Leavy J (2004) Prevalence of parenthood in adults with mental illness: implications for state and federal policy, programs, and providers. In: Manderscheid RW, Henderson MJ (eds) Mental health, United States, 2002. Center for Mental Health Services, Maryland, pp 120–137

Nicholson J (2009) Guest editorial: building an evidence-base for families living with parental mental illness. Australian e-Journals for the Advancement of Mental Health (AeJAMH) 8(3). ISSN: 1446-7984

Nicholson J, Deveney W (2009) Why not support(ed) parenting? Psychiatric Rehabil J 33(2):79–82

Sherman M (2007) Reaching out to children of parents with mental illness. Social Work Today 7 (5):26

Suggested Readings

Parenting Well (Resources for Healthy Families): http://www.parentingwell.org/
The Temple University Collaborative on Community Inclusion: http://www.tucollaborative.org/resources/resources.html#parenting
Seeds of Hope Books: http://www.seedsofhopebooks.com/about-our-books.html
Children of Parents with a Mental Illness (COPMI): http://www.copmi.net.au/
Children of Mentally Ill Consumers (COMIC): http://www.howstat.com/comic/Home.asp
Recovery Innovations: http://www.recoveryinnovations.org/
Royal College of Psychiatrists: http://www.rcpsych.ac.uk/expertadvice/parentsandyouthinfo/parentscarers/parentalmentalillness.aspx
The Blue Polar Bear (A downloadable book for children who have a parent with dual diagnosis): http://www.community.nsw.gov.au/docswr/_assets/main/documents/dualdiagnosis_polar_bear.pdf

Reaching Back for Reason and Resilience 46

Cheri Bragg

Cheri is a 46-year-old mother from Connecticut. In this chapter she explores her experience as a daughter of a parent with a psychiatric label, as well as the understanding that has come in part from her work with the Daughters and Sons Initiative. She discusses her relationship with her mother over the years and hopes to offer insight into the development of strength and resiliency in both herself and her mother.

I must admit that although I hear the word "resiliency" all the time that I had to look up the formal definition in order to find a starting place to talk about my experience as a proud "Daughter" (a term preferred by many of my fellow "Daughters & Sons" who have experienced being the child of a parent with a psychiatric label).

According to Wikipedia: **Psychological resilience** is an individual's tendency to cope with stress and adversity. This coping may result in the individual "bouncing back" to a previous state of normal functioning, or simply not showing negative effects. A third, more controversial form of resilience is sometimes referred to as 'posttraumatic growth' or 'steeling effects' where in the experience adversity leads to better functioning (much like an inoculation gives one the capacity to cope well with future exposure to disease). Resilience is most commonly understood as a process, and not a trait of an individual.

Recently there has also been evidence that resilience can indicate a capacity to resist a sharp decline in other harm even though a person temporarily appears to get worse. A child, for example, may do poorly during critical life transitions (like entering junior high) but experience problems that are less severe than would be expected given the many risks the child faces.

It is this last explanation that I can most relate to.

My father has, on more than one occasion, stated that "Your mother can take care of herself!" Now this might seem odd, given more explanation. My mother has been labeled "seriously mentally ill" for decades. She has resided, for the most part, in state mental institutions from the time she turned 28 until her mid-60s, and from then on, in nursing facilities. I've had people tell me that she "must have been very ill" for the hospital to keep her during the national trend of deinstitutionalization. She has had some serious sounding diagnoses and words attached to her over the years: schizophrenia, hallucinations, delusions, bipolar disorder with psychotic features…hardly things one might equate to an ability to take care of oneself.

But sometimes it depends on what you are looking for. If you are looking for deficits, my mother's records certainly hold the right buzz words. If you are looking for strengths, on the other hand, you might have to speak to her yourself or to family or friends, or a compassionate caregiver, to hear about those. My father no doubt remembers some of my mother's strengths from her early days: that she was a good student, typed over 100 words per minute, ran on the track team, and liked to dance. She was even runner-up in a local beauty contest! He also remembers that she once "eloped" (ran away) from the State hospital in Connecticut arriving in New Mexico to visit her first child's grave without so much as a dime in her pocket. I can't imagine the fortitude it must have taken to complete this trip! I don't remember realizing that she had run away. I do remember receiving her postcard, adorned with her sketch of cacti, with the cryptic message "Rebekah is fine with me!" meaning that a previous discussion about choosing the biblical name of Rebekah had her approval, a secret we alone shared.

I also remember my mother patiently teaching me to read before Kindergarten. We would take the bus to the elegantly adorned G. Fox & Co. department store in downtown Hartford to purchase the next "Sally, Dick & Jane" book in the series, a special treat. Although she never drove, she took us to museums, the circus, book stores, and libraries to expose us to any community enrichment program offerings that she could find. Though her times with us at home were short and always measured, she taught me to cook and bake, to write proper term papers, and all about the Bible and her view of Christianity. Her knowledge, patience, and love seemed endless. These experiences, along with those my father gave me, I know are truly gifts and I cherish them today.

Upon reflection, even when things were not going so well for her, she still showed her courage and strength by knowing and asserting her rights and standing by what she knew to be the truth/her reality. The way she calmly and logically spoke to the policemen who were sent to pick us up, wandering the streets. Although her descriptions of "spirits" floating down the hallway of our home was scary to me, she also took the time to relay the meaning she attributed to these experiences, something that gave me a frame of reference to process them by rather than face them alone. When she told me things that might be confusing, I easily believed her, something not uncommon for young children to do with their primary caregiver. I believed she had been born a boy and was really Jesus Christ for instance. I suppose that at some point, on some level, I knew not to re-voice these opinions, but I don't recall giving them much thought. That was just my mom and I loved her. I was confident that she loved me too. Her love was a stabilizing factor in my life. I remember praying together that she would find sandals for my sister and I on the amount of money she had to spend. Then, when she took us walking in the streets of Hartford, pressing coins into the hands of children and anyone she deemed to be "poor" saying "God Bless You," I was proud of her! It felt like we were doing important work as she read me the Bible stories about the widow who gave the last two coins she possessed at church offering. Her message about giving unto others I have tried to incorporate into who I am today.

Many people have suggested to me, often without words, that I should be "over it"—that this experience happened to my mother, but not me. This is preposterous. We experienced both good and bad times together: As when I happily learned to cook by her side, and when she experienced stress that led to anxiety, paranoia, delusions, or psychosis, I, too, often walked by her side, experiencing it through her words and actions, mainly through the eyes of a developing child. What most people don't understand is that most of the impact came not by exposure to mental health "symptoms" or human expressions of stress, but rather by the response (or lack of response) by systems (mental health, school, etc.). Just because my grief was "invisible" to professionals and other adults around me, doesn't mean it wasn't real or impactful. Researchers knew the damaging effects of early, traumatic family loss, yet no one acknowledged my experience. In fact, many people would be more comfortable if I didn't talk about my experiences, as if I don't deserve to process them, as if they should be left "in the past." An amazing MAAFA (pro nounced MA-AH'-FA) influence production entitled "The Sankofa Experience" that I had the great honor to witness this year gave me pause to reflect. The term 'MAAFA' is a Kiswahili word from the Swahili language that defines the catastrophic event experienced by millions of African people during the Transatlantic Slave Trade or Middle Passage Journey from freedom in Africa to bondage in the New World. It can also mean "great disaster," "the great suffering," and "the great catastrophe," not unlike the meaning the term "Holocaust" has to Jewish people. Although I most certainly could not relate from the point of view of being of African heritage, I was able to relate on the broader level of human suffering. I cried, to my colleague's gentle teasing, from start to finish, "feeling" the portrayal of suffering. I am sure I was not alone—anyone who has experienced trauma and suffering would have been deeply touched that night. My ongoing outrage is that while my friend bought $40 V.I.P. tickets to sit toward the front pew of a city church, months later we paid $70 for a far less superior show in a "known" venue. Why was this story of suffering not playing at the big venue in my State? Surely, it would fill the place and bring down the house! Why hadn't I learned more of this history during my own school years? If such a well-known movement is still struggling to "tell truths" in large venues, what chance does the movement, in its infancy, that I belong to stand?

I am more heartened by exploring the meaning of the word Sankofa, an Akan word from Ghana that translates in English to "Reach back and get it." In terms of African-American history, many state "We must go back and reclaim our past so we can move forward; so we understand why and how we came to be who we are today." There are two Akan symbols for Sankofa; one resembles a heart and the other a bird with its head turned backward reaching to get an egg off its back, symbolizing taking from the past that which is good and bringing it to the present to make positive progress through knowledge. I think this is something that many Daughters & Sons strive to do both individually and collectively. To make sense of our own individual suffering in order to move forward personally; to make sense of our collective and systemic suffering in order to grow and strengthen our small, but powerful movement into something that is recognized, something that has the power to move systems, to make positive change in the present, and to make the path a little easier for those Daughters & Sons and their parents who come after us. But how to do so when many of us are still suffering? Perhaps the key is in first reaching back to understand and learn from our personal and collective resilience...

Today, my mother does not directly acknowledge me as her daughter. As a daughter, I am invisible. She does this without any intent to harm. I have heard many stories about why she believes this: from someone telling her that my whole family died in a car accident when I was 11 or that the hospitals did this to "help" patients get over the long-term "loss" of their loved ones, to explanations of delusions, both clinical and humanistic. Whatever the reason, as an adult, I had to come to a degree of peace with this. It is her way of coping and I honor the strength and resilience it shows, despite the loss I feel. Usually I just sit silently "taking" her explanations of why I am someone else's daughter. When I feel brave, I may softly disagree. Perhaps both are my own strength and resilience.

I never used to think of myself as "strong" or "resilient." Today, in my mid-40s, I will tell you that I feel emotions "intensely," both my own and those of others, and I cry easily. Not long ago, I would tell you that I was "oversensitive" or "weak," certainly never "strong." It wasn't until a few years ago when a colleague, Robert E. Davidson, a fellow "Son," heard my story during an educational course delivered to mental health providers that I even began to entertain that I might be anything but "weak" and "emotional." I had just shared with the class the painful memory of when I first became aware that my mother thought we were dead. I remembered with vivid detail the smokestacks that meant we were nearing the hospital grounds always corresponding with the sinking of my emotions. I remembered my sister, my mother's sister and her mother, and myself sobbing as she told us why we were all "spirits" and that we needed to go away. I retold the memory of how, in that awful moment, my mother, seeing that my sister and I were despondent, softened her message saying that "It's not the children's fault." Giving voice for the first time to an event packed, for me, with such raw, emotional pain, I easily slid into my "stance of shame": eyes and head downcast, shoulders hunched, tears flowing. The group was silent, and I immediately shifted back to my "professional role" of facilitator and moved the presentation on to the next person. What I didn't expect was the gift of my colleague, after class, looking at me and stating "How strong!" and smiling. I was immediately caught off guard. "Who, me? Strong? You CAN'T possibly mean ME?" And yet those words stuck with me. For the first time in my life I was given the gift of seeing my experience from another perspective. A positive one. I had never thought of myself and my experience in that light before. I had not only survived, but I had sought out information. I had sought out the unmatchable experience of connecting to others with the same lived experience. I was not complacent, but enraged that little to no change had taken place on this issue in over 40 years. I had made the decision to surround my entire life with the issue of mental health in hopes that I could make the journey a little easier for the next mother/daughter/son/family. Yeah, I guess you must have to have some kind of strength and resiliency to handle the things I'd tasked myself with, plus the ghosts of my past, all at the same time when I had become a single parent myself.

A recent experience really brings this idea home for me. For years, my mother lived in institutions during which time she often chased us off wards and returned the letters and money my father attempted to send her. Years passed this way. My sister and I grew up. Despite my father having the same address and phone number he had always had, hospital records indicate "Whereabouts of family unknown." Later I would learn that she was the last patient to leave the State hospital, not by her choice. That same year my son was born.

A few years later, after taking the only family class I could find on mental illness, I began a quest to find out where my mother was after hearing that the hospital had closed. I secretly made a list of all of the state hospitals and any local hospital wards. I was well versed in the limits of confidentiality and HIPPA, so I decided to tell anyone who answered the phone that I was looking for my mother and that I knew they couldn't tell me she was there, but they could tell me if I could leave a message. I think my resolution finally convinced a man who answered my third call to say "What message would you like to leave?" Eventually an astute doctor at the nursing facility she later transferred to insisted I be asked to be her new conservator of person which I gladly accepted. Over the years, my mother and I formed a trusting, solid relationship. Although I was not her daughter, she referred to me as "The best conservator in the world!"... not a bad second.

Unfortunately, the nursing facility conditions went downhill. Despite this, my mother insisted that she could not leave because she had signed a "contract" when she came there and she could not break her contract. We explored this together at length and I saw that often she would rather that I said "nothing" because she feared retribution and I couldn't blame her.

Finally, events happened that would change everything. The facility had my mother hospitalized 2 years ago stating that she was psychotic (she was not) and the head nurse screamed at me over the phone when I refused to have her forcibly medicated. The residential home and hospital agreed with my mother and me and sent her back to the nursing facility where "miraculously" she did just fine for another 2 years. During her absence, her room was repainted, carpets pulled up and flooring installed, and half to three-quarters of her belongings were thrown out. Come to find out a public health inspection had happened. I was furious at the abuse of power, the loss of her personal belongings, but my mother insisted over and over again that I not make any waves that would cause them to hospitalize her again, and instead set about throwing out even more of her belongings. Against my better wishes, I relented.

When a new social worker tried to hospitalize her yet again, this time via a P.E.C. (physician's emergency certificate) by a policeman, I knew it was an opportunity for her to move to a better setting. The time frame was less than 2 weeks, but the fight took everything I had. The emergency room helped by telling my mother that the nursing facility would not take her back. This meant, in my astute husband's estimation, that the facility had broken the contract, not my mother. My mother astounded me by remaining fairly calm, even though we tried to initially help her fight for her rights by stating that she knew she was not a threat of harm to herself or others nor "gravely disabled." As it turns out, the moment the facility said they would not take her back from the emergency room, she was considered "gravely disabled" as she had no means to take care of herself by walking out of the hospital. After hearing that the facility would not take her back, she was open to hearing about other housing options. That last week I learned how nursing facilities say that they are full when really they don't want to admit you. I also learned that some social workers will lie to families and say that they have tried calling other facilities when they haven't. We were successful in keeping her out of two facilities that we knew from personal experiences had rats, unchanged light bulbs, and untimely deaths. The pressure to discharge her within the days that insurance pays is enormous. On the last day, while simultaneously trying to work, I was faced with only one option. Unfortunately my mother had heard a rumor that this particular nursing facility only gave residents 17 cents per day and despite my explicit request to inform her immediately about discharge plans, the staff ignored this request and instead told her just 10 min beforehand. Arriving there to try to make the transition smoother, I was told she had just been informed and was summoned to try to help her call for legal assistance. Unfortunately, the legal assistance, which had told ME that I had NO CHOICE but to discharge her when the time was up, told my mother that once her conservator of person had made a decision, she had to go. My mother was understandably angry. At the same moment, the previously friendly and patient ambulance workers became angry and impatient with my mother's refusal to go willingly. They did not want to have to lift her from her wheelchair. I frantically told her I would meet her at the new nursing facility after going to get some of her belongings. She quickly yelled "I don't care where you go!" My mind whirled as I backed down the hallway, making my escape as old memories of watching my mother being "forced" into an ambulance leapt from the recesses of my brain. I cried in the car trying to call the state staff member who had been working with me to try to get her into less restrictive housing. The friendly ear helped me regain my composure enough to fetch her belongings, but upon arriving at the new nursing facility, I was told that my mother was still a little angry. Sure enough, when I tried to give her some of her things, she angrily started pronouncing my name in odd ways, telling me to "Never come back!" I was crushed.

I retreated. I sobbed in my car in the parking lot. Emotionally drained, I took to bed that evening, sleeping fitfully, awakening often with nightmares. This was, of course, one of my biggest nightmares. The relationship that I craved with my mother, the relationship which we had worked so hard to reinvent over the years, was gone in a moment. I woke in a haze, voicing to my husband the panic I felt: I felt like "the world was ending"—that "nothing would ever be okay." He left for a conference we were supposed to attend together telling me to get some more rest and that everything would be okay. Still devastated, but better rested, I awoke a little later having to attend to driving my teenage son around town for some errands.

"Losing" my mother again devastated me, but rising to the demands of my own motherhood rallied me physically at least. I functioned over the next several days, deciding to give my mother some time. Honestly, I wasn't ready to risk rejection again so soon.

Then came the phone call from the housing specialist. She had visited with my mom. My mom still wished to leave, but had settled in and, to my relief and surprise, wanted me to come visit saying she wanted to apologize in person for the way she had treated me. I truly had thought our relationship had suffered an unrecoverable blow, and here my mother had "bounced back" so quickly after a huge change. Upon visiting, she was in a wonderful mood having gotten to know her new roommate, a sweet person whom she liked immediately. I had the chance to tell her how sorry I was about how the staff had treated her and empathized with how it must have seemed like she had no choice after all of our efforts to give her one. She said that was exactly how she felt, that she felt completely understood, and that she was sorry for telling me to "go away," quickly inserting that "It's just how I react." We gently leaned our heads together in mutual understanding.

My mother had taught me another lesson in strength and resiliency. Despite the potentially devastating move she had just experienced, through the total loss of control and choice, she still was able, after a brief period of decline, to bounce back better than ever. It made me rethink my own panic about our relationship. We've both been through very different experiences. My mother has been through more torturous situations as an adult than I could ever imagine. I have been through some childhood system trauma that many cannot understand. The gift and lesson of this experience is that I should have more faith in my mother and in our relationship, developed slowly, but surely; in our resiliency, both shared and unique. And, perhaps, a little more faith in me.